T0314149

# WHEN MEDICINE GOES AWRY

Case Studies in Medically Caused Suffering and Death

Medical error often results in disability, pain, and suffering, and it is the third leading cause of death in hospitals. Despite its frequency, medical error has been largely invisible to the mainstream public. Within the medical system itself, medical error is often understood as the result of an isolated case of malpractice.

*When Medicine Goes Awry* argues that the causes of medical error are not an anomaly but rather the outcome of a number of factors at play, ranging from political to social to economic. *When Medicine Goes Awry* dismisses the common blame perspective associated with medical malpractice, instead asserting that medical error is – and will continue to be – inevitable, given the relentless and expanding processes of medicalization. Shedding light on the ways these forces lead to medicine going awry, the book examines seven well-known cases of medical error. Taking an in-depth look at both patients and medical care providers, Juanne Nancarrow Clarke offers a novel approach to medical error or mishap that applies sociological research and theory to the larger societal forces contributing to a taxing and endemic medical problem.

JUANNE NANCARROW CLARKE is a professor emeritus of sociology at Wilfrid Laurier University.

# WHEN MEDICINE GOES AWRY

## Case Studies in Medically Caused Suffering and Death

Juanne Nancarrow Clarke

UNIVERSITY OF TORONTO PRESS
Toronto Buffalo London

© University of Toronto Press 2022
Toronto Buffalo London
utorontopress.com
Printed in the U.S.A.

ISBN 978-1-4875-0835-7 (cloth)    ISBN 978-1-4875-3807-1 (EPUB)
ISBN 978-1-4875-2581-1 (paper)    ISBN 978-1-4875-3806-4 (PDF)

**Library and Archives Canada Cataloguing in Publication**

Title: When medicine goes awry : case studies in medically caused suffering
    and death / Juanne Nancarrow Clarke.
Names: Clarke, Juanne N. (Juanne Nancarrow), 1944–, author.
Identifiers: Canadiana (print) 20210375531 | Canadiana (ebook)
    20210375566 | ISBN 9781487508357 (hardcover) | ISBN 9781487525811
    (softcover) | ISBN 9781487538071 (EPUB) | ISBN 9781487538064 (PDF)
Subjects: LCSH: Medical errors. | LCSH: Medical errors – Case studies. |
    LCSH: Medical errors – Prevention. | LCGFT: Case studies.
Classification: LCC R729.8 .C53 2022 | DDC 610 – dc23

We wish to acknowledge the land on which the University of Toronto
Press operates. This land is the traditional territory of the Wendat, the
Anishnaabeg, the Haudenosaunee, the Métis, and the Mississaugas of the
Credit First Nation.

This book has been published with the help of a grant from the Federation
for the Humanities and Social Sciences, through the Awards to Scholarly
Publications Program, using funds provided by the Social Sciences and
Humanities Research Council of Canada.

University of Toronto Press acknowledges the financial support of the
Government of Canada, the Canada Council for the Arts, and the Ontario Arts
Council, an agency of the Government of Ontario, for its publishing activities.

Canada Council    Conseil des Arts
for the Arts    du Canada

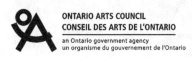

ONTARIO ARTS COUNCIL
CONSEIL DES ARTS DE L'ONTARIO
an Ontario government agency
un organisme du gouvernement de l'Ontario

Funded by the    Financé par le
Government    gouvernement
of Canada    du Canada    Canadä

# Contents

# Preface

This book is based on a number of noteworthy and well-publicized instances of what could be called medical errors. All reflect negative outcomes in the provision of health care. They were all identified from headlines and lead stories in the national media of Canada over a number of years. Many of them resulted in special inquiries or inquests. Yet they represent just a small sample of errors that have occurred during the same time in Canada.[1] Such medical errors are ubiquitous. Some errors affect one person only. Others affect many people and over many years. Some result in death. Others result in disability, ongoing pain, and suffering. A few may lead to fortuitous but beneficial discoveries.[2] The effects of some may be minor, invisible, or non-existent. Some occur in the hospital. Some happen in the community or in the doctor's office. We do not know the true incidence of medical errors or the devastation they cause. We know they exist. In fact, we know that one reliable estimate is that error is the third leading cause of death in hospital (Johns Hopkins Medicine, 2016). This figure does not include death resulting from mistakes in the provision of medicine occurring in the community or clinic.

I became especially interested in this topic when I initially learned from television and newspaper reports about Brian Sinclair. You may remember that he was the Indigenous man who died after waiting thirty-four hours in his wheelchair in an emergency room in a Winnipeg hospital. I found it very hard to believe at first. How could this have happened? I remember wondering: Is this the state of anti-Indigenous racism in our country? Were even nurses and doctors willing to overlook a suffering patient because of racial discrimination and stereotyping? Or, what was the explanation for this egregious outcome in health care provision? I decided to look into it further, initially just out of interest. As I read about Brian Sinclair and his death, I began making notes, and then I started to try to understand the situation in more depth. I became curious about the larger topic of medical mishaps. Once I had read a bit more, I started to develop a sociological case regarding medical error. I decided to examine another situation and then another. Finally, I realized that I had something I wished to say in a book. It was based on an argument that I had not seen made. It challenges and expands upon the two prevailing theories of error: the blame and shame, and the systems viewpoint. It reflects on major sociological critiques of medicine in the modern world: medicalization and, increasingly, pharmaceuticalization. It points to the fundamental role of the social determinants of health for understanding the incidence of disease and the receipt of appropriate medical care.

The fact that medical error was anything but a rare and anomalous event was largely unknown until the publication of *To Err Is Human: Building a Safer Health System* in 2000 by the Institute of Medicine in the United States (Kohn et al., 2000). The media reflected this view of medical error. I compared stories about medical error in popular mass magazines during three intervals: 1980–89, 1990–99, and 2000–14 (Clarke, 2016). The number and the content of the stories differed significantly from time to time. During the first decade, there were very few stories, and error was represented as an occasional, unique, and horrific event. In the next two and a half decades and progressively over time, medical error was represented as unexceptional. It was portrayed as if it were so frequent that it could be found in all segments of the health care system, across all stages of life, and from pre-diagnosis to death. Readers were exhorted to individually take responsibility for managing the risk of being a victim of error. They were told to continuously, assiduously monitor dangers everywhere in the medical care system. I linked this changing representation of medical error to the medicalization of everyday life in the context of the expansion of neoliberalism and the enlargement of the sense of everyday risk. I expand these ideas through the case studies found in this book.

The cases in the book illustrate contemporary sociological ideas about what constitutes a medical mishap or error. There are seven cases discussed. They are all historical cases, but as you will see, and as I document, most of the circumstances that enabled their occurrence persist today. The cases are in the past, but the causation endures. After this preface, the book is divided into four parts. The first part is the introduction. Then the first four chapters are from the viewpoint of a particular harmed patient – Brian Sinclair, Ashley Smith, Vanessa Young and Marit McKenzie, and, finally, Amy Tan. They constitute the second part of the book. The third part of the book looks at three cases that focus on error in the work of an individual health care provider. They include Dr. Charles Smith, nurse Elizabeth Wettlaufer, and Dr. Norman Barwin. The final and fourth part of the book is the conclusion. Each case adds a particular part of the argument to the story that I am telling about medicine going awry. The story is complex and involves a number of different factors. It covers aspects of both physical and mental illness. In the following, I offer a very brief introduction based on a few headlines derived from national media and related to the cases examined.

## Brian Sinclair

Ignored to death: Brian Sinclair's death caused by racism, inquest inadequate, group says

– Aiden Geary, 2017, *CBC News*

Homeless man's family feels marginalized at inquest

– Patrick White, 2009, *The Globe and Mail*

Housekeeping, but not nurses, called after Brian Sinclair threw up in the Winnipeg ER where he died

– The Canadian Press, 2013, *National Post*

In the case of the Indigenous man, Brian Sinclair, all of the headlines, while accurate, represent only a part of the story and give us a limited picture of medical error.[3] In the first headline, the error seems to be the result of the callousness of the relevant system – the health care system. In the second, the problem may be the insensitivity of the judiciary system, along with members of the audience of the inquest. The first headline implies that the staff were racist. The second headline also underscores the role of social exclusion in Mr. Sinclair's family's experience at the inquest into his death. The third headline focuses on the malfunctioning of the nurses as compared to the housekeeping staff in particular. Together, they reinforce the image that Mr. Sinclair's death was an isolated incident and that his case was an aberration caused by a unique confluence of events and the particulars of an incident of anti-Indigenous racism in a specific location. Particular changes in the provision of medicine and the organization of the inquest are at the heart of the solution implied by the news stories in this case.

How did medicine go awry here? I had to ask how an Indigenous man could be ignored in a busy emergency room and for so long. What, if anything, did the fact that he was described as homeless have to do with the situation in the ER? Why was housekeeping involved but not the medical staff? These questions led me on a search for answers.

In the chapter on Brian Sinclair, I show how his death could have been predicted and how such events will continue until certain fundamental social, economic, and political changes occur. Medicalization and racism both played fundamental roles in Brian Sinclair's death. Various other aspects of the social determinants of health were major causes in the death of Mr. Sinclair.

## Ashley Smith

Jail cell death of N.B. teen "entirely preventable": Report

– *CBC News*, 2009

Ashley Smith's inhumane death

– *The Globe and Mail*, 2009

Troubled teen died in prison "needlessly"

– Richard J. Brennan, 2009, *Toronto Star*

The headlines about Ashley Smith emphasize the preventability of her death. The CBC story, for example, attributes her death to systemic problems in the provision of health care and points out that she had never received a comprehensive psychological assessment while in federal custody. That she was kept in solitary confinement is mentioned as a contributing cause. *The Globe and Mail* article focuses on the idea that she was mentally ill. She was not a "killer or a hardened criminal," the article asserts. *The Globe and Mail* reiterates the fact that she was residing in a solitary cell measuring 6 feet by 9 feet when she died. Richard Brennan's article in the *Toronto Star* also emphasizes that she was mentally ill and in solitary confinement. Again, these headlines simplify the causes of Ashley Smith's death. All of the stories suggest that more and better care for mental illness is a part of the solution. Additionally, they point to the destructive effects of solitary confinement within prisons.

Reading these headlines and stories, I was compelled to ask: What exactly could have prevented Ashley's death? If it was preventable, why wasn't it prevented? What was the role of what was labelled her mental illness in her death? What sort of health care did she receive? Why was she in a prison and in solitary confinement rather than in a treatment facility?

The argument I make takes issue with the idea that more mental health care is always a solution. I argue that medicalization obfuscated the continual psychosocial harms to Ashley Smith during her years in custody. I also look to a number of the social determinants of health such as Ashley's gender for understanding and explanation.

## Vanessa Young and Marit McKenzie

Calgary teen was slowly dying and didn't know it
> – Diana Zlomislic, 2013, *Toronto Star*

Family of teen never told of drug warnings
> – *CBC News*, 2001

"This is what Marit wanted": Calgary teen saved lives by donating organs
> – Emma Jones, 2021, *National Post*

The first headline about Marit McKenzie emphasizes how invisible the symptoms that killed her were until it was too late. The story emphasizes that Marit was well and energetic until the weeks before she died, when she started feeling tired and out of sorts. Her parents noticed, and her mother took her to the doctor. Her blood work was normal, and the doctor did not link the fatigue to blood clots, a known side effect of the medication the doctor had previously prescribed. The second headline reports that Vanessa Young's family had never been informed that there were serious warnings associated with the drug she was taking for an eating disorder. The final story ignores the complex causes of Marit's death and focuses on the fact that her death resulted in organ donation to prolong the life of another.

How did medicine go awry here? How could a teenage girl be slowly dying in front of her family and friends without anyone suspecting how sick she was becoming? What was the pharmacy legally expected to do, if anything? Why are warnings about the side effects of drugs at times ignored by doctors, pharmacists, and patients?

I show how both of these deaths were predictable and the result of many factors, including primarily pharmaceuticalization under medicalization. Both young women may have turned to medicine to solve personal or social problems. I also document the ways in which the relative power of the pharmaceutical industry vis-à-vis the Canadian government was implicated in these untimely and sudden deaths. In addition, I explain how the particular social identities of the two young girls played a part in their deaths.

## Amy Tan

"I am in this for the long haul": Writer Amy Tan's frustrating struggle with Lyme disease highlights the controversy on diagnosis and treatment

– J.J. McCoy, 2003, *The Washington Post*

The case chosen to illustrate a new diagnosis is that of Amy Tan, an American, which reflects the point of the argument made in the chapter: although people in Canada experienced symptoms of Lyme disease, it was not acknowledged as existing in Canada for many years. Initially, people in Canada had to go to the United States to be tested, receive a diagnosis, and have access to the prevailing treatment regimen. This disparity reflects the political and economic forces operating behind diagnoses. The story in *The Washington Post* about Amy Tan is a long one. It was the only time her case made the headlines to my knowledge and using my search strategies. It describes some of the frightening, changing, and multisystem symptoms that Amy Tan experienced over a long period of time before she finally found a diagnosis and treatments for her Lyme disease. She went to doctors representing a variety of specialties, including a primary care doctor, a neurologist, a cardiologist, an endocrinologist, a sleep specialist, and even an orthopaedic surgeon to find help for the way she was feeling. The story describes how immersed in social issues and politics the diagnosis was. There were different complex concerns and opposing sides to the controversial diagnosis. The sides disagree about specific features of diagnoses and about a number of other issues, including whether or not long-term antibiotic prescription is legitimate or not. Some do not believe in chronic Lyme disease. Others do. Labs and lab tests for the diagnosis are mired in inadequacies, including false positives, on the one hand, and false negatives, on the other.

I asked questions such as the following: Why is getting a diagnosis for Lyme disease experienced as such a struggle? What explains the long time to acquire the diagnosis? Why were so many different types of specialists involved in the search for help? In what ways and for what reasons is Lyme disease considered a controversial diagnosis, and why are there such opposing ideas about treatment?

I argue that this fraught search for a diagnosis is typical of new diseases, especially those with multisystem and multi-organ involvement. I identify medicalization as an underlying source for this searching. More specifically, relying on evidence-based medicine for diagnosis, a key aspect of modern medical practice, is problematic both in this case and those of other new diseases. I consider the influence of the political economy on diagnosis and treatment, and reflect on how Tan's social position might have worked in her favour in her relatively productive trajectory of diagnosis and treatment.

## Dr. Charles Smith

Tribunal revokes licence of discredited pathologist Charles Smith
– Tom Blackwell, 2011, *National Post*

Staff was in crisis, chief pathologist testifies
– Kirk Makin, 2007, *The Globe and Mail*

Ex-chief coroner knew of issues with pathologist but took little action
– The Canadian Press, 2007, *CBC News*

The stories about Dr. Charles Smith accentuate that he had long been found to engage in problematic behaviours. He had been discredited, but he was not adequately monitored or chastised because of confusion in the authority structure of the unit within which he worked. Furthermore, because there were few specialists in his area of work, he would not have been easily replaceable. There were staffing difficulties. The first story focuses on the suffering caused by Dr. Smith and reiterates, through quotes from some of those he harmed, that the "slap on the wrist" he received was a totally insufficient punishment. The story in *The Globe and Mail* focuses on the crisis in the pathology department in which Dr. Smith became caught up. The CBC story emphasizes again how egregious Dr. Smith's errors were but also spreads the blame and chastises the chief coroner for not acting on repeated prior warnings.

Here I had to ask: What did the pathologist do to have his license taken from him? Was it really his fault or was it the fault of the lax authority structure of the pathology unit? Why didn't anyone stop him? Was Dr. Smith the only one who ought to have had his license removed?

I add to the media explanations and show how such problems are inevitable in new specialties with few trained practitioners and still fewer published and relevant studies. I also point to the lack of adequate monitoring, which is, at the best of times, tenuous and uneven. Medicalization is again an underlying cause of the acceptance of Dr. Smith's errors over many years. The social identities of the accused and accusers are important here too.

## Elizabeth Wettlaufer

"Systemic vulnerabilities" let killer nurse Elizabeth Wettlaufer keep on killing – Report
> – Kate Dubinski, 2019, *CBC News*

Nurse charged with murdering eight Ontario nursing home residents
> – Moira Welsh, 2016, *Toronto Star*

Nurse was fired prior to murder charges; dismissed for misusing drugs, warrant says
> – J. Sims, 2017, *National Post*

Nurse Wettlaufer was the subject of many headlines. The CBC story emphasizes the ninety-one recommendations of the Gillese Inquiry. In particular, it notes the need for more funding for long-term care. It argues for more full-time and fewer part-time staff. The *Toronto Star* story focuses on the problems in the funding of long-term care institutions. The story in the *National Post* emphasizes that Wettlaufer had been fired for mishandling insulin prior to her arrest. These critiques are correct and do help explain why Elizabeth Wettlaufer's murders had not been observed until she herself confessed. They may even help explain why the many deaths were not seen as remarkable. These issues are aspects of the whole story. They implicate continuing issues in long-term care.

I wondered about the systemic issues that could allow Wettlaufer to murder and continue to do so over time at her workplace. Was the fact that the murdered were elderly a part of the explanation? Was Wettlaufer addicted to drugs, and if so, why wasn't this discovered and acted upon earlier? These are a few of the questions raised by this case.

I add to these arguments in showing how medicalization was fundamental to understanding Elizabeth Wettlaufer's repeated murders over many years. I document problems in long-term care and the significance of ageism in the ongoing murders.

## Dr. Norman Barwin

Disgraced fertility doctor's clinic broke federal rules as far back as 1999
— Amanda Pfeffer, 2020, *CBC News*

Fertility lawsuits name Ottawa doctor: Two families want to rule out possibility Barwin was sperm donor
— Andrew Duffy, 2010, *Ottawa Citizen*

Sperm donor mix-up: Where do these two girls come from?
— Amber Kanwar, 2010, *The Globe and Mail*

The first story about Dr. Barwin stresses that there had been problems in his practice for many years. The next two stories focus on the impact of the fertility doctor's errors on the offspring born as the result of interventions by his clinic. They underscore the outstanding question regarding unknown sperm donors and whether they could possibly be the doctor himself. Again, the headlines highlight the possibility that Dr. Barwin was a "bad apple" who had been able to avoid a malpractice suit and the loss of his licence for many years.

Here I wondered how a doctor could go on breaking rules for such a long time and not be stopped. Was it possible that his own sperm had been used accidently, as he claimed, in impregnating some of his patients? I wondered about the impact of these awful mistakes on the lives of the families who had chosen him as a doctor when they experienced fertility issues.

I explain how some social factors and other medical system errors contributed to these dreadful mix-ups. Medicalization is implicated in the continuance of Dr. Barwin's sloppy and unethical practice for decades. The social location of doctors may also play a role here.

## Summary

All seven cases emphasize different issues that may lead to medical mishaps and error. They incorporate both mental and physical illness. At first glance, they all seem unique. There do not appear to be obvious commonalities. They are similar in the sense that a medical care provider or a patient has suffered and been harmed. However, the type of harm differs. The causes are said to differ. There are men and women among these cases. One person, in particular, was described as a member of a racialized minority. One error occurred in the emergency room of a big city hospital. One occurred in the criminal justice system. Two happened in the community under the jurisdiction of doctors and pharmacists. The final patient case took place over many years and across geographic and specialty medical perspectives. The doctors represent different specialties, including those as different as pathology and fertility. The pathologist's job is mostly lab based, and the fertility doctor's patients needed help conceiving or were donating sperm for use at a later date or for others who wanted to conceive. The nurse worked with (mostly) elderly people in long-term care, a seemingly low-risk non-acute health care environment. Four of the patients discussed in the book died as a result of a specific medical error. One of them was murdered. The last, Amy Tan, did not die but had to search and search for a very long time to get a diagnosis and treatment. The health care providers are described as "bad actors." All of the cases are presented in the mass media as unique cases. I document the underlying similarities in all cases and demonstrate that they are all part of the same underlying sociological principles, including medicalization, pharmaceuticalization, and the social determinants of health. The introduction explains these concepts in detail.[4]

# WHEN MEDICINE GOES AWRY

Case Studies in Medically Caused Suffering and Death

# Introduction

This book is about medicine going awry or, in other words, medical mishap or error. Broadly speaking, medical errors are calamities that occur in the provision of health care. The errors in this book are of diverse types and consequences. They focus both on negative outcomes for patients and faulty or even unethical medical care by professional physicians and one nurse.

Although they are quite different in cause and consequence, I use the term "medical error" because it reflects the fact that the event causing harm occurred within the delivery of medical care. As such, all of the cases can be considered medical error whose remedy is related to medicine and health care.

Medical error is now recognized to be the third leading cause of death in hospital (Makary & Daniel, 2016). It is also associated with death, sickness, and disability for an unknown number of outpatients. In the past, medical error had been largely invisible, but when observed, it had been viewed through an individualizing blame and shame perspective. It was understood as anomalous and the fault of one bad actor or decision. More recently, error has been discovered as endemic, and health policy interventions have been introduced. These new policies are based on a medical systems perspective regarding error identification, causation, and elimination.

The argument of this book extends beyond both the blame and shame and the medical systems perspectives. It asserts that medical errors will continue to be inevitable, given the relentless and expanding processes of medicalization, because medicalization assumes the beneficence of allopathic medicine's goals and functioning. It tends to resist critical thinking. The definitional power of medicalization over many aspects of life obfuscates the serious ongoing and challenging limits in medical science, medical practice, medical systems organization, and pharmaceuticalization. The dominance of medicalization also obscures the powerful impacts of the social determinants of health, including social inclusion.

The argument I am making is complex. Ultimately, I am trying to add to the explanations for medical error and therefore help to address it. There are major concepts that need to be discussed to understand the case that I am making. They are medical error; medicalization; medical systems, practice, and research issues; pharmaceuticalization; and the social determinants of health. This introduction describes each of these concepts in some detail, with historical context. I will first explain some highlights of contemporary thinking about medical error. I will investigate ideas about the perspectives on the reality and the causes of, as well as the remedies for, medical error. I will then explain the meaning and the history of medicalization. I will offer an operational definition of medicalization that is the bedrock of the argument in the book. I will discuss the inherent limitations of medical practice, research, and systems organization, as well as pharmaceuticalization, and finally, the importance of the social determinants explanation of health, illness, and death. I end this introduction with a very brief overview of the case studies I use to demonstrate the central arguments of the book.

## Medical Error

The Institute of Medicine's Committee on the Quality of Health Care in America published *To Err Is Human: Building a Safer Health System* in 2000 (Kohn et al., 2000). This document was momentous at the time. It proposed that medical errors were a significant problem. It documented the resultant widespread morbidity and mortality to the American people. It demonstrated that medical error was so frequently a cause of death in the United States that it surpassed deaths from breast cancer, motor vehicle accidents, and AIDS. This finding only reflected errors that resulted in death. It did not include errors that solely led to morbidity or disability. It was restricted to errors that occurred within hospitals and excluded those that occurred in the community as the result of outpatient care.

The report, *To Err Is Human: Building a Safer Health System*, and the newly available statistics initiated a national policy discussion on the topic of medical error in the United States. It became "a call to arms" (Jensen, 2008, p. 309) for error prevention. The growing awareness of an intolerable error rate in medicine led to new policies and practices. It repudiated the previous individualization of the problem of errors as infrequent, deviant, and the fault of particular individuals – the "blame and shame" method. It argued instead that errors are inevitable and normal, just as accidents are normal, in complex systems. Using the normal accidents theory (Perrow, 1984; Clearfield & Tilcsik, 2018), the text proposed that the way to prevent and mitigate errors was through a systems, rather than an individualized, approach. The report advocated the creation of a safety culture in hospital practice that would encourage the reporting and monitoring of error. This recommendation was designed to inspire learning from mistakes and making changes in the operation of medical care systems.

The approach to error and its reduction within the paradigm laid out by the report assumes that it is possible to simply and objectively define errors. They are considered obvious and understood by health care practitioners. In this sense, medical error is viewed as a clear and non-controversial idea. It is assumed to be straightforwardly observable and amenable to widespread and easy agreement. The distinction is frequently made between errors and near misses. Statistics on the rate of error in various locations over time are calculated and published. They become benchmarks for error reduction policies. There are lists of such errors as under- and overdosing with medications, confusing patients or drugs, and mistaking the location of a site for surgery. However, estimates of the incidence of medical error differ widely, depending on the measurement system used. They vary depending on which health care practitioner (for example, a nurse or a doctor) is doing the observing. Generally, all error measurements are highly likely to be based on under-reporting (Baile & Epner, 2015) and can be ten times as large as stated (Classen et al., 2011). By the most reliable calculations, medical error is likely the third leading cause of death in the United States and Canada (Charney, 2012; Leapfrog Hospital Safety Grade, 2013; Makary & Daniel, 2016).

Researchers studying medical error from outside the field of medicine think that the idea of what constitutes medical error is complex, nuanced, and variable. Charles Bosk (2005), for example, distinguished four types of error. He studied the work of surgeon interns and noticed how surgeons differentiated among technical, judgmental, normative, and quasi-normative errors. He said that all four types of error were a fundamental part of one aspect of medical practice – learning to be a surgeon. Senior surgeons easily forgave and even expected the first two types of errors (technical and judgmental). The last two (normative and quasi-normative) were thought to be serious and to reflect deficiencies in the surgeon in training. Technical errors, such as poor stitchery, are expected as an inevitable part of learning and accepted as necessary in the early stages. Judgmental errors are mistakes of timing and include either failure to act when surgery would be desirable or, by contrast, acting before surgery is optimal. Senior surgeons simply excuse such errors as a necessary part of the learning process. On the other hand, the last two types of error involve ignorance, or the misinterpretation, of the norms and culture of the group and of the surgeon in charge. They involve failure to abide by the group rules and procedures. Surgeons in training are held culpable for these behaviours. These errors are considered to be difficult to fix even with increased training. However, they are unlikely to be the sorts of errors that patients are concerned about. They may not be the kinds of errors through which patients are harmed.

Furthermore, acknowledgement and recognition of error is often problematic (Jain, 2013). Regardless of the type of error detected, doctors have tended to respond with denial, discounting, and distancing (Mizrahi, 1984, p. 135). Denying doctors use justifications such as "medicine is an art and thus mistakes are unavoidable." Discounting medical error involves suggesting that the mistake was beyond anyone's control and instead was the result of the relentless disease process or the fault of the individual patient, for example. Whenever denial or discounting fails to work, staff may simply distance themselves from the error. Doctors tend to be afraid of litigation, embarrassed and unclear about the best way to report error (Jain, 2013). A culture of non-disclosure prevails (Jain, 2013).

The definition of error depends on the observer or interpreter of error. Weingart and colleagues (2005) found that many errors identified by patients during their medical care were not identified by the hospital or medical centre incident reporting systems or in the medical record. Thus, what patients consider errors may be different from those incidents that various health care workers consider to be errors. The definition of error reflects the norms, attitudes, and beliefs into which group members are socialized (Paget, 2004). Patients often focus on psychosocial slights and harms, and consider delays, poor communication, and lack of information as errors (Rathert et al., 2012; Weingart et al., 2005; Paget, 2004). Physicians, nurses, and others in the medical system tend to view error as evident in an incorrect medical action.

The blame and shame approach to error has had the problem of encouraging errors to be hidden and ignored. It has also, at times, targeted individuals who were just acting as everyone in the system did, yet were singled out and blamed. The focus on errors as systems problems is not without complications either. There are potentially significant negative and unintended consequences of the emphasis on errors as systems failures. First, the meaning of system and what is included and excluded varies considerably. Second, the systems approach may result in doctors, nurses, and other health care personnel feeling that they hold no or very little responsibility for error because, after all, it results from systems failures. As Waring says, "this line of thinking serves to mitigate individual wrongdoing and protect professional credibility by encouraging doctors to accept and accommodate the shortcomings of the system, rather than participate in new forms of organizational learning" (Waring, 2007, p. 29). Third, the systems approach to medical errors may be vexed by what Rittel and Webber (1973) call wicked as compared to tame problems. Wicked problems are difficult to delineate, check, or resolve. Tame problems are easily defined and have relatively clear remedies. Wicked problems recognize that systems are constantly moving and changing, and that monitoring must be ubiquitous and continuous. They are inextricably linked to other problems and solutions. Thus, solving one problem, preventing one error, or promoting one solution at a time can lead to the replacement of the first problem by a second problem. Burns (2008), for example, showed how attempts to change the system for the majority can lead to particularly intransigent problems for the more vulnerable persons in a system. A fourth problem with the systems approach is that error is only one of the dimensions of quality of care. The many others include concerns such as pain reduction, comfort, felt support, and so on. Thus, focusing on error reduction can lead to the neglect of other emergent systems challenges and innovations.

Bosk (2005) also argued that the systems perspective on error has other inherent and serious drawbacks. For example, it requires "teamwork" among different medical care providers. But "teamwork" is "based on interpersonal communication, collaboration, coordination, seeking qualified assistance when needed and accepting colleague supervision, knowledge and expertise" (p. 518). These all require a basic level of accepted equality and mutuality among health care providers. But these values are problematic on account of the hierarchical structure of the medical system in which, for instance, physicians tend to have power over others such as nurses and various levels of nursing assistants (Zelek & Phillips, 2003). Medical culture is based on the assumption of the particular acumen of the individual doctor and his or her active and independent decision-making. Furthermore, the contemporary allopathic medical culture may be more likely to be error prone because of its commitment to aggressive intervention and control, even in the face of uncertainty (Freund et al., 2003).

None of this is to say that the intention of medicine or health care professionals is to do harm. In the vast majority of cases, the opposite is likely true. It is probable that most health care professionals choose their occupations because they want to help people who are suffering (see Wouters et al., 2014, for one study of motivation of applicants for medical school). Yet the reasons for medical error are often human and social reasons. All of us make mistakes as individuals, often daily. Individual mistakes are one part of the reason for medical error. Focusing on the mistakes that individuals make has certain benefits in that it can locate and possibly fix the habits, education, and training insufficiencies of individuals. It can thus work towards preventing future mistakes by the same people. Such a focus can also route out health care workers with mental health or addiction issues, or other similar personal problems that need to be addressed. Alternatively, a systems perspective also has many benefits. It can draw attention to and address widespread issues, such as the needless spread of germs resulting from a simple lack of handwashing or an easily mistaken and confusing labelling technique.

The argument I am making is not one that rejects these other two models of medical error causation or their strategies for improvement. Each is an important component of improving medical care. My argument goes beyond them and takes a different tack on the problem of error. Instead, I offer the theory that medical error is inherent in the contemporary medical system because of medicalization and its expansive definitional power. Such definitional power means that we tend not to use our analytical thinking capacities. We tend to be unquestioning in our reliance on medicine and pharmaceuticals. Medical error results from a culture, a society, a polity, and an economy that uncritically promote medical solutions to an ever-wider range of problems. Moreover, a medicalized perspective tends to ignore the powerful effects of social determinants of health, which would involve social changes to eliminate poverty, homelessness, racism, and the like and would go a long way to reducing the numbers of people who are sick and in need of medicine.

## Medicalization: A Brief History and Overview

Medicalization is a ubiquitous process in the modern world. By this, I am referring to the increasing power of allopathic medicine to define the terms of engagement with everyday life. It occurs when more and more of life comes to be considered relevant to medical research and practice. The idea of medicalization points to the expansion of preoccupation with problems in bodily bio-logical functioning. It includes a growth in classifications of mental illnesses. It encompasses the proliferation of early detection tech-nologies and the widespread adoption of the imperatives of health promotion and prevention activities. Medicalization implicates the specific power of medical practitioners to use their tools, tech-nologies, and worldviews in shaping the way we live our lives. It corresponds to our willingness to internalize and adopt the mes-sages of the benefits of medicine, early detection, health promo-tion, and prevention, and to make engaging in them integral to our self-images as good citizens. Medicalization has been taken up by for-profit pharmaceutical, laboratory, and medical device corporations. In many ways, we have come to see our bodies and minds through the veil of biology and medicine. Such a viewpoint paves the way for the increased tendency to turn to pharmaceuti-cal solutions. Medicalization is also associated with an increase in categories of illness to which medical research and treatments can be assigned. It is connected with an intensification of the social control powers of medical definitions of reality over everyday life. Things previously considered to have been under the authority of the church, the law, the family, or the community have moved within public consciousness and actions into the realm of medicine. Medicalization takes a fundamentally individualizing stance. It is designed to fix or change one body at a time. As such, it eschews a focus on community supports and interventions.

Medicalization is a particular problem because its benefits are accompanied or overshadowed by its damages. One of the first critiques to point out the dangers of the overextension of mod-ern medicine was Ivan Illich's (1976) book *Medical Nemesis: The Expropriation of Health*. To Illich, a Catholic priest, medicine was inherently iatrogenic. By this, Illich meant that medicine invariably caused disease, death, and disability. The practice of medical care, he argued, caused these harms by its very processes of diagnosis and treatment. Medicine was fundamentally error ridden. With myriad statistics and arguments, he documented the impacts of three types of medical iatrogenesis on society: clinical, social, and structural iatrogenesis. Clinical iatrogenesis occurred when medical care or treatment directly caused sickness and death. One example of clinical iatrogenesis would be a harmful side effect of a prescribed medication. Alternatively, iatrogenesis was social when health policies reinforced inequities and other invidious social phenomenon that lead to sickness, death, and suffering. For example, women are encouraged, by the lack of supportive and preventative health and social policies, to take antidepressants to cope with the aftermath of sexual assault. In this way, sexism and inequity between the genders is perpetuated. Structural iatrogenesis ensued when a reliance on medicine led to the breakdown of the ability of people to care for themselves and each other, while they tended to rely on medical systems instead. Iatrogenesis, for Illich, was not limited to the fact that specific medical interventions sometimes caused illness. It was broader. It was that the whole medical enterprise, because it restricted the ability of individuals to choose a good and moral life involving self and community care, was an error-ridden yet increasingly uncritically accepted aspect of life.

Others since Illich have taken up the case that medicalization casts a dark and sometimes dangerous shadow over the provision of health care. Peter Conrad is a sociologist who has written critically about medicalization over many years. His and colleague Joseph Schneider's analysis of the medicalization of "social problems" has been highly influential (Conrad & Schneider, 1980). They noted that medicalization was observable in the ways that medicine worked as a social control mechanism to manage, demarcate, and provide a remedy for all sorts of social behaviours in areas that might formerly have been considered relevant to the law or to morality. They argued that actions such as alcohol and drug addictions and homosexuality, previously considered to be signs of moral failure, were increasingly likely to be seen as sicknesses and subject to medical intervention. They observed that this tendency to medicalize social problems often hid other interests. For example, they contended that hyperkinesis (now called attention deficit disorder [ADD]) and attention deficit hyperactivity disorder (ADHD) had been discovered as diseases only after the finding that a certain class of amphetamine drugs had a powerful calming effect on extremely busy and active children. The availability of the new pharmaceutical, Ritalin, and the way it changed the unwanted behaviours of children, was instrumental in the development of a new diagnosis, which led to the categorization of certain behaviours in some children as diseased. That this strategy for managing unwanted behaviour was successful also meant that other, non-medical and non-pharmaceutical, ways to minimize the troubling, possibly just childish actions tended to be ignored.

Opioid addiction and its associated suffering and death are a contemporary case in point. In 2019, close to 50,000 people in the United States died as a result of opioid-involved overdoses, according to statistics from the National Institute on Drug Abuse (2020). Eleven Canadians lost their lives every day in 2017 for the same reason, according to statistics from the Canadian government (Government of Canada, 2019). More than 14,000 people in Canada died from opioid overdoses between 2016 and 2019 (Cecco, 2019). Many of these people became addicted initially as a result of legal medical prescription of medications in response to surgery or based on self-reports of chronic pain (Cecco, 2019). However, the prevalence of the experience of pain grew as the advertisement for the medications expanded. Today, the opioid addiction epidemic occurs most heavily among the poor and the racialized (Saloner et al., 2018). Pain medication became a means to cope with social suffering and not merely physical symptoms.

Irving Zola, another sociologist, focused on the idea that medicalization was the result of the increasing power of the medical profession (Zola, 1972). The essence of medicalization was the creeping process whereby more and more of life comes to be of concern to physicians. He portrayed medicalization as an expanding attachment process with the following four components: (1)

the expansion of what in life is deemed relevant to the good practice of medicine; (2) the retention of absolute control by the medical profession over certain technical procedures; (3) the retention of near-absolute access to certain areas by the medical profession; and (4) the expansion of what in medicine is deemed relevant to the good practice of life. The first area of medicalization is the change from medicine as focused on a narrowly defined biological model of disease to encompass the social, spiritual, and moral aspects of life. In addition to bodily symptoms, the entire lifestyle of the patient becomes subject to medical surveillance through the broad dictates of medicine. The expansive edifice of testing in the interests of early detection (and intervention) is one case in point. Mammography and prostate-specific antigen (PSA) testing are two clear examples of the proliferation of what is now called preventative medicine or early detection. The second component of medical power refers to the fact that a doctor is permitted to do things to the human body that no one else has the right to do. Doctors are able to cut the body up through surgery, prescribe pharmaceuticals, admit to hospital, and refer to a specialist or another doctor. Doctors are the gatekeepers to numerous associated services and provisions. The maintenance of nearly absolute control over a number of formerly "normal" bodily functions is the third component. Here, Zola argues that processes such as aging, pregnancy, and childbirth, once considered normal, are now understood through the gaze of medical specialties such as gerontology, gynaecology, and obstetrics, and associated with pathologies. The last component is the expansion of what in medicine is seen as relevant to a good life. Health promotion prescribes advice to people regarding an increasing array of the components of everyday life. Thus, the good citizen is one who abides by an expanded list of medically derived rules. There are now healthy ways of eating, sleeping, exercising, communicating, and even having sex.

The theories discussed so far are among the earliest critical reflections on the growth of medicine. Conrad returned to a consideration of medicalization research over the years. In "The Shifting Engines of Medicalization," Conrad (2005) argues that, despite the many changes in the understanding of medicalization, the central idea remains. "The essence of medicalization became the definitional issue: defining a problem in medical terms, usually as an illness or disorder, or using a medical intervention to treat it" (p. 3). What has changed, Conrad argues, are the causes of the continuous growth of medicine. Conrad reasons that medicine is less about the growth in the power of the medical profession and now more rooted in the pursuit of commercial, political, and market interests. Other social theorists such as Coburn (2006) and Foucault (2006) agree with this assessment. Foucault says about doctors: "These professionals are more and more aware that they are being turned into almost mechanized intermediaries between the pharmaceutical industry and client demand, that is, into simple distributors of medicine and medication" (p. 18).

Thus, while medical doctors are still the primary gatekeepers in the system of diagnosis, they are now subservient to and constrained by larger social and economic forces including governments and health insurance, hospital administrators, and pharmaceutical, media, and advertising companies. The future of medicine itself is increasingly subject to developments in such highly specific and expertized areas as genetics, biotechnological innovations, and those that occur in the realms of pharmaceuticals and various high-tech and digital medical devices. They encompass the replacement and harvesting of various "natural" or manufactured body parts for transplant into another body. These highly technical innovations are transforming medical practice and removing the locus of expertise from the physician and placing it onto other specialized and highly trained scientific entrepreneurs and enterprises. This shift frequently involves the incursion of profit-making initiatives. Changing payment schemes such as national medicare and powerful health insurance companies are altering the financial autonomy of the doctor. The increases in social organizing, advertising, and consumer power, along with the economic reliance on managed/insured care, have led to the decline of the power of the medical practitioner. Furthermore, it is essential to recognize that medical care is also patient driven and mutually constructed by the patient in interaction with the doctor (Rose, 2007). That direct-to-consumer advertising is an effective tool for motivating people to go to doctors and seek particular remedies (for example, advertised medications) is a case in point (Zaitsu et al., 2018).

Foucault's work adds complexity and nuance to the discussion of how medicalization becomes a part of culture and social relations (Foucault, 1988, 1994, 2006). He focuses on the ways that medicalization is deployed to distinguish the normal from the abnormal through the pathologization of the non-normal. Medical discourse has been used as a bludgeon, a tool that, through its dominating and reflexive knowledge/power discourses, has led to the very identity of the modern person as a medical subject. Through this introjection of discourses, people learn to govern themselves and see themselves as well or ill, in part, in the terms set forth by medicine. Citizens, by absorbing and internalizing circulating discourses, come to think of themselves partially as bodies existing in states of health or illness and in need, or potential need, of medical intervention or disease prevention. For example, with respect to feelings of anxiety, people have come to think of themselves as requiring medications because of their neurochemistry or neurochemical selves (Rose, 2003). These technologies of self are internalized messages activated as people self-govern (and sometimes resist) in the interests of the prevailing medical power and knowledge.

Adele Clarke and colleagues (2003) have built on the previous ideas about medicalization. They term what was called medicalization as "biomedicalization" to underscore the "increasingly complex, multisited, multidirectional processes of medicalization" (p. 161). Biomedicalization has emerged from the political and economic context characteristic of today. This contemporary political economy is often termed "neoliberalism." Neoliberalism signals the move over the past forty years or so to value markets and capitalist economic growth over governments for supporting the well-being of citizens and societies. Neoliberalism encompasses five basic principles: (1) minimal governmental intervention in the markets; (2) an assumption that markets are fundamentally good and have the potential to solve social, economic, and political problems; (3) an acceptance of risks as an inevitable accompaniment to unfettered economic growth; (4) the promotion of individualism and self-responsibility over communal care; and (5) the acceptance of the resulting inequality as a necessary cost for market-based progress (Ayo, 2012).

The new medicalization or biomedicalization is complementary to neoliberalism. In fact, there is a way in which biomedicalization has intensified in the neoliberal context (Conrad, 2005; Clarke et al., 2003). Its expression corresponds to the growth of privatized or profit-making health care, the pharmaceutical and medical device industries, genomics, and so on. Today medicine comprises a significant component of the gross national product (GNP). In 2018, it was 10.9 per cent of the GNP in Canada, while in the United States, it was 16.9 per cent (Canadian Institute for Health Information [CIHI], 2019, p. 35). Furthermore, medicalization is increasingly a global phenomenon (Clarke, 2016; OECD, 2015).

In sum, while medicalization proceeds unabashed, the interests and power of the medical profession no longer lead the process. Corporate economic interests frequently initiate and sustain increases in medicalization. Citizens, too, increasingly seek medical interventions as they aspire to improve their bodies and minds through wide varieties of treatments designed to improve moods, sleep better, lose weight, and enlarge or shrink breasts, tummies, and other body parts. Today, medicalization processes have enlisted medicine to make individuals "better than well," according to Carl Elliott (2004). Highlighting the corporatization of medicine and its growth are concepts like disease mongering (Payer, 1992) and selling sickness (Moynihan & Cassels, 2006).

The spread of medical definitions of reality can be seen in many places. I would like to illustrate through one small example the prominence of "diagnostic inflation" in mental illness (Kudlow, 2013). The *Diagnostic and Statistical Manual of Mental Disorders* (DSM) is the "bible" or dictionary of mental illness (see American Psychiatric Association, n.d.). It lists all the diagnoses considered acceptable at any time and lays out their symptoms. This empirical clarity and specificity was intended to provide consistency in diagnosis for medical practitioners, insurance companies, and governments. It has also been useful for monitoring and costing diagnoses and treatments over time. The first edition of the DSM was published in 1952. It was 130 pages long and included 106 mental disorders. The DSM-II was published in 1968. In 1980, another revision to the DSM was made by a group of expert psychiatrists working together to try to come to agreement and to represent the different types of suffering they saw in their practices. The DSM-III was 494 pages long and had 265 diagnostic categories. The DSM-IV, published in 1994, was 886 pages long and included 297 disorders. The most recent DSM-5, published in 2013, is "about the same length" but has added new diseases and removed others (Grohol, 2013). Critics say that now there is a disease for everyone and a drug treatment for most of us and for many aspects of life (see Bolton, 2013, for example). The dramatic growth in the types of mental illnesses overtime is one specific illustration of medicalization.

Medicalization is both directly and indirectly related to medical error. Its influence is direct to the extent that it leads to an expansion in the unquestioned relevance of medicine to everyday life. Its influence is indirect to the extent that it obfuscates the limits of medical science, medical practice, medical systems, and pharmaceuticalization. It is also indirect in the extent to which the investments in the medical care system – in early detection, health promotion, and disease prevention – block monies being spent on promoting equality and inclusion through investments in the social determinants of health and in community-based interventions.

## Medicalization Processes Obfuscate the Inherent Limitations of Medical Science and Medical Practice

### Limits of Medical Science

Science is a highly valuable and important means to discover, describe, and explain the world. Music, art, and literature comprise other means. Some people believe in religion and supernormal events as a way to understand underlying truth. Science, though, is thought to have a more reliable and objective window into the workings of the universe. Since the enlightenment, science, as a means of knowing, has become pre-eminent. It is considered to be of value in particular because it supersedes reliance on magic, idiosyncratic morality, superstition, and the unlimited power of the church and autocratic authority. Science may stand for secular pragmatism, rationality, objectivity, and universal generalizations. But science in practice is not always entirely based on principles such as these. Science too has biases, subjectivity, illogical presumptions, and statistically quirky findings.

Learning about science begins early in Canada. The importance of empirical observation, mathematical skills, reasoning, and logical thinking are a fundamental part of the curriculum from grade school through high school and college. We Canadians perform relatively well on cross-country comparative tests. Our scores on science literacy are eighth out of sixty-five countries and fall well above the overall Organisation for Economic Co-operation and Development (OECD) average. We are ahead of the United States and the United Kingdom (Loughran et al., 2011). Despite this rate of science literacy, only 11 per cent of Canadian students score well enough on the international science assessment tool, PISA, to be likely to pursue advanced education in science or engineering (Loughran et al., 2011). This finding suggests that Canadians may know more than the average student around the world, but the vast majority could not be considered sophisticated at scientific knowledge and thinking, which may sometimes lead to unwarranted acceptance of medical authority and the science upon which it is based.

To begin any discussion of medical science, we have to be sure that we understand the meaning and the importance of the fundamental building blocks of the scientific method. The definition and measurement of the basic concepts must be valid and reliable. In short, validity refers to the extent to which the concept under consideration (for example, diagnosis) is well defined, clear, and excludes other concepts. A valid concept is one that accurately and precisely specifies and describes the subject matter under discussion. Validity is never absolute. It is never perfect. It is always an approximation. Reliability refers to the extent to which a concept (or diagnosis) is the same when measured/observed by different observers or by the same observer over time. Robust and accurate reliability depends on the assurance that the repeatedly measured concept is valid. Perfect reliability is elusive, which means that specific diagnoses and treatments are necessarily subject to inevitable slippage or error.

These two concepts, validity and reliability, along with the idea of probability are the basic building blocks of a trustworthy medical science. Probability logic, too, has inherent limitations. It is only able to assert the likely correctness of a finding by failing to reject a hypothesis. Probabilistic reasoning can only assert that y follows x with a known or estimated degree of error. It is never certain. Thus, in this and other ways, medical science, the firm foundation for medical practice, is always constrained by some degree of subjectivity and error, even when of excellent quality. Perfect truth in science is by definition elusive and tenuous.

The essential function of medical science is embedded in the cause and effect model, in the determination of causality. Causality is fundamental because the task of medicine is to diagnose, mitigate, and/or eliminate the disease state or the disability from the individual. The treatment, in other words, is designed to cause a change (for the better) in the medical or health problem. The classic "design" of medical research to determine causality is the simple two group double-blind experimental study, sometimes called the randomized controlled trial (RCT). There are always at least two groups in this design, the experimental and the control group. Both groups are measured before and after the administration of the independent variable. The groups should be equivalent before the administration of the independent variable. The experimental group is administered the independent variable, and the control group does not receive it. Instead, the control group participants receive the placebo, which should be exactly like the independent variable except that it is inactive. This design allows the researcher to ensure that the independent variable is administered after the initial measurements are taken and after equivalence between the two groups is demonstrated. Thus, any change in the dependent or outcome variable is logically due to the implementation of the independent variable. While there are other components necessary for the assurance of a causal connection, these are the basic elements of the RCT.

Randomized controlled trials are one of the basic tools required for the development of a medical practice that is established on evidence. Formally, medical practice today is guided by what is called evidence-based medicine (EBM; Masic et al., 2008). Evidence-based medicine, thought the ideal by many who evaluate medical practice, is founded on "the conscientious, explicit, judicious and reasonable use of modern, best evidence in making decisions about the care of individual patients" (p. 219). It requires the ongoing evaluation of guidelines for practice that are built upon the continuing assessment of the research. Such research is conducted in a wide variety of different areas and corresponds to the different medical specialties as well as to the variety of basic biological and associated sciences.

All medical research is not considered to be equal. Instead, there is a hierarchy of medical knowledge ranging from that based on the most rigorously tested and robust investigations, such as the RCT, to the most casual and insubstantial inquiries. In addition to validity and reliability, scientific findings need to be evaluated for clarity, logic of design, sample size, statistical power, sample socio-demographics, and other particulars. Longitudinal designs observe changes (or their lack) over time, whereas cross-sectional designs observe effects at one time only. Different conclusions are appropriate to each of these designs. Survey designs, cohort designs, case studies, and a variety of other research blueprints are in themselves of varying degrees of value in determining reliable, objective, and universal truths. Within EBM, the scientific findings presumed to have the greatest value are meta-analysis and systematic reviews. These designs both summarize and evaluate a series of studies that all address the same topic. If the findings are consistent from study to study, they are considered to be of greater value than if they are inconsistent. After these two types of designs, the next best research design is an individual experimental design. We have briefly discussed the RCT, but there are a number of other experimental designs that can be used. The essence of all of them is the determination of causality. Other designs that do not test for causality, such as case studies, are considered to be of less value in deciding on practice guidelines.

Science and evidence have developed and altered over time and will continue to progress and change. Findings (or scientific truths) will be modified and hopefully become increasingly robust as scientists ask more questions about the functioning of the human body; as ever-more rigorous, objective, and elegant research studies are funded and executed; and as more research outcomes are published in widely read peer-reviewed journals. Implicit in this process of progress is that science is never complete. Knowledge of the world is not comprehensive or conclusive. Science proceeds through a focus on one small and finite investigation at a time. Scientific knowledge is always at one "stage" or another, from the beginning or early stages to widely, but not perfectly, accepted latter stages. EBM can only be based on the current knowledge base, and it is necessarily always under construction, change, and refinement. If science is always under construction and open for improvement, it is also reflective of various errors along the way. In this way too, medical science is imperfect.

*The Development of the COVID-19 Vaccine*

With the spread of the pandemic COVID-19, knowledge of research designed to develop a vaccine has become a matter of public knowledge and the basis for international health policy. A brief examination of the classic designs used in developing the various vaccines for COVID-19 may be instructive. Vaccine discovery and testing involved experimental designs in which some people received the new product designed for COVID-19 (the experimental group) and some people received a placebo (the control group) that was administered like the new product in every way (via a "shot" in the arm) except that it contained inactive ingredients. The outcome measure, or the dependent variable, was complex and manifold, and included all of the following component variables: the diagnosis of COVID-19 or not, its severity, and its likelihood of leading to hospitalization and/or death. The clear advantage of this design is that both the experimental and the control groups can be matched and should be equivalent with respect to any factors that could potentially interfere with the outcome measurement of the effectiveness and safety of the new product. The ideal is that both groups are fundamentally the same in terms of all such possibly competing causes of COVID-19 as age, the presence of underlying disease conditions, work or living within congregate settings, density of workplace or home space, and the like. Equivalence can be achieved by random assignment to the control and the experimental group or explicit matching of the two groups on all the variables thought to affect the likelihood of a COVID-19 diagnosis. There is always the possibility of error in matching or equivalence.

This ideal design is, however, not perfect. It is subject to many possible sources of measurement and sampling error as well as mistakes in inference. Another major issue that threatens the potential value and reliability of the findings is the length of time taken after the administration of the vaccine to measure for its effectiveness and/or side effects. We still do not know if or when a booster shot might be necessary. We do not know how effective the vaccine developed for one strain of COVID-19 will be for the inevitable variants that will develop over time. Another important issue is determining the level of statistical significance required for confidence in the research findings. This decision is a somewhat subjective one that researchers make, and it permits either more or less (inevitable) error. The other important issue in the use of any new treatment is safety and the level of risk that is acceptable. Here, too, arises the question of how long to investigate the safety of the new treatment. The safety data for the vaccines adopted around the world demonstrated a risk level and time period that were considered satisfactory. However, there still could be some unknown long-term negative consequences.

There is always a possibility of fraud or perceived or real conflict of interest in any research design. The chance of such problems is heightened when the research is done by an organization that may benefit financially or any other way by the development of the treatment. The discovery, testing, development, and manufacturing of COVID-19 vaccines were, in many instances, under the jurisdiction of pharmaceutical companies, which poses obvious, or at least perceived, threats of conflict of interest. In the case of the development of vaccines for COVID-19, there was a great deal of debate about how it was managed. As late as January 2021, the *Canadian Medical Association Journal* was calling for greater transparency among the members of the decision-making bodies who might and might not have lucrative financial ties to the pharmaceutical companies that discovered and were then to manufacture approved vaccines (Traversy et al., 2021). Some argued that decision-making bodies should include underserved populations who were more likely to have been diagnosed with COVID-19 (van Daalen et al., 2020). There was a call for greater transparency on this and other matters that were viewed as problematic and a potential source of conflicts of interests by some scholars (Lexchin et al., 2020).

**Further Limits of Medical Science**

Other limits to medical science occur when the stated and ostensible values of scientific research are ignored or violated. Numerous examples can be given of the problem of conflict of interest in research, and there are also examples of fraud and "cooked" data. For instance, Dr. David Healy, a renowned Welsh psychiatrist and an expert on antidepressant drugs, was hired in 2000 by the University of Toronto and the Centre for Addiction and Mental Health (CAMH) to head up a new research clinic. The university had courted him for two years. He had finally accepted the offer. His family had visited Toronto as he considered the move. Then, he flew over to Canada from Wales to hire staff, buy furniture for the new clinic, and give a short speech. During the speech, he raised a concern that he had about an increase in suicide rates, in the order of approximately 1 in 1,000, for some people on the antidepressant drug Prozac. He had already published this finding and was not the first researcher to suggest that some depressed people may have serious and negative side effects from a particular antidepressant, Prozac. However, after this speech, the offer of the position at the University of Toronto and the affiliated CAMH was rescinded. Controversy ensued. Some argued that Dr. Healy was fired because of a conflict of interest between him and the university funding formula. What he found in his research, published, and said publicly threatened the reliance of the University of Toronto on funding from pharmaceutical companies in general and particularly from Eli Lilly, the manufacturer of Prozac (Healy, 2002).

Published medical research is not immune to fraud or mistakes of various sorts. Retractions of published research provide a window into the frequency of this problem. A study of 2,047 retracted peer-reviewed articles, published in diverse biomedical and life sciences journals indexed through PubMed, found a variety of types of problems that led to retractions of once published research. In 21 per cent of the cases, the retractions were due to errors. In more than 67 per cent of the cases, the retractions were the result of researcher misconduct of various sorts, including fraud, plagiarism, and duplicate publication (Fang et al., 2012). Furthermore, there is evidence that the rate of retractions may be increasing (Steen, 2011).

Research, however imperfect, is at the best of times a substantial contributor to excellent health care. It is important, however, to acknowledge its inevitable limitations. In the next section we discuss how medical practice falls short of perfection.

**Limits of Medical Practice**

Medical practice is also susceptible to error, because it is based on all the potential limits and omissions of biomedical research already discussed plus the issues raised by practice. Practice is, in fact, built on the foundation of imperfect medical science. There are, however, numerous additional potential concerns related to the work of the doctor and the practice of medicine (Goold & Lipkin, 1999; Kaba & Sooriakumaran, 2007). Medical practitioners are not perfect. Doctors are no more perfect than you and I. They make mistakes. They are more or less attentive, careful, and painstaking on some days than on others. As am I. Diagnosis is an objective, logical, and empirical process, but it is also subjective and the result of experience, intuition, and possibly even – at some points – luck.

Doctors may be unaware of certain new diseases or treatments. They may be unaware of the exclusions and the side effects of popular and conventional remedies. Pharmaceutical company representatives, local medical culture, or personal religious beliefs, among many other issues, may unduly influence doctors and affect their work. It is conventional among some physicians to use drugs, at times, for conditions for which they have not been approved. This practice is called off-label prescribing. For this and other reasons, medical practice does not consistently reach its idealistic goals of being based on scientific findings and evidence.

Diagnosis is a process built, in part, on the interaction between the patient and the doctor. Patients are not perfect communicators. They may remember irrelevant symptoms and forget those that are the most significant. They may change their perceptions and then perhaps, over time, add new symptoms. Patients differ in their cognitive abilities. Some are more capable of describing and reporting changing bodily signs than others. Sometimes patients may want to hide symptoms or behaviours from their doctors. For example, people who are addicted to drugs or alcohol may not want to share their problems with their doctors. Some patients go to a number of doctors, swapping stories until they get what they think they need or want.

Sometimes words mean something different to a patient than to a doctor. For instance, doctors may ask patients whether their pain is stabbing or sharp or throbbing and so on, and patients may not know how to distinguish these various options. At times, there may be just plain "bad chemistry" between a doctor and a patient, leading to misunderstanding. Gender issues, including sexual attraction or repulsion, can cloud the mind of the doctor or the patient and affect interaction. In these and numerous other ways, communication between doctors and patients may be flawed and lead to faulty diagnoses.

The essence of the medical encounter is the assignment of a diagnosis, on the one hand, or a "clean bill of health," on the other. Some health problems are easier to diagnose than others. Compare, for example, a broken bone with cardiovascular disease. The first is relatively clear and easy to observe with an X-ray. The second is more complex. It involves the weighing of a number of different variables such as blood pressure, cholesterol counts, resting heart rate, and so on for an accurate diagnosis. Many diagnoses are tentative and at least somewhat uncertain. Symptoms can wax and wane, and disappear completely on their own or morph into other symptoms. A particular diagnosis may be given because it is a necessary feature of a form to be filled out so that the doctor can get paid or the patient can be given legitimacy or compensation for missing work. A tentative diagnosis can be given as a stopgap for immediate reassurance for the patient and family. A diagnosis may be rejected by a patient because it might result in restrictions and responsibilities. For instance, a diagnosis of a sexually transmitted disease may require the naming and contacting of all prior sexual partners in order that they can be tested and that the contagious disease not be spread further. Those who receive such a diagnosis may attempt to resist it. Sometimes symptoms are on the border between pathology and good health. What this situation means is that the patient may have some of the relevant signs or symptoms but not all of them, and the doctor may have to decide whether to diagnose a disease or leave the diagnosis for a time to see whether the symptoms become full-blown or disappear. Diagnostic error is recognized as a serious problem. Strategies to minimize this type of error are being developed (Abimanyi-Ochom et al., 2019).

In addition to the clinical encounter between the doctor and the patient, lab tests may be added into the process of diagnosis. They, too, may be in error. There are both false positives and false negatives. Tests have a variable degree of sensitivity. Lab tests are not always perfectly objective measures. In the end, a diagnosis is a convenient label, a way of talking about a constellation of reported problems or observed anomalies as if they were a unit for which a remedy is possible.

Diagnoses arise from a social context. Clinical experience is another aspect of a social context. Younger or less experienced doctors may be poorer diagnosticians. Or, because of their knowledge of more recent research, newer doctors may be better diagnosticians. Diagnostic skills may change over time. Doctors who begin with poorer abilities or credentials or because they lack the intuitive gift may never improve, but others may become outstanding over time. Skills may also deteriorate over time. Patients have no way of assessing to which category their own physician belongs. Doctors may be quick diagnosticians or slow. They may take all information into account. They may be too busy or bored. They may work in teams, in clinics, or on their own. They may be willing to consult with others about what they perceive to be a difficult case or they may not. Their business model or government and insurance company funder may allow for shorter or longer visits. Some doctors will only entertain one set of symptoms at a time. Finally, and generally speaking, there is no mechanism for easily double- checking or verifying a diagnosis.

Cultural differences between doctors and patients, and indeed between doctors and other doctors, may also alter the quality of health care (Ferguson & Candib, 2002). Newcomer doctors bring with them certain assumptions and implicit learning about, for example, such culturally sensitive arrangements as sexuality and gender roles. These assumptions may vary from those of the mainstream culture in the receiving society. They may lead to confusion, poor care, and even conflict at times. Newcomer patients, too, must negotiate health care in the midst of often conflicting ideas about such topics as privacy, family, and gender. Culture can be particularly significant when it comes to religious or moral preferences and laws. Birth control, abortion, homosexuality, and transgender issues are examples of such cases. Medical practitioners always come to their work and to their patients with their own deeply embedded sense of right and wrong and the taken-for-granted. These ideas can affect care in significant and yet largely unknown ways. Socio-demographic and economic characteristics of doctors along with those of patients can also have an effect on care (Bertakis, 2009; Saha et al., 2003). For example, the gender of a doctor as well as gender discordance versus concordance with the patient can influence health care provision. Other socio-demographic characteristics such as age, racial identity, and cultural or ethnic background of doctors, and as compared to their patients, can also play a role in care (Schieber et al., 2014; James, 2017). For example, when fibromyalgia occurs in men, their descriptions of their physical symptoms are more likely to be taken seriously. Women with the same symptoms are more likely to be sent for psychiatric help (Arout et al., 2018). Equity and inequity between patients and doctors are ongoing issues that affect most aspects of the doctor-patient relationship and the care received by the patient (Verlinde et al., 2012).

Medical practice is also constrained by external forces such as payment systems and their restrictions. Government-covered services may face more oversight than those services that are paid for privately. Different insurance companies have different policies with respect to the services they cover. Practice is affected by whether the doctor is working alone or in a clinic. The pressures and decisions of country doctors and those working in remote communities may differ from those of city doctors. The presence of colleague networks for referral alters the responsibilities and the practices of doctors. Physicians who work for corporations may have different issues and potential conflicts of interest to contend with than those who are in private practice. Emergency room doctors have all the time and workload challenges of the urgency of an acute-care hospital and frequently face the inadequacies of long-term care and chronic care systems in their daily work.

The work of the doctor has been influenced by patient use of the internet (Kaba & Sooriakumaran, 2007). Additionally, there has been an increase in litigiousness, so that doctors, especially those in some specialties, sometimes tend to practise defensive medicine. The newer model of care called patient-centred medicine has brought with it some particular challenges to the authority of the doctor (Goold & Lipkin, 1999). Electronic medical records already do and will increasingly affect patient care and autonomy (Alkureishi et al., 2016). Many physicians have commented on the particular challenges of working during the COVID-19 pandemic, and the phrase "moral distress," pointing to the suffering of the health care practitioners working during the pandemic, has become a common descriptor of working during this trying time (Kanaris, 2021).

## Limits of the Medical System

Medical system factors contribute to the quality of health care as well. For example, doctors who work alone or in solo practice have all the responsibilities of running a small business (including hiring, firing, and training staff, and managing accounts and payments), along with providing health care. This arrangement may lead them to feel they have more control and more autonomy, and therefore to consider that they have greater job satisfaction. However, they may be overwhelmed because they are responsible for their patients on a 24/7 basis. They may be isolated from others and thus fail to stay informed about new practice issues. They may be more or less likely to prescribe drugs or to suggest surgery or to refer to a specialist. On the other hand, some may give exceptional service, and their patients may be more likely to feel special and known by their doctors. Certain research has found that patients fare better in group practices, as measured by their likelihood of readmission after hospitalization (Riverin et al., 2017).

Payment methods can also affect practice (Blomqvist & Busby, 2012; Gosden et al., 1999). Salaried physicians may take more time with each patient than those who work fee for service. Those working fee for service may need to see a certain number of patients for a certain delimited period of time in order to pay their bills. In a situation lacking universal health care coverage, patients who rely on insurance may be denied service by their insurance provider, even though it is recommended by doctors. Patients in a universal coverage environment may be denied certain types of interventions because of their cost, their experimental nature, or wait times. Universal health care insurance covers more conservative treatment as a general rule. Doctors themselves may be more or less risk averse and thus more or less likely to recommend new and experimental treatments in favour of the proven and therefore financially covered treatment interventions.

The overuse of the emergency room (ER) is a growing problem (Cowling et al., 2013; Villani & Mortensen, 2013). It is the result of both the lack of family practitioners in some locations and also the simple perceived convenience of not having to take time off work or make an appointment ahead of time. It is occasionally because symptoms arise late at night. Sometimes this overuse results in very long wait times in the ER and may even lead to chaotic or inadequate health care. There is already a lack of long-term care beds across Canada, and this situation is expected to get much worse as the baby boom generation ages (Conference Board of Canada, 2017). The lack of long-term beds often leads to crowded emergency rooms and very expensive care, which robs the health care system of dollars that could be spent on such things as home care or hospice or palliative care.

Another system problem is relying on evidence-based medicine (EBM) when faced with a new disease. By definition, a new disease is one without any evidentiary base, either for recognition or for treatment. While EBM is logically the source of the best information about disease and treatment, it relies on published and peer-reviewed journal articles. Each article is generally the outcome of research studies, which may take many years to conceive, garner funding for, execute, and then write up and get published. In the case of new diseases, particularly those that involve multiple bodily systems, there will not have been time for this process to unfold.

Ongoing monitoring of medical practice may not occur frequently enough. At any one time, a certain percentage of health care providers should not be practising because they are offering inadequate care. The goal of the Canadian Medical Protective Association (2017) is to evaluate every doctor every ten years. However, a lot can go wrong in ten years in the ability of a doctor to offer safe and effective care. Such failures and inadequacies may very well be unknown to medical authorities or to patients.

Specialties have proliferated (Weisz, 2006; Gritzer & Arluke, 1989). While concentrating expertise in novel ways to represent the development of new knowledge and practice may be a very good thing in the long run, in the short run, there may be only a very few doctors who are adequately trained for the specialist job they choose or are asked to do. Labour force issues, reflecting the number of doctors with different specialties in different geographic areas, can potentially limit and bias the availability of excellent and safe health care provision. Another problem is the growing reliance on specialists who focus on one organ or one system at a time when, ironically, chronic illnesses, which are often defined by multi-bodily system or organ involvement, are growing as life expectancy extends.

There are significant power differentials among the differing occupational groups within and between hospitals (Zelek & Phillips, 2003). These power differentials are mirrored by large differences in income, both among the different personnel in any particular setting and between settings. The quality and safety of care may differ depending on the remuneration of the worker. These and other medical system issues have powerful effects on patient diagnoses and outcomes.

## Pharmaceuticalization

Pharmaceuticalization is defined by Abraham (2009) as "the process by which social, behavioural or bodily conditions are treated or are deemed to be in need of treatment with medical drugs" (p. 934). The concept of pharmaceuticalization has been elaborated by a number of sociologists (see, for example, Fox & Ward, 2009; Williams et al., 2009). In these discussions, the process of pharmaceuticalization is considered as both an aspect of medicalization and as separate, with its own independent causes. Pharmaceuticalization essentially refers to the social and cultural processes involved in the translation of problems in human living into problems with pharmacological solutions. It is, like medicalization, an expansive process, one wherein more and more of life is designated as susceptible to and benefitted by the introduction of various chemicals into the body. Abraham (2010b) points to the popular explanations offered for the growth of the pharmaceutical option. The primary one is that developments in biomedical research have led to more and more specificity and assurance about the value of drugs in certain circumstances. In this explanation, pharmaceuticalization is an expanding process because of its power to positively affect health. The process, in this view, reflects increased knowledge and discovery. However, Abraham (2010b) says that this explanation is not tenable because the significant rates of growth in drug utilization are not correlated with therapeutic advances in specific enhancements in related areas of health. In fact, improvements in health statuses have been declining, even while the utilization of pharmaceuticals has been increasing (Abraham, 2010b). Furthermore, there is evidence of significant roles in the expansion of drug solutions played by advertising, drug company promotion, and the diminution of the powers of states vis-à-vis the pharmaceutical industry (Abraham, 2010b, 2010a). Busfield (2006) points to another factor in the growth in the power and influence of pharmaceuticals. It has to do with the industry's control over both the processes and the findings of science pertaining to drug development. Williams and colleagues (2011) add to this analysis by directing us to think about the ways that drugs have been increasingly developed with enhancement and not cure or mitigation of symptoms in mind. In this instance, they are talking about the way that certain drugs are less about disease amelioration and more about improving life quality. For instance, antidepressants are not always or necessarily prescribed to people with the disease of depression but are sometimes prescribed to people who say they want to feel better or better than well, according to Peter Kramer (Stossel, 2016). Medical professionals increasingly use pharmaceuticals for cognitive enhancement (Enck, 2014). Further, pharmaceuticals are sometimes prescribed in the interest of anticipated health futures. The mass media have also contributed to pharmaceuticalization and to the sense that drugs are widely available and able to solve myriad problems through widespread advertising.

Pharmaceutical companies, Conrad (2007) suggests, now, in fact, market more than drugs. They market and thereby create new diseases. Moynihan and Cassels (2006) have been particularly vocal proponents of this view, which calls pharmaceutical advertising and drug promotion "selling sickness." This campaign happens, they argue, as pharmaceutical companies describe ordinary mild suffering and bodily or behavioural anomalies as endemic and as seriously problematic. In turn, they offer ready-made solutions. In addition, there is an extensive expansion of interventions based on ideas such as prevention and risk (Moynihan et al., 2002). Many of these drugs, such as Vioxx, have been withdrawn from the market because their use became associated with health problems (Sibbald, 2004).

## Limits of Pharmaceuticals and the Pharmaceutical Industry

The pharmaceutical industry is a central component of an expanding network of corporations that manufacture and deliver aspects of medical care and medical care products, supplies, and services for a profit. In addition to pharmaceuticals, this list includes medical devices, tools, and technology. The growth in privatization that this trend represents is a significant part of globalization under neoliberalism (Usher & Skinner, 2012). Drugs compose the second largest expenditure in the health care system today, coming only after hospitals. This share of the health care budget signifies a substantial growth in reliance on medications over the past few decades (CIHI, 2019). In fact, the percentage of monies dedicated to pharmaceuticals has been one of the fastest growing components of the health care system (CIHI, 2019).

In Canada, prescribed drugs increased as a piece of the total health care budget an average of 10.6 per cent per year between 1985 and 2005, and 7.6 per cent from 2005 to 2010 (CIHI, 2019). They encompassed 17.6 per cent of the total spent by the health care system in 2016. According to data compiled by the OECD (2018), pharmaceutical spending comprised a significant driver of the overall cost of health care. In Canada, where we congratulate ourselves on our national health care coverage, only 40 per cent of the cost of prescribed medications is born by the government, and the rest is an out-of-pocket or private insurance expenditure (Canadian Foundation for Healthcare Improvement, 2011).

As pharmaceutical spending has increased in Canada, the industry has grown in power both here and around the globe (Statista, 2018). As a consequence, we can have less confidence that all drugs available in Canada have been thoroughly tested and are safe. Instead, it appears that a conflict of interest may be at the heart of funding for drug regulation and safety in Canada and elsewhere. Regulatory and overall health care budget declines at Health Canada have meant, in practical terms, that the pharmaceutical industry "is now providing a substantial fraction of the money needed to run the drug regulatory system" (Lexchin, 2013, p. 285). This shift may result in a situation in which Health Canada is in a weaker bargaining position than the industry. The safety and effectiveness of drugs in Canada may be declining because responsibility for testing new drugs has increasingly been given to the profit-driven industry (Silversides, 2010). One illustration of the potential dangers of unsafe drugs is that approximately a third of all emergency room visits among people over sixty-five in the United States are due to adverse drug reactions (Budnitz et al., 2011).

The balance of power between the Health Products and Foods Branch and the pharmaceutical industry has been moving towards the industry as Canadian government policies have generally moved to the ideological right, with an emphasis on relying on neoliberalism and market principles to govern growth, productivity, and ultimately safety. Most government regulations are inadequate, with the result that (1) half the drugs now on the Canadian market have never passed modern tests regarding safety or effectiveness; (2) even where regulations are in place in the industrialized world, substandard drugs are being marketed and distributed overseas; and (3) drug companies seem to have a monopoly on the information available to doctors as well as on the side effects of various drugs (Clarke, 2016).

There is considerable evidence that drugs are frequently overprescribed in Canada. We take the beneficence of prescription drug use for granted. However, the situation is more complicated. For example, evidence suggests that about half of the antidepressants in use do not work except as placebos (Smith, 2012). Off-label use of pharmaceuticals is routine. This practice means that medications are used for conditions for which they have not been approved and for uses for which there is no or very little published evidence. While off-label prescribing may be justifiable in a situation in which there is no alternative (such as pain reduction in end-of-life care), the off-label use of medications may be especially problematic when such treatment is discretional and for minor problems or aspirational desires, such as to have clearer skin or bigger muscles.

Another serious limitation regarding the safety and efficacy of drugs available to Canadians lies in the numerous conflicts of interest that have been reported between researchers and the pharmaceutical industry, as well as between doctors/doctors in training and the industry. We briefly discussed the case of Dr. David Healey earlier. But there are many other examples of the problems of conflict of interest. Such problems mean that the evidence upon which diagnoses and treatments depend may be biased in favour of the interests of pharmaceutical companies (Roseman et al., 2012). Conflicts of interest can lead to changes in study design that favour one outcome or another and the probability that results will support the use of a sponsor's drug, whether or not results will be published, how findings are interpreted, and so on (Roseman et al., 2012).

Ultimately, because research is cumulative, the existence of any one biased study in a sense prejudices all subsequent research on the same topic. However, researchers have to rely on pharmaceutical funding to some extent, as the amount of government funding is not sufficient to provide monies to all of the labs and researchers working in biomedical fields. Because of this problem, journals require that authors indicate whether or not they have received industry funding in their publication, which allows readers the opportunity to assess the potential effects of conflicts of interest in any particular study. This requirement has been in place for several decades now. Once awareness of the problem of conflicts of interest emerged and was documented, science journals began to require disclosure. However, explication of conflict of interest is still not a requirement for some medical journals.

Drug companies are also allowed to advertise their products directly to consumers in the United States and New Zealand. Although advertising directly to consumers is illegal in Canada, Canadians consume considerable advertising through the mass media emanating from the United States. Advertised drugs are more likely to be requested from the doctor and are more likely to be prescribed by doctors where consumers are reached by American mass media (Donohue et al., 2007; Friedman & Gould, 2007; Hollon, 2005). There are serious costs as well as some benefits from direct-to-consumer (DTC) advertising according to research. The negative effects include the spread and up-take by the public of misinformation, as well as an expansion of unnecessary drug use and unjustified diagnoses. This expansion can both cause side effects and increase the likelihood that newer and more expensive drugs will be used (Almasi et al., 2006). Another negative effect of DTC advertising is that the request for a medication from a doctor can result in the prescription of the requested drug without a full physical examination (Almasi et al., 2006). On the positive side, doctors say that they see patients they would otherwise not see and can sometimes find diagnoses that they would not have had a chance to observe. Doctors have also reported that having patients come in to their offices, even if it is merely to request a medication, can lead to better discussion of the patient's health and the opportunity to provide health education (Parekh et al., 2012). Another potential benefit is that patients may be more likely to take their prescription if they trust mass media sources of information and thus feel confident about the beneficial effects.

Pharmaceutical companies advertise directly to doctors, medical school professors, and medical students. These corporations also attempt to indirectly influence doctors and medical students to favour their products through sponsoring conferences, paying for holidays and dinners, buying new computers, and the like. Ranking of Canada's seventeen medical schools found that twelve achieved a failing grade in respect to their conflict of interest guidelines and policies. Marked out of twenty-four, the majority garnered less than twelve points because they neglected to ban things like taking gifts from, and ghostwriting for, pharmaceutical companies (Glauser, 2013; Shnier et al., 2013). A recent survey found that about one half of the physicians in the United States who were studied received various sorts of payments from pharmaceutical and medical device corporations. These gifts amounted to 2.4 billion dollars in 2015. At least 700 physicians in the United States received more than one million dollars each from pharmaceutical companies (Ornstein et al., 2019). Such conflicts of interest have been shown to affect prescribing habits (Mozes, 2018).

## Limitations Due to the Social Determinants of Health

There is a consistent and positive relationship between good health and higher socio-economic status. This statement represents a basic finding in the perspective called the social determinants of health. Social conditions are fundamentally linked to health outcomes. Consequently, in a society such as Canada, people who have more wealth tend also to be healthier, and people who have less wealth tend to be in poorer health. How does this process work? Why would relative economic advantage in a society be connected to good health and a lower location in the economic structure with illness? There are several different explanations. Dennis Raphael (2002a, 2002b, 2016, for example), especially, has helped to outline the different explanations of inequality and health, and their consequences for Canadians. The most obvious link is that health is associated with the availability of basic material goods and services. This viewpoint is called the materialist approach. From this perspective, human health depends fundamentally on available, accessible, and good-quality nutritious food and water; good transportation systems and infrastructure, including public transit; consistent, safe, adequately remunerated, and satisfying work; and appropriate and affordable housing, early childhood care provision, and other essential components of life. Without these, health is compromised and challenged. Income is central to attaining these material goods.

A second explanation for the link between inequality and health has been called the neo-materialist approach. This perspective acknowledges the importance of a basic level of material adequacy but then looks at the relative distribution of material and social goods across society. The argument in this explanation is that, once material adequacy is in place, then perceived social equity becomes crucial to health for all (see, for example, McLeod et al., 2003). Societies with progressive redistribution policies designed to ensure the social welfare of their populations, such as unemployment insurance, generous leave policies for sickness, pensions, compassionate care, benefits and advocacy for the disabled, early childhood education and care programs, universal education, and a basic guaranteed annual income, are more likely to have a population with lower infant mortality, longer life expectancy, and longer disability-free life expectancy (OECD, 2018). Living in a society characterized by inequality has negative health consequences for people all the way up and down the status hierarchy (Chang & Lauderdale, 2009; Bryant et al., 2011).

A third explanation for the links between social determinants and health serves to explain how the neo-materialist theory might work at the level of individual social-psychological functioning. It focuses attention on the impacts of inequity and highlights the importance of social inclusion/exclusion to the ongoing daily internal psychological and social processes of life for people as social beings in a community. Inclusion enhances health and well-being. Marginalization, exclusion, discrimination, and stigmatization decrease health and well-being. Experiences of inclusion/exclusion vary by such social conditions as race, gender, age, and Indigenous status. Both being included and including others have health benefits. The perception of inclusion also impacts individual health (Hartung et al., 2015). "Though there is no singular definition of social inclusion, there is general understanding that a socially inclusive society is one in which people feel valued, their differences and rights are respected, and their basic needs are met so that they can live in dignity, and have their voices heard. An inclusive society is one in which people are able to meaningfully participate in social, economic, cultural, and political systems" (Mamatis et al., 2019, p. 1). The experience of being included through the ability to take civic action and to be involved in political reform and change is essential to good health. Social cohesion is enhanced by inclusion and is indeed another powerful predictor of health (Marmot, 2018). Social exclusion is associated with about eight times higher mortality rate among women and twelve times higher mortality rate among men (Marmot, 2018).

Figure 1. Medicalization Model

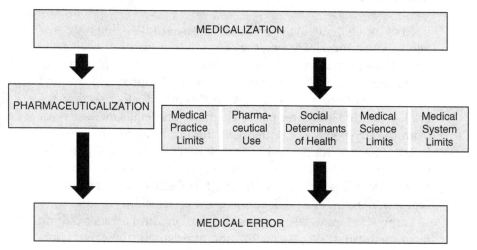

The social determinants of health are important to consider in any attempt to reduce medical error. Attention paid to inequities would mitigate against many people needing to visit doctors, take medications, be hospitalized, or use the ER. Greater equality and fewer people experiencing poverty or other vulnerabilities would result in less sickness, fewer accidents, and less disability. Greater equality would result in longer life expectancy, less disability, better perceived health, less chronicity over a lifetime, and fewer infectious diseases (Government of Canada, 2018).

In the following section, I briefly introduce you to the case studies of medical error. Together, my explanations of these cases will buttress the claim that medicalization, through its emphasis on medical definitions and interventions, obscures the importance of recognizing the limits in medical and pharmaceutical usage. It also supports an emphasis on medical benefits that may subvert attention from the social determinants of health. Figure 1 provides a visual representation of the relationships used in this book to explain medical error.

## The Case Studies: A Very Brief Overview

Each of the chapters in the book uses a case study to illustrate how all of these issues, including the social determinants of health; the limitations to medical science, practice, and systems; pharmaceuticalization; and medicalization are potential sources of error and may cause suffering and death. After this introductory section, the book is divided into three parts. The first part details medical error from the perspective of patients, including Brian Sinclair, Ashley Smith, Vanessa Young and Marit McKenzie, and Amy Tan. The second part addresses medical error focusing on health care providers, including Dr. Charles Smith, Elizabeth Wettlaufer, and Dr. Norman Barwin. The final section is the conclusion.

I argue that these case studies all reflect medical errors resulting from medicalization. Medicalization affects both the experiences of patients and those of medical providers, because it encompasses the capacity to focus uncritically on the benefits of the medical system while ignoring related issues. The case studies point to fundamental sources of the limitations of our unquestioning reliance on allopathic medical care. The case studies argue that we fail to understand the limits of medical science, medical practice, medical systems, and pharmaceutical use at our own peril. Good health outcomes also depend on a consideration of the role of the social determinants of health in illness. These, too, need to be addressed in an effort to diminish medical error. I will return to the explanations of ongoing, inevitable, and predictable medical error in the conclusion.

# CASE STUDIES, PART 1

## Focusing on the Patient Victim of Medical Error

# chapter one

# Brian Sinclair: Waiting and Waiting until Dying in the Emergency Room

## The Issue

Brian Sinclair is the name of the Indigenous man who died while waiting for simple medical assistance in an emergency room (ER) in Winnipeg. He had remained, in his wheelchair, for more than thirty-four hours. Eventually, he died of a treatable bladder infection while slumped in his seat. During this time, many other patients came, were treated, and went home or were admitted to hospital. He died among busy nurses and doctors, security guards, cleaners, and other hospital personnel. Over his long stay, other patients-in-waiting, their companions, and casual visitors surrounded him as he became sicker and sicker and, finally, non-responsive.

By the time the medical staff took notice of Brian Sinclair, thirty-four hours after he first arrived at the ER, he was dead. Rigor mortis had already set in. Although the doctor who examined Brian Sinclair after he was identified as possibly not breathing could not estimate the exact time of death, he was sure that Mr. Sinclair would have been dead for at least several hours. The national news picked up on this story. Mr. Sinclair's death was followed by an inquest under the Fatality Inquiries Act, to which eighty-two witnesses were called, including medical and social care providers, administrators and various other hospital personnel, as well as a number of civilians who had observed some of the events of the weekend in the ER where Brian Sinclair's death occurred (Provincial Court of Manitoba, 2014, pp. 188–90). The findings of the inquest were presented to the public. Mr. Sinclair's death was ruled as accidental. Sixty-three recommendations for changes in the emergency room and in the health care system more generally were made so that this sort of event would never be repeated (pp. 182–7).

I remember hearing this story on the news and being shocked. How could such a thing happen in Canada in 2008? Could it occur today? This chapter will discuss some of the causes of the death of Brian Sinclair. For details surrounding aspects of Brian Sinclair's life, both before and at the time of his death in the ER, I rely partly on the inquest report that detailed many problems with the health care system and the particular hospital and emergency room during the fateful time of his death (Provincial Court of Manitoba, 2014). But Brian Sinclair's family and others argued that this focus missed the point. Instead, they said, Brian Sinclair's death was caused by a history of racial prejudice and discrimination, which led him to be in the ER on that fateful weekend (Geary, 2017). I ask, then: What was the role of racism in this tragedy? And what was the role of medical system error? I question who or what was to blame. I describe how the system worked, but failed to work for Brian Sinclair. I ask to what extent his death was the result of medical error, just an accident, or due to something else. This chapter looks at Brian Sinclair's death from a broad and sociological perspective. It was considered an accident and thus not predictable. I will argue that, while this particular event was not precisely predictable, outcomes such as this one should have been expected and, furthermore, we ought to expect comparable events unless significant changes occur. I note that the inequities in the social determinants of health that played a role in Sinclair's death continue today.

In the final medical analysis, Brian Sinclair died of acute peritonitis (Provincial Implementation Team, 2015, p. 1). This illness is neither a rare nor complex problem. It would have been easily treated with antibiotics had he been assessed and cared for soon after he had arrived at the hospital. Many health care personnel, including nurses, aides, doctors, and the ER security guards, observed Brian Sinclair. Some noticed that he had been sitting in essentially the same place through one shift and then seemed to be in the same position during the next shift and day. Still, however, none of these health care personnel walked over to the Indigenous man in the wheelchair to ask how he was feeling and whether he needed anything. It appeared that he was never assessed, never triaged; nor was his name written in the formal log indicating that he needed care. There were at least seventeen members of the ER staff who noticed Mr. Sinclair (Kubinec, 2013). However, he had never been formally assessed.

The videotape of the emergency room provided some suggestions as to what might have happened when Mr. Sinclair entered and languished in the ER (Rollason & Welch, 2014). Sometime after Brian Sinclair entered, the triage aide was seen on the video recording of the ER to bend down and talk to him for about thirty seconds. Then the aide seemed to go on to do the same thing with another person who had entered the ER immediately after Mr. Sinclair. This second person was quickly assessed and cared for by the staff. Brian Sinclair was not. A short time later, Mr. Sinclair was seen taking a letter in an envelope out of his pocket, looking around (perhaps for someone to whom he might be able to give it), and then putting the letter back in his pocket. Next, the ER video camera caught him wheeling himself to find a place away from the triage aide to wait for care. At this point, he looks fairly energetic. Later, he was seen buying potato chips from a machine. Over time, he vomited a few times, and a member of the cleaning staff and then a security guard are seen offering him a washbasin, on one occasion, and a kidney basin, on another. Towels and a yellow caution tape were placed around his wheelchair so that no one fell or slipped in the fluids from his vomit. Eventually, he appeared to fall asleep, with his head bent down off to the side and his baseball hat covering his face from the camera above. He did not appear to remind anyone that he needed service. He never seemed to assert himself. He sat quietly on his own, getting weaker and weaker and finally dying.

The inquest report on Brian Sinclair's death essentially took the medical systems approach to error for an understanding of how and why Brian Sinclair died. Even though a few individuals are described as failing to do their jobs adequately, the ultimate problem that led to this unnecessary and tragic death was systemic according to the report (Provincial Court of Manitoba, 2014, p. 181). This chapter will discuss and illustrate what this systems approach to medical error looks like in the case of Brian Sinclair. We will examine systemic problems such as waiting times within the functioning of ERs across Canada. We will investigate the over-investment in allopathic high-tech medicine as compared to long-term care and community living alternatives for those with chronic and complex care needs and various different types of abilities. We will then look outside the medical care system for other possible explanations of Mr. Sinclair's death and other deaths and harms. In particular, we will look at the role of the social determinants of health, particularly racism and the history and present status of racial injustice that characterizes the relationship between the Canadian state and Indigenous people, in Mr. Sinclair's death. We will begin this section of the chapter in the days, weeks, months, and years leading up to Mr. Sinclair's death.

## Brian Sinclair's Life in the Year Leading Up to His Death

In the year before his death, Brian Sinclair's health status changed dramatically. He essentially became a ward of the province; under this status, he was called a Committee (ward) of the Public Trustee (Provincial Court of Manitoba, 2014, p. 8). By this term, he was understood by the state to be its responsibility. This designation was because he needed help with daily living activities and ongoing medical care after losing his legs. In the winter of 2007, when Brian Sinclair was forty-four years old, he was evicted from a rooming house. He searched for a place to sleep out of the cold and tried to get access to a church. The church was locked. He was unable to gain entry. It was cold, and he was tired. He collapsed and fell asleep. "He was found, literally frozen to the wall of the church. As a result, he required a bilateral amputation of both legs above the knee" (p. 60). While recovering from this surgery, Mr. Sinclair developed a difficult-to-control bladder infection. Ultimately, this infection led to the insertion of a permanent catheter and the requirement that it be regularly cleaned and changed. This new situation made Mr. Sinclair unable to fend for himself. He became dependent on others and on ongoing health care for his survival.

After the amputation of his legs and for about a year prior to his death, Brian Sinclair was living in a personal care home – a place called Quest Inn. This was his home, a Winnipeg Regional Health Authority assisted care residence. Although Quest Inn was normally designed for short-term stays, there were no other housing options available for Mr. Sinclair. He had health monitoring and some support at Quest Inn (as described in the next paragraph), but it was essentially a residence and not a medical care facility. Whenever Mr. Sinclair needed further medical care, he had to go to the Health Action Centre (HAC) or the hospital ER.

To help him manoeuvre through the complexities of living without legs and to provide ongoing regular health monitoring and catheter care, he had a number of different state-supported "workers" who were attached to him through the Quest Inn. One, called his integrated support worker, described him as "relatively contented" (Provincial Court of Manitoba, 2014, p. 5) during their time together in his last year of life. This worker and Mr. Sinclair usually spent a few hours a week, twice a week, together in the personal care home, in coffee shops, going to medical appointments, and engaging in various activities. Brian Sinclair was described as enjoying helping others and doing voluntary work at the Siloam Mission. The mission provided meals, clothing, and other services to Winnipeg's poor and homeless community. Brian Sinclair went to the mission virtually every day, where he hung out with his brothers, Bradley and Russell.

Mr. Sinclair apparently spent his time at the Siloam Mission serving others by table washing or offering greetings at the door. His integrated support worker underscored a picture of Mr. Sinclair as a generous, kind, and thoughtful man. He sometimes brought his support worker fruits and vegetables from the mission and "would literally give his shirt or jacket to someone in greater need than he" (Provincial Court of Manitoba, 2014, p. 6). He was said to enjoy "doing volunteer work and socializing with friends" (p. 5) at the mission. His integrated support worker also suggested that Mr. Sinclair "did not fully appreciate his vulnerability" (p. 6). At times, Mr. Sinclair was known to strike out at others, especially when questioned about his substance use.

In addition to his integrated support worker, who visited regularly and engaged with Brian Sinclair in informal social activities, Mr. Sinclair also had a health care attendant whose responsibility was to see him three times per day, a laundry/bathing worker who was to call on him once a week, and a registered nurse who was to visit every two weeks. It had been difficult to find alternative housing for Mr. Sinclair because he was both "vulnerable" and "fiercely independent" (Provincial Court of Manitoba, 2014, p. 5). He was also described as having "untapped potential" (p. 19). He did not want to live in a nursing home and yet was apparently "not competent to make medical decisions for himself, manage his own finances or his own disposition (discharge) plans" (p. 10). Furthermore, "he had no desire to live with the white man" (p. 14). Because he had a Foley catheter (an indwelling thin sterile tube that was inserted into the bladder to drain the urine), he needed ongoing medical care. The catheter had to be changed every four to six weeks and cleaned regularly, at least every two weeks. In the absence of such ongoing care, Mr. Sinclair was vulnerable to bladder infections, which, left untreated, were known to potentially lead to very serious illness and death.

On the morning of his death, Brian Sinclair's home care nurse said that she felt something didn't look right with his catheter (Provincial Court of Manitoba, 2014, p. 29). She reported at the inquest that she had told him to go to the hospital but did not think his medical situation was an emergency, and at the time, he seemed fine (p. 30). Not much later in the day, however, when Mr. Sinclair went to the Health Action Centre (HAC) to get a cab to the hospital, he was described as "disheveled and malodorous" (p. 30). Although he was supposed to have been cared for by a number of service workers, according to the staff at the HAC, he seemed to have been neglected. His catheter had last been changed on 11 July, and he died on 20 September. That length of time is considerably longer than the recommended limit of four to six weeks between catheter changes (p. 30).

According to his home care nurse, the explanation for the overly long time since the catheter had been changed was that Brian Sinclair was "non-compliant" (Provincial Court of Manitoba, 2014, p. 9). He was seldom home when she went to attend to his catheter, even though she called and left messages with the Quest Inn to ask him to stay and wait for her arrival. As a consequence, she had "put a hold" on her services for him (p. 9). She said she could not do her job with him because he was not usually where she thought he should be or where she had asked him to be. The nurse had asked the nurse practitioner at the HAC to care for the catheter. The nurse practitioner had apparently agreed to do so but soon left for another job. In the meantime, the HAC did not have a chart for his medical care, and the home care nurse did not follow up to ensure that the nurse practitioner had been able to care for the catheter.

## Brian Sinclair's Earlier Life

Who was Brian Sinclair? Until he was eight years old, his mother and father raised him, along with eight brothers and sisters, on Fort Alexander First Nation. He was "kind and helpful," according to his sister, and an "excellent student" (Provincial Court of Manitoba, 2014, p. 3). His father was of mixed heritage, Indigenous and European, and was described as a good provider and a successful fisher and logger. His mother was an Indigenous woman who had been educated in a residential school. When Brian was eight, his family moved to the North End of Winnipeg, where his life began to change. In the first place, he and his brothers took up with other neighbourhood kids and started to sniff solvents. Then, when he was twelve, his mother and father separated. The Manitoba Child and Family Services took him into care for about a year; afterwards, he and some of his siblings were returned to live with his father in Winnipeg.

Brian Sinclair was very close to his father until his father died when Brian was in his twenties. Then, he and two of his brothers,

Bradley and Russell, moved into a boarding house together (Provincial Court of Manitoba, 2014, p. 3). When the landlady sold the boarding house, he and his brothers moved into a different boarding home, from which they were later evicted. After that, they "moved around a lot" (p. 3). Still, Brian was known to have shown exemplary courage and altruism when, for example, he "risked his life to save the occupants of a burning house" (p. 4). Although the description of his life from this time forward is sketchy, it appears from reports based on later stages of his life that Brian and his brothers intermittently sniffed solvents and drank excess alcohol.

## The Weekend Brian Sinclair Died in the ER

The waiting room of the ER had been newly redesigned about a year prior to Mr. Sinclair's death. Some of the nurses who worked there had been worried about what they considered to be design flaws in the layout. In particular, they were concerned because the nurse who was responsible for triage, for ensuring that the most serious patients were seen first and checking on the progress of waiting patients, had an obstructed view of the waiting room. Not only were waiting patients sitting in chairs that faced away from this desk but also many of the chairs upon which patients and their companions sat were very high. The view was thus blocked. The nurses had complained to management about this problem in the year before Mr. Sinclair died. The administration had asked them to wait a while and use the space as it was before they reorganized it. The staff was not satisfied. The nurses said the room was as long as a football field (Provincial Court of Manitoba, 2014, p. 59). Partly as a result of not being listened to, the staff morale was low (pp. 110–11).

There was another design issue that also had consequences for Brian Sinclair's unnecessary death. The emergency room had both back and front entrances and exits. People could and did easily come and go without being triaged or assessed by the health care staff. The ER was often used as a place for people who lived in nearby shelters and boarding homes and wanted to come in out of the cold or heat during the daytime to sit a while and watch television or chat. The nurses sometimes fed these visitors and gave them something to drink to make them more comfortable. This compassion and kindness to people who regularly used the ER for shelter because there was nothing else available to suit their needs may have contributed to the circumstances of Mr. Sinclair's death.

On the day that Brian Sinclair went to the hospital, he had wheeled himself to the Health Action Centre, where he was described as "obviously in distress" (Provincial Court of Manitoba, 2014, p. 30). A nurse and a doctor there saw him. They reported that he was cognitively "OK" but foul-smelling and partially covered in dried feces (p. 30). The medical staff determined that he needed to have his catheter changed. They were not able to do so. They lacked the equipment necessary for creating and maintaining a sterile field and could not safely lift him from his wheelchair. Thus, they decided to send him to the ER with a letter explaining what the problem was and asking that his catheter be changed. They described him as calm, coherent, and motivated when he left the HAC for the ER unaccompanied. At this point, he was not "critically ill" and stable (p. 39). Staff at the HAC did not call ahead to say that Mr. Sinclair was on his way or follow up in any way. They had sent a letter with him detailing his needs and assumed that he would be able to get to the hospital on his own and present the letter to the ER staff.

Brian Sinclair did take a taxi, and he arrived at the ER safely. However, he was never medically assessed there. The triage aide appeared to have neglected to note that Mr. Sinclair had arrived at the ER and needed service. This aide did not appear to write the specifics of Mr. Sinclair's name and complaint down for the triage nurse to investigate. Once he finished with Mr. Sinclair, the aide immediately talked to another person who needed care (Provincial Court of Manitoba, 2014, p. 55). He appeared to write this person's name down, and the nursing staff saw the next patient quickly.

On the weekend that Mr. Sinclair died, there was a 20 per cent shortage of staff and a greater number of patients than was usual (138 versus 120) and thus normatively expected. The ER was even busier than usual. In this chaotic atmosphere, it was difficult to determine whether the people sitting throughout the waiting room were patients, family members, friends, or just people inside to rest, watch television, and maybe get a bite to eat (Provincial Court of Manitoba, 2014), p. 59). Typically, in the ER one could see and hear people who were moaning, screaming, vomiting, and sometimes intoxicated. At the time of Mr. Sinclair's death, there was no policy requiring that staff keep track of who was in the waiting room for rest, warmth, food, drink, or even bus tickets and who was there for medical treatment. On this particular weekend, both shifts were characterized as "horrendous" (p. 59). As well as the people waiting to be seen, there were six patients in beds who had been admitted to hospital but for whom a permanent hospital bed had not yet been found and twenty-three patients who had been admitted but were without even a temporary bed.

All these issues contributed to Brian Sinclair's death: the over-crowding of the ER, the unusually high number of patients in the ER, the back-up of admitted patients without beds to which to go, the impeded sight lines in the ER for the care-providing staff, the failure of the administration to act quickly on the complaint about the obstructed view by the nurses, the aide's (seeming) failure to record Mr. Sinclair's presence in the ER, and the multiple function-ality of the ER as both a day shelter and a place for the assessment and care of medical emergencies.

The numerous and varied assumptions made about Brian Sin-clair fit within this context of the multi-use of the ER and a lack of clear special demarcation between pre-triaged and post-triaged patients, companions, and casual visitors. Among the assumptions made were that Mr. Sinclair had already received treatment or that he was just a drunk who was "sleeping it off" (Provincial Court of Manitoba, 2014, p. 64). It is important to note that there was no record in the previous six years of Brian Sinclair ever being in the ER because he was intoxicated. Nor was there any evidence that he had ever had to be removed because of intoxication (p. 79). Some people reported that they thought he was homeless and simply seeking shelter. Some assumed that he was waiting for a bed in another area of the hospital or waiting for further medical atten-tion. Later, some other explanations for ignoring Brian Sinclair included the idea that he had seen medical staff and was now just resting, seeking shelter, or that he was waiting for the attention of another nurse. He was passive, and he did not appear to be a security threat. He was easily ignored. The staff were busy working with other individuals who had been properly triaged and cared for in the order that they had appeared in the ER asking for help.

In this context, it was non-medical people, civilians as well as security guards, who were concerned enough to draw Brian Sinclair's well-being to the attention of various medical staff. One woman approached a security guard to say that she thought he was dead: "He was like a person frozen in time" (Provincial Court of Manitoba, 2014, p. 67). The guard replied: "I explained to Debbie that he is a regular patient and that is the usual position you would find him in when intoxicated" (p. 67). The civilian (Debbie) tried again and said: "I'm dead serious. Someone needs to go out there" (p. 101). Another civilian reported that "he certainly thought that Brian Sinclair required medical attention" (p. 83). He noticed Mr. Sinclair almost immediately when he entered the ER. He said he noticed "right away because [Mr. Sinclair] seemed distressed, fidgeting and rolling back and forth in his wheel chair" (p. 83). This civilian sat beside Sinclair and called him "buddy" but did not get a response. Then the civilian went to ask the nurse for help. At another point, a different security guard told the triage aide that Brian Sinclair did not look good and was vomiting. He also asked a nurse if Brian Sinclair was OK. The nurse replied: "Yes, he has been treated and has gone home and returned" (pp. 92–3).

There are numerous problems that the health care system needs to address that have come to light as a result of the inquest into Brian Sinclair's death. Some individuals failed to do their jobs. The design and everyday use of the emergency room as a shelter, although motivated by kindness, contributed to the problem. The lack of a clear viewpoint from behind the triage desk obfuscated the sight lines of the staff and prevented them from seeing the whole space. A number of support staff from the community and "home care" failed to follow up on Brian Sinclair, even though he had been deemed unable to fend for himself. It was an unusually busy weekend, and the emergency ward was understaffed.

A number of people were just waiting in the ER in order to be admitted to the hospital, and a number of others were waiting to be discharged into the community with ongoing care. These and other problems were brought to light from the inquest. They begin to explain why an unnecessary death occurred. They do not, however, explain why it occurred to an Indigenous man, Brian Sinclair. Advocates, including Brian Sinclair's family, argued that the ultimate cause was racism (Brian Sinclair Working Group, 2017).

## Racism and Indigenous Canadians Today

The specifics of Brian Sinclair's story may well be where the idea of racism, raised by Sinclair's family among others, must be taken into account. Racism is said to be defined as "a set of attitudes and behaviours in which social groups are identified, separated, treated as inferior or superior, and given differential access to power and other valuable resources" (Goldner et al., 2016, p. 190). The perniciousness of racism is exacerbated because it gets under the skin of the person who is labelled as being of a certain denigrated category. Internalizing racial epithets can cause distress (Delgado, 1982; Sanders-Phillips et al., 2009). Racism may also be detrimental to the well-being of the person with the racist attitudes (Sue, 2010).

Racism is often both ubiquitous and invisible to the perpetrators (Sue, 2010). Nevertheless, health care professionals are affected by and exhibit culturally available stereotypes and stigmatic attitudes in interactions with others (Paradies et al., 2014). These may be racist, sexist, homophobic, or other such simplifications that have negative consequences. We all make judgments in the "blink" of an eye (Gladwell, 2005). We make our lives manageable and have smooth interactions with others partly through the construction of quick or instantaneous judgments about them. Sometimes our assessments pertain to a simple large category placement: "this is a male" or "this is a female." Such categorization is often accompanied by our gender-based assumptions and expectations or varieties of sexism. Sometimes our judgments reflect subcategorical notions such as "she is a tall woman" or "he is a short man." We streamline interactions through stereotypes that we attach to certain characteristics. These stereotypes reflect social values and hierarchies or ranks of types of people into which we order and organize our cognitively created social worlds. Observational, survey, and experimental research have demonstrated over and over again that health care personnel, including doctors, nurses, and others in the system, as social beings, are encumbered with the same sorts of biases that prevail across societies (Paradies et al., 2014). Racism is one such bias or stereotype that undoubtedly played a pivotal role in the life experiences of Brian Sinclair and is an ongoing issue in Canadian society. The United Nations and other international social justice bodies continue to document how Canada is failing Indigenous people (Union of BC Indian Chiefs, 2015).

## Indigenous Canadians, Social Determinants of Health, and Health Status Today: The Latest Statistics

There were approximately 1,673,780 people of Indigenous descent in Canada in 2016, according to Statistics Canada. They comprised about 4.9 per cent of the population of Canada (Statistics Canada, 2018). The label "Indigenous" includes First Nations people (about 60 per cent), Metis (about 33 per cent), and Inuit (about 4 per cent). Indigenous people living in Canada are a part of the global total of more than 370 million Indigenous people around the world (United Nations, 2010). Within Canada, there are substantial provincial differences in the proportions of Indigenous people. Indigenous people make up more than 18 per cent of the population of Manitoba, where Brian Sinclair's death occurred (Statistics Canada, 2017b), which is about four times the average percentage of the other provinces. The number of Indigenous people is growing rapidly, and the average age is younger than that of non-Indigenous people in Canada ("Manitoba's Aboriginal population," 2013). The rapid growth of the population is largely due to natural increase. Both the birth rate and life expectancy are increasing. Still, however, Indigenous people live shorter lives than other people living in Canada and experience a considerably higher birth rate. The Indigenous birth rate is four times that of non-Indigenous people in Canada (Kirkup, 2017). The average age among Indigenous people is 32.1, which is about a decade younger than the average in the rest of the population (Statistics Canada, 2017a). This figure speaks to the relatively high birth rate. It also speaks to the shorter life expectancy. These factors are reflected in the fact that Indigenous communities tend to have a much greater proportion of people under thirty years old than other communities.

The status and the experience of Indigenous people in Canada are most likely affected by the microculture of the city, town, or reserve area within which a person lives. About 60 per cent of Indigenous people in Manitoba live on reserves. There are sixty-three different nations in the province ("First Nations in Manitoba," 2021). In this context, the history of Manitoba is particularly shrouded in a painful past of conflicts between Indigenous and other peoples, which includes the significant and violent rebellions under the political leadership of Louis Riel on behalf of the Metis against the Canadian government in the 1870s and 1880s (Read & Webb, 2012). This and other historical social and economic factors have played a role in the status and circumstances of Indigenous people in Manitoba and contributed to ongoing racism and profound inequities associated with Brian Sinclair's tragic death.

Today in Manitoba and across Canada, Indigenous people face numerous challenges. Many of the very names used by Canadians to label and to address Indigenous people are denigrating slurs, such as savages, redskins, halfbreed, squaw, buck, brave, and papoose, that reflect racism (Vowel, 2016). The present situation of Indigenous people has been profoundly affected by the colonial history and structure of Canada (Truth and Reconciliation Commission of Canada [TRC], 2015). The first encounters of Indigenous people with the colonial European and British settlers were overwhelmingly violent. Those who were not killed by the ravages of the diseases brought from Europe to North America were forcibly moved to remote lands that lacked resources. In turn, they signed treaties that were supposed to guarantee their rights and obligations. The colonial powers claimed the resource-rich lands as their own. The settlers passed the Indian Act in 1876 to control the futures of the First Nations. Subsequently, the cultures of Indigenous people were attacked. The colonial powers built residential schools designed to assimilate the children into the mores, languages, and cultures of the settlers. In the 1960s and beyond, Indigenous children were taken from their homes to be adopted and fostered by white people in what has been called the "Sixties Scoop."

The present life of Indigenous people is built upon this brutalized past, resulting in significant deficits in the social determinants of health. There is systemic discrimination against Indigenous peoples across all areas of social life, including policing and criminal justice, education, health care, employment, and income possibilities. People on reserves continue to face environmental challenges, including the lack of potable water and adequate sanitation. In addition, there is continuing need for economic development on reserves (Employment and Social Development Canada, 2019). The median income for Indigenous people in Canada is $25,526; for non-Indigenous people in Canada, it is $34, 604 (Kirkup, 2017). Furthermore, almost one quarter of Indigenous people exist below the Canadian poverty line. Indigenous people are also more likely to be homeless and to be dependent on social assistance. Around 20 per cent of Indigenous people live in homes that need significant repairs. Clean water for drinking and cleaning is still missing on a significant number of reserves (Levasseur & Marcoux, 2015).

Significant inadequacies in the levels of the social determinants of health in populations contribute to morbidity and mortality rates (Canadian Institute for Health Information [CIHI], n.d.; Government of Canada, 2019). Deficits lead to increases in both acute and chronic illnesses for men, women, and children. The racism at the root of the profound inequities both exacerbates the effects of the other social determinants of health and is a direct social determinant and cause of illness on its own (Rotenberg, 2012). Indigenous people tend to have lower levels of education; they are more likely to be poor, to live in substandard housing, and to have to rely on contaminated water and insecure food supplies, and less likely to be employed (Rotenberg, 2012). In consequence, they are less likely than other people in Canada to say that they experience excellent or very good health and more likely to suffer from a chronic condition that limits their activity (Garner et al., 2010).

The health-related behaviours of Indigenous people in Canada tend to be more problematic than those of non-Indigenous people (Rotenberg, 2012). They are more likely to smoke cigarettes (Ryan et al., 2015). Indigenous men, women, and children are less likely to be physically active and more likely to be obese (Rotenberg, 2012). Indigenous children are much more likely to be taken away from their parents and taken into the "care" of the state (Clarkson et al., 2015). The long-term negative consequences of being taken into "care" are hard to determine, but one study found that 65 per cent of Indigenous people using illicit drugs in Vancouver and Prince George had been through the child welfare system (Clarkson et al., 2015). Having been through the child welfare system was also associated with being homeless, selling sex, self-harm, and thinking about and attempting suicide (Hwang & Hopkins, 2015).

The rates of drug and alcohol addiction are higher among Indigenous people (Currie et al., 2015; National Collaborating Centre for Aboriginal Health, 2013). They are more likely to be homeless and to depend partly on shelters where they risk violence (Daiski, 2005). In addition, people who live "rough" (otherwise known as homeless) are more likely to have seizures, skin diseases, chronic respiratory diseases, and a number of other specifically related health conditions (Hwang & Hopkins, 2015). Another study found that 80 per cent of Indigenous people using illicit drugs said they had experienced racism and discrimination (Currie et al., 2015). They also reported that they had faced post-traumatic stress disorder and prescription drug problems. However, it must be noted that there are significant differences within Indigenous communities. Thus, those with higher levels of education and higher incomes are less likely than other Indigenous people to smoke and drink heavily (Currie et al., 2015).

In consequence of these various socio-economic limitations, coupled with racism, Indigenous people experience higher rates of a wide range of major health problems than other populations living in Canada. Overall, First Nations adults under seventy-five years are more than twice as likely to die from what Statistics Canada terms "avoidable causes" ("First Nations adults," 2015). For example, they are more likely to die from tuberculosis, pneumonia, and breast cancer. These diseases are particularly avoidable, preventable, and delayable with early detection. Indigenous people are approximately four times as likely to have tuberculosis (Andermann, 2017). They also experience "high maternal morbidity and mortality; heavy infectious disease burdens; malnutrition and stunted growth; shortened life expectancy; diseases and death associated with cigarette smoking; social problems, illnesses and deaths linked to misuse of alcohol and other drugs; accidents, poisonings, interpersonal violence, homicide and suicide; obesity, diabetes, hypertension, cardiovascular, and chronic renal disease (lifestyle diseases); and diseases caused by environmental contamination" (National Collaborating Centre for Aboriginal Health, 2013). Across the country, the death rates from all causes are higher in the First Nations population.

Crucially too, Indigenous people are more likely to use ERs for drop-in health care than other people living in Canada (Gershon et al., 2014). This pattern is likely linked to less stable housing and relationships, including with a doctor. Reliance on the ER for care is a poorer health care option than a family doctor. It can lead to the development of complicated comorbidities and health challenges. Emergency rooms are equipped and staffed to deal with acute events. Yet many treatable problems are chronic and in need of ongoing management and medical support. Furthermore, even though Indigenous people may be more likely to use the ER, they do not report feeling accepted there. Instead, when in the ER, they describe themselves as feeling like an underclass and unworthy of treatment (Tang & Browne, 2008). Brian Sinclair was the likely recipient of a variety of undesirable racist social stereotypes and discrimination during his last time in the hospital ER. He also suffered from most of the negative social determinants of health, including poverty, insecure housing, and family breakdown, being taken into care by the state as a child and in adulthood, and welfare dependency.

Brian Sinclair was also likely stereotyped because he was in a wheelchair. His wheelchair was a visible representation of his vulnerability (Galli et al., 2015). People in wheelchairs tend to be viewed negatively and are subject to discriminatory attitudes and behaviours by others, even others in wheelchairs. Health care workers, too, see people in wheelchairs as somehow less deserving, less whole, less human. "The use of a wheelchair immediately and profoundly affects how a person is perceived" (p. 1239). Brian Sinclair may also have been, in the immediate situation of the ER, subject to racist stereotypes by the nurses, doctors, aides, security guards, and some civilians. There is evidence that, beginning in medical school, racist stereotypes of Indigenous people prevail both among doctors and "down" throughout the medical care system among nurses, aides, and so on (Ly & Crowshoe, 2015; Paradies et al., 2014).

Health care workers belong to societies, and their opinions often reflect the views held by other people in those societies. There is confirmation, for example, of negative and discriminatory attitudes of health care providers towards people with mental illness (Razali & Ismail, 2014; White & McGrew, 2013), people with intellectual disabilities and those with physical disabilities (Dinsmore, 2012; Lewis & Stenfert-Kroese, 2010), people with medically confusing or unexplained symptoms (Shattock et al., 2013), people who abuse substances (Puskar et al., 2013) or who possibly use and abuse drugs (Monks et al., 2013; Morgan, 2014; Silins et al., 2007), older patients (Meiboom et al., 2015), people with HIV/AIDS (Chambers et al. 2015), LGBTQ people (Carabez et al., 2015; Eliason et al., 2011), and people who self-harm (Kool et al., 2015).

Negative attitudes and stereotypes among health care workers have thus been linked to a wide variety of socially denigrated differences embodied by patients. It is important to note that this finding occurs regardless of the personal goals and good intentions of individual health care workers, most of whom likely chose their caring and healing focused jobs in large part to be of service and help to others who are sick and suffering. The beneficence of the nurses in the ER at the Winnipeg hospital is a case in point, as they were kindly feeding and providing drinks to homeless and insecurely housed people in the ER waiting room.

## The Truth and Reconciliation Commission Report

The four major reasons for this ongoing inequity that we will consider include the legacy of colonialism, the experiences of residential schooling, the Sixties Scoop, and ongoing governance and land claims issues. The Truth and Reconciliation Commission of Canada (TRC) report offers a timely, incisive, and historical account of some of the bases of inequities between Indigenous people and others in Canada from the time of confederation (TRC, 2015). The report documents and illustrates how the colonial and assimilative policies of Canada constituted a complex, exhaustive, and lengthy genocide through assaults to the culture, languages, spirituality, and a myriad of other practices and conditions of First Nations people. It documents the ways that genocide was an essential component of the very foundation of Canada as a nation. Canada's first prime minister, John A. Macdonald, reflecting the colonialist and Christian views and values of the time, called the First Nations people "savages." He used this characterization to rationalize a range of violent and abusive actions that undermined the identities, lands, safety, health, health care, education, and so on of First Nations people. Macdonald is quoted as saying, in justifying his educational and residential school policies for First Nations people: "When the school is on the reserve the child lives with its parents, who are savages; he is surrounded by savages, and though he may learn to read and write his habits, and training and mode of thought are Indian. He is simply a savage who can read and write" (TRC, 2015, p. 2).

The TRC (2015) report documents the many causes and results of governmental racism against Indigenous people, including destroying their systems of governance, taking away their land, writing treaties that the Canadian government did not intend to keep, and so forth. It was all done with the ostensible goal of assimilating the Indigenous people to the European colonizers' way of life, values, and religious practices. The European ways of life were seen as far superior and eminently worthy of dissemination across the "new" land. As late as 1969 with the "White Paper," the Canadian government "sought to end Indian status and terminate the Treaties that the federal government had negotiated with First Nations" (p. 3).

Central to this effort to eradicate the "savage" from First Nations children was the movement of these children, often unwillingly, forcefully, and without warning or options, from their reserves and from their parents in a mass grouping into the back of a truck, on a boat, or an airplane. Authorities appointed by the government gathered children from their homes and schools and took them into residential schools. The apprehension of Indigenous children happened across the country in many different places and over more than a century. The federal Indian residential school system was in place from 1867 to the 1990s. At the residential schools, the children were taught in English. They were taught in a language and with a curriculum that seemed irrelevant and even oppressive to many of the children. Many references in the curriculum were to ways of living and values of which they had no prior experience and little or no interest. Many children were sexually and physically abused. Their cultures, their families, and their fundamental worldviews and values were denigrated repeatedly. This disparagement included a wholesale repudiation of their parents and communities.

In many cases, the residential schools were "dangerous and harsh" (TRC, 2015, p. 4), siblings were separated, marriages were often forced, food was scarce and even, as described by former students, disgusting. Several of the thousands of witnesses to the TRC talked about being hungry all the time and hating the food. It often lacked nutritional value. Fundamental spiritual practices such as the Potlatch and the Sun Dance were banned, as was the use of the children's native and local languages. Even siblings were forbidden to speak to one another in the language of their communities and families. Often siblings were prevented from seeing one another or talking at all. Those in residential schools were taught that the ways of the white European colonizers and settlers were much superior to their own way of life. Their caretakers, including religious functionaries such as priests and nuns, and other teachers and staff in turn denigrated and abused these vulnerable children, their families, and cultures. The physical spaces of the schools were often derelict, isolated, poorly maintained, drafty, and too cold in the winter or too hot in the summer. Many lacked adequate ventilation and sanitation.

It is estimated that at least 150,000 students passed through this residential school system (Bousquet, 2021). By 1930, there were eighty such schools operating across the country. Some continued until the last residential school was closed in the late 1990s. The children were often left traumatized, sick, or dead as the result of their time in residential school. More than 6,750 statements from survivors of residential schools, their families, and others with knowledge of the experience of the residential schools and their legacy were presented to the TRC. These presenters offered substantiation of the suffering experienced during residential schooling. They documented the long-term tragic effects of this policy of forced removal of children from their homes and communities. These policies are not just of historical interest, however. They have had long-lasting and negative impacts on the health and well-being of First Nations people for several generations, and the legacy continues up to today. These policies constitute the implementation of many forms of symbolic and real verbal and physical violence by the Canadian state against Indigenous people (Potvin, 2015) and represent the background to the continued racism that exists today. Still, however, most Canadians had no idea about the existence of the residential schools, let alone their dreadful conditions.

The policies also help to explain why it was Brian Sinclair, a First Nations man, and not me, who died after hours of being ignored in the ER in the Winnipeg hospital in 2008. This racist legacy had long-term devastating effects on Brian Sinclair, who as a little boy was known as good in school and kind to others. There may have been a direct and powerful impact on Brian Sinclair from his mother's time in a residential school. Many of those who attended residential schools and their offspring have suffered intergenerational trauma (Menzies, 2020). They had had no experience of good parenting or being loved as they were growing up. Thus, the toxic legacy of racism as well as his family heritage of residential schooling helps to explain Brian Sinclair's substance abuse, his poverty, his vulnerable health status, the amputation of his legs, and a multitude of other factors that led to his death.

There were many direct impacts of the colonial policies on health. Children in residential schools were five times more likely to die compared to non-Indigenous children (Potvin, 2015). "The main causes of death were tuberculosis, influenza, pneumonia and other respiratory illnesses – diseases for which the primary causes are malnutrition, squalor and inadequate ventilation; in other words, destitution" (p. 258). Children at residential schools became ill and died from contagious diseases at a far greater rate than children in the general population across Canada (Leung, 2015). Many children died with no known cause and/or were buried in unmarked graves. Oftentimes, even the parents of these dead children did not know what caused their death or where they were buried. Sexual and physical abuse, as well as separation from families and communities, caused lasting trauma for many others. The effects of this trauma were often passed on to the children of the residential school survivors and sometimes to their grandchildren. Residential schools also posed a threat to the mental health of students through the pervasive assumptions and assertions they made about the inferiority of Indigenous peoples, cultures, and languages.

The legacy of the colonialist and racist attitudes that were at the very foundation of Canada have profoundly affected race relations and the status of Indigenous people in the province of Manitoba and across Canada. There has been a particular concentration of harm in the capital city of Winnipeg, where Brian Sinclair died waiting for care in the ER (Macdonald, 2015). I have mentioned that, when Brian and his family moved from the reserve in the north into the city, they moved to the North End of Winnipeg. As noted, this area was shaped by the violent heritage of the conflict between the forces of the colonial systems of government and the Metis and First Nations people, as evidenced in the story of Louis Riel.

Winnipeg is physically divided into the North End and the rest of the city by the Canadian Pacific (CP) rail yards. On one side, the North End, life is hard, and on the other side, it is largely different. The majority of people in the North End are Indigenous (First Nations), Metis, or Inuit (Macdonald, 2015). The average income is less than one half that in the rest of the city. Two of the three poorest postal codes in Canada are in the North End of Winnipeg. One-third of North End children drop out of school before finishing grade nine. There is a "shameful state of life for many Aboriginals in Winnipeg, where disdain for poor, inner city Natives has long bubbled just barely beneath the surface" (Macdonald, 2015). According to MacDonald (2015), Winnipeg tweeters communicated the highest proportion of racist tweets of six Canadian cities known for hate crimes. Furthermore, the Manitoba Children and Family Services routinely take one-sixth of the children of Indigenous parents into "care" away from their parents. This "care" sometimes results in children being housed alone in hotels. In 2014, there were sixty-five children taken away from their parents residing in hotels. It is difficult for Indigenous people to find a place to rent. One-third of those who had responded to an advertisement for a rental property were turned away with the comment that the apartment or home was already rented. The hospitalization rate resulting from violence in the North End is seven times that of the rest of the city. Generations after residential schools, the effects are still evident in Winnipeg, in the ER, and in the death of Brian Sinclair.

## Discussion: How Did Medicine Go Awry in the Case of Brian Sinclair?

The immediate cause of Brian Sinclair's death was the lack of urgent, appropriate medical care. He died because he was not treated for an easily manageable bladder infection in a timely manner. He died because he was not triaged according to the protocol of the ER. The triage aide apparently did not note his name and problem on the list of patients waiting for care. While other staff noticed him over his long wait in the ER, they apparently thought he was either "sleeping it off" or waiting to be moved into the hospital. No one with medical authority recognized that he was in distress until it was too late, and he was dead in his wheelchair. That weekend, the ER was exceptionally busy. It was understaffed. The morale of the nursing staff was low because their repeated complaints to hospital management concerning their blocked sightlines in the ER waiting room were unaddressed. There were other design features of the ER that limited their ability to see the full waiting room. The ER had become the daytime shelter for a number of homeless people. The nurses even welcomed these indigent people by kindly offering them drinks and snacks. The television was generally on, so people who were cold or wanted a place to go for any other reason would come in to sit and watch.

But why am I arguing that Brian Sinclair's tragic death is, in part, an outcome of medicalization? Certainly, as detailed above, there were many medical system mistakes and poor decisions that contributed to Mr. Sinclair's death. However, the problem of medicalization that I want to emphasize here is the overinvestment in medicine, characteristic of medicalization's tendency to encroach on more and more of everyday life, including the overuse of ERs across the country. Further, the over-reliance on medicine has meant that many people are languishing within hospitals, using hospital beds as they wait for more appropriate care in other places such as long-term care and rehabilitation institutions. This decision has meant that social and health policy supports the hospital and acute medical care system at the expense of other levels and types of care. There was no long-term care institution available to provide Brian Sinclair with a safe or adequate home. In his case, investment in the hospital sector meant that there was no culturally appropriate alternative care option for Mr. Sinclair. He had to rely on a patchwork of services and providers who failed him.

The very fact, however, that Brian Sinclair was in a situation in which he had become homeless, lost his legs, and needed health care intervention was because he, similar to Indigenous people across the country then and now, had innumerable challenges to surmount in the areas of the social determinants of health.

In particular, he lived in the North End of Winnipeg, a city and a community with an especially racist culture, in a province in which relations between Indigenous and non-Indigenous people remained particularly fraught. Although he had apparently been a very good student as a child on the reserve, his family move to the city and to a neighbourhood where illicit drugs were prevalent led to his early drug use and the failure of the school system to fully engage and support his abilities and gifts. It ultimately led to his lack of education or training for a job. He grew up in poverty. This fact alone would have likely led to inadequate housing, poorer quality food, unsafe neighbourhood environments, and a probable lack of accessible sports and leisure facilities. All of these deficits, undergirded by the racial discrimination in his social life, subjected Brian Sinclair to much poorer chances for a fulfilling and happy life. They ultimately led to his homelessness and the fact that he found himself sleeping outside on such a cold night in Winnipeg that he froze and had to have his legs amputated. This situation led to his need for a catheter, and an infection in the catheter led to his final and deadly trip to the ER.

## Conclusion

The case of Brian Sinclair illustrates the importance of eradicating inequities and racism through the introduction of social and health policies. There has been some movement towards acknowledging the racism against Indigenous people that is evident in the very founding as well as the continuing practices of Canada. This shift is evident, for example, in the national call for, and funding of, both the report of the Truth and Reconciliation Commission of Canada (TRC, 2015) and that of the National Inquiry into Missing and Murdered Indigenous Women and Girls (National Inquiry, 2019). Both took years of research and resulted in hundreds of recommendations altogether. However, most recommendations remain just that, recommendations (Graham, 2020; Martens, 2019). Human Rights Watch (2017) in its *World Report 2017* has called out Canada regarding the violation of the human rights of Indigenous people in Canada and the particular situation of women and girls, details of which are specified in the section on Canada.

Our tragic loss of Brian Sinclair's life also reflects the need to demedicalize care and provide options for long-term care and rehabilitation. COVID-19, the pandemic that swept the world beginning in 2020, shone a brilliant and harsh light on the dreadful inadequacies in long-term care. More than 80 per cent of all the deaths in Canada occurred in long-term care. This statistic speaks to many issues related to the quality of the services, some of which will be explored in Chapter 6 on Elizabeth Wettlaufer.

# chapter two

# Ashley Smith: The (Mis)Treatment and Death of an Incarcerated and Troubled Youth

### My Life

My life I no longer love
I'd rather be set free above
Get it over while the time is right
Late some rainy night
Turn black as the sky and cold as the sea
Say goodbye to Ashley
Miss me but don't be sad
I'm not sad I'm happy and glad
I'm free where I want to be
No more caged up Ashley

Wishing I were free
Free as a bird

– Ashley Smith, age 18, New Brunswick Youth Centre (as cited in Ombudsman and Child Youth Advocate, 2008, p. 2)

## The Issue

Ashley Smith is the nineteen-year-old who strangled herself while being observed by her prison guards. Ashley was supposed to be on suicide watch in the Grand Valley Institution for Women, a federal prison for adult females operated by Correctional Service of Canada. There had already been numerous occasions at Grand Valley when Ashley had tied a ligature around her neck so tightly and for such a lengthy period of time that she turned blue, had trouble breathing, and broke blood vessels before the staff physically intervened (Kilty & LeBlanc, 2012). Because of Ashley's long history with self-strangulation, the warden of the Grand Valley prison had asked her guards not to intercede the next time Ashley tied a ligature around her neck. They were told not to offer assistance until she lost consciousness. This plan for Ashley was based on the opinion recently offered by a psychologist that Ashley was playing games and not suffering from a mental illness ("Ashley Smith inquest," 2013a). Ashley likely believed that the guards would come to her aid as they had always done in the past. She did not know that her management plan had changed ("Black out," 2011). This time, when no one intervened, she died or, as the inquest into her death found, was murdered ("Ashley Smith death," 2013).

In the days before she died, Ashley had asked to be transferred to a psychiatric facility. The transfer did not happen. Instead, the guards were told that she was not serious about her request or her need. According to videotape evidence, the guards stood outside and watched Ashley lose consciousness and die. Then they entered her cell. Three guards were eventually charged with criminal negligence causing death. The warden and deputy warden were fired. In the end, the criminal charges were dropped, but Ashley's family sued the Correctional Service of Canada for 11 million dollars. They settled out of court for an unknown figure (*Fifth Estate*, 2010b). The final report of the inquest called Ashley's death a homicide and not a suicide (Correctional Service of Canada, 2014). However, in the end they did not successfully charge any of the personnel who had been involved at the time of her death.

Ashley was and had been under the care of the state and the ministrations of the medical care system from the time she was fourteen. She had spent most of that time in provincial and, finally, federal detention. She was assessed repeatedly and diagnosed with numerous mental illnesses over her time in custody. How did medicine go awry? In this chapter, I ask what role medicine and medicalization might have played in Ashley Smith's death. In the following sections, you will learn more about the story of Ashley

Smith's life before and during her time in custody. I will offer you a more nuanced and critical understanding of how we failed Ashley with our medical practice and some of the torturous actions engaged in by the criminal justice system and buttressed by the medical care system. I will describe how some of the limitations inherent in the epistemology of mental health diagnosis and treatment facilitated Ashley's suffering. You will read about the problematic effects of criminalizing people, especially children and young people with mental health issues. The chief social determinant of health explored in this case is that of gender. I ask how much of Ashley's pathologization resulted from her non-gender-conforming behaviours.

## Early Life in Ashley's Family and Community

Ashley was born on 29 January 1988 in New Brunswick and was adopted by Coralee Smith when she was five days old. Her adoptive mother married Herbert Gober three years later. According to her mother, Ashley had a happy and active childhood (*Fifth Estate*, 2010c). She didn't seem different from the other kids: "she babysat, played basketball and hockey, learned to kayak and never really got the hang of cross-country skiing" (Zlomislic, 2009). But when she was in her pre- and early teens, Ashley, according to her parents, changed from a happy child to a defiant teenager who would not obey the family rules. By the time she was fifteen years old, Ashley had been in front of the court fourteen different times. Each appearance was for a relatively minor but frequently aggressive incident of acting out, such as creating a disturbance at the local mall and trespassing. Two of her biographers, authors of the book *The Life and Death of Ashley Smith*, tell the story as follows: "Puberty brought out a more intense, rebellious side of Ashley Smith. A natural prankster, she started taking her jokes too far. She 'played chicken' in the street with oncoming traffic. She crank-called her neighbours and strangers. She had a salty tongue. Teachers described her as disrespectful, refusing to follow their rules" (Zlomislic & Vincent, 2013).

During these early teen years, Ashley was repeatedly suspended from school for belligerent behaviour (*Fifth Estate*, 2010c). In March 2002, when Ashley was fourteen years old, her Mom sent her to a psychologist. This psychologist said that Ashley did not have a mental illness, just behavioural problems. The school made an effort to work with Ashley to manage her behaviour in school. They attempted to integrate her for half days. In addition, Ashley was enrolled in an intensive support program and had a youth worker assigned to spend time with her. The youth worker was expected to help Ashley transition in and out of school and to prevent her from acting out. This intervention seemed to benefit Ashley for a while. Apparently, there was a satisfactory rapport and connection. Ashley enjoyed spending time with her youth worker. In fact, the youth advocate for the province reported that this intervention was the only successful publicly supported initiative that had ever provided noticeable benefit. Nevertheless, Ashley did not or could not continue to control her actions. In May 2002, she followed a teacher home and repeatedly hit the teacher's door until the police were called. Again, she was suspended from school (*Fifth Estate*, 2010c).

In September 2002, Ashley started high school, but she was suspended almost immediately. In total, Ashley was involved in seventeen incidents involving suspensions from September to November 2002. The school reported that her behaviours included bullying other students, talking back to teachers, and in general exhibiting a disrespectful attitude towards others. She refused to comply with school rules. Ashley was sent to another psychologist who thought that Ashley might have some "neurological deficits" (Zlomislic & Vincent, 2013). As treatment, he recommended behaviour modification. By November, Ashley was in court again, this time for creating a disturbance. She was put on probation and asked to do community service work for a year and a half. Her parents took her to another psychologist, who said that Ashley "had some kind of conduct disorder" (Zlomislic & Vincent, 2013). Then, a subsequent psychiatrist "advised her to lose weight and get treatment for her acne" (Zlomislic & Vincent, 2013).

In December 2002, Ashley was transferred to an alternative high school. She was quickly banned from the school bus because of misbehaviour. Her mother had to drive her to school. She was soon in more serious conflict with her parents. She was acting out at home in many ways, including making expensive long-distance telephone calls on her home phone. Her parents were also upset that she seemed to be looking at questionable, possibly pornographic websites.

## Youth Custodial Care

In March 2003, Ashley was in court again. This time, the court decided that Ashley could no longer be managed at home. The alternative high school was no longer enough. The court ordered a thirty-four-day assessment at the Pierre Caissie Centre, a youth treatment centre in Moncton, New Brunswick. The centre was to evaluate Ashley's behaviour and mental health, and then work with Ashley's parents, her probation officer, and the school to reintegrate Ashley into her community once again. No formal diagnosis was made, but in the notes describing diagnostic impressions, Ashley was said to possibly have attention deficit hyperactivity disorder (ADHD), a learning disorder, borderline personality disorder, and narcissistic personality characteristics (*Fifth Estate*, 2010c). The police were called to the centre twice because she assaulted staff. She was discharged seven days early because of her aggressive and intimidating behaviour towards the other children and the staff. The Pierre Caissie Centre apparently could not diagnose, help, or even manage fifteen-year-old Ashley.

Ashley's aggressive behaviour continued after she had left custodial care and returned again to her community and family. Almost immediately, in April 2003, Ashley was sentenced to the New Brunswick Youth Centre (NBYC) for a month. She now had to live 150 miles from home. "She packed for youth jail like a kid going to camp. She brought a SpongeBob SquarePants address book, a Walkman, headphones, a colouring book, a rhyming dictionary, vanilla body wash, blue plaid pajamas, three pairs of

socks, four pairs of underwear, jeans and just a few hoodies" (Zlomislic & Vincent, 2013).

The innocence evident in the choices she made of things to take
away with her was soon obliterated. Almost immediately, Ashley
was repeatedly in trouble at NBYC. In November 2003, at the age
of fifteen years and ten months, Ashley stopped any kind of formal education (Ombudsman and Child Youth Advocate, 2008).
She began a long trajectory in which she spent the majority of the
rest of her life in custody. She was often unbathed or unshowered
and dirty. She was frequently kept in very small isolation cells.
She was generally separated from her peers. Although there was a
legal limit of five days in isolation, Ashley apparently spent two-
thirds of her time, for the next three plus years, in solitary confinement (Zlomislic & Vincent, 2013). This punitive isolation was in
retaliation for her numerous breaches of institutional policy. She
refused to obey the rules, used foul language, and interrupted
staff. Staff laid hundreds of institutional charges against Ashley.
She was found guilty of every one of them. Many were based on
seemingly trivial infractions such as interrupting and cussing. She
refused to follow the orders given by the guards and other workers. She wrote numerous letters to the authorities within the institution advocating for others and for herself. She wrote asking for
more fresh fruit and fewer muffins, weekend newspapers for the
unit, and new communal headphones.

As well as institutional charges reflecting infractions of the policies of the youth centre, Ashley also amassed a series of minor
criminal charges when the staff called the local police on her at
least twenty-four times (Zlomislic & Vincent, 2013). Staff tried to
contain her within the institution. To do so, they used a number of
questionable and aggressive practices. She was pepper sprayed,
tasered, and tied in personal confinement (or "wrapped"). All her
complaints about being mistreated and wanting better food and
amenities for herself and others were ignored. She engaged in
continual resistance to her circumstances. She pulled fire alarms.
She covered her cell windows with toilet paper so the guards
could not see in. In turn, she was punished again and again. She
registered a complaint against the staff, saying that they used
extreme force on her. It was apparently disregarded. Instead, she

was vilified, rejected, and described as an extreme high-risk prisoner (Zlomislic, 2009).

Ashley asked for anger management classes but was refused them, ironically, because of her angry and aggressive behaviour. Within a couple of weeks in custody, Ashley had more than thirty incidents noted in her record, including repeatedly threatening to harm herself (Zlomislic & Vincent, 2013). Her aggressive and self-harming behaviour continued when she left the facility and went home. She was repeatedly returned back to the centre over a three-year period. She was described as bullying and vulgar in her interactions with staff and the other youth. In total, more than 800 incidents of misbehaviour were documented over the three years Ashley spent in and out of the NBYC, including repeated attempts to harm herself (Carlson, 2013).

The security and care offered by NBYC was based on modern standards. The centre used a therapeutic community model. The physical layout included a central building and four interlocking cottages, each with two units and twelve beds. There were a number of recreational, educational, and support activities offered. It included a gym, a library, a woodworking centre, an art room, a space for horticulture, a computer lab, and educational facilities. There were medical services and nursing staff available. The philosophy of the centre was based on a form of community self-help (Ombudsman and Child Youth Advocate, 2008, pp. 12–14). Days were highly structured, and there were clear rules and associated sanctions for disobedience and rewards for good behaviour. Individual change was to be encouraged by learning to follow the rules in order to get more and more privileges in turn. The structure was hierarchical so that the girls worked their way to the top by engaging in appropriate behaviours and gaining authority as role models to the others along the way. There were two group meetings a day. The one in the morning was an opportunity for the leaders and group members to point out when they had observed good or bad behaviour in themselves and others. The one in the evening was more like a peer "encounter" group in which participants challenged one another. The idea was that peer pressure would encourage the girls to conform and increasingly follow the rules and gain authority and privileges. This model of rehabilitation did not work for Ashley.

In the face of continuing problems with Ashley at NBYC, in April 2005 a judge ordered that she be sent to Restigouche Hospital for psychiatric testing. The psychiatrist who examined her at this hospital concluded that Ashley could control her behaviour when she chose to do so. He said she understood her responsibilities (Ombudsman and Child Youth Advocate, 2008, p. 19). She was not deemed to be mentally ill but wilful. She was returned to NBYC, where she carried on getting into trouble and being repeatedly sent back to an isolation unit. She amassed more institutional charges for failing to follow the rules of her incarceration. These charges continuously lengthened her stay.

By July 2006, after spending nearly four years in and out of youth custody and having been moved nine times among institutions and in and out of school, Ashley was still described as out of control (Ombudsman and Child Youth Advocate, 2008, pp. 21–2). She did not have a consistent diagnosis or treatment plan. None of the mental health professionals had been able to provide a robust explanation for her behaviour. No one was able to offer the care or treatment that Ashley needed. The diagnoses were multiple and inconsistent.

As she approached her eighteenth birthday, Ashley indicated that she was opposed to being transferred to adult prison. In an affidavit, she said that she wanted to but could not control her outbursts. She asked for help. At the time, as evident in the following quotation, Ashley sounded remorseful and said she wanted to do something productive with her life: "I would never intentionally hurt anyone" (*Fifth Estate*, 2010c). Finally, as she "aged out" of youth services, she was to be transferred to adult custody. She was terrified of this transfer and hired a lawyer to fight the decision. She lost her case and was moved to the first of a number of different adult facilities, beginning with the Saint John Regional Correctional Centre.

## Adult Correctional Institution

Ashley Smith's final destination was the adult correctional institution Grand Valley Institution for Women, where, it was argued, there would be lots of programs available to help her. She was then transferred back and forth to other institutions for various assessments seventeen times during her eleven months in federal adult custody (Office of the Correctional Investigator, 2014). Again, much of the time she was in solitary confinement.

Notes found in Ashley's journal indicate that she did not know why she did what she did but that it made her life not worth living (*Fifth Estate*, 2010c). Here is an example of a note found in her journal. Her desperation and self-loathing are evident.

> If I die I never have to worry about upsetting my Mom again ... It would have been nice to stick my head in the lawn mower blade ... I really did have to hold back the urge. Maybe next time I will give it a try ... Most people are scared to die. It can't be any worse than living a life like mine. (quoted in *Fifth Estate*, 2010c)

The journal entry goes on and on about wanting to die and how she might be able to do it successfully.

> Maybe I will use a brand new pair of socks. Fresh for me. No, I don't f***ing deserve a new pair of socks. I will use the old dirty ugly ones ... Time is running out. My chances are getting fewer and fewer. F*** I give up! I'm done trying. (quoted in *Fifth Estate*, 2010c)

Within a year, Ashley was dead. Some call her death a homicide. Some call it suicide. It was officially ruled a homicide. In the following sections, I discuss some of the larger issues that led to Ashley's continually repeated incarceration and the failure of the state to educate Ashley and provide her with compassionate care, diagnosis, and treatment during her life in custody.

## What Went Wrong?

### Many Contradictory Diagnoses and Treatments

Diagnosing mental illness is not necessarily easy or straightforward. There is usually no obvious physical injury or evident biological variance as there is in the case of a broken bone or another similarly observable and measurable anomaly in the body. As of yet, there are no lab tests that would clearly demarcate the presence or the absence of psychiatric disorders. There is no blood test and no brain scan that would definitively indicate a mental illness such as a personality disorder, for example. The quality of diagnosis, as is true of any measurement, should be continuously assessed and evaluated. The two primary means for evaluating measures and, by extension, diagnoses are reliability and validity. Of these, validity is the most fundamental. A valid diagnosis is one that is accurate and true. It represents to the underlying phenomenon being identified. Thus, a valid measure of depression is one that is able to distinguish depression from anxiety or from sadness, for instance. Reliability relates to the fact that the measure (or diagnosis) is consistent or is able to accurately differentiate the specific diagnosis repeatedly over time within the same person or a different person with the same behaviours or characteristics.

There were numerous disparate and even contradictory diagnoses offered for Ashley. There was never a consistent or valid diagnosis. The diagnoses were not reliable. They ranged from the psychiatrist who said her problem was that she was overweight and had acne, to the psychiatrist who said she might have ADHD, to wilful and controllable disobedience, to various personality and learning disorders, such as a borderline personality disorder and narcissistic tendencies. Other assessments said she had adjustment disorder, oppositional defiant disorder, borderline personality disorder, and a cyclic mood disorder (Ombudsman and Child Youth Advocate, 2008, pp. 14–16). Some said that there was nothing wrong with her and that she could change her behaviour if she wanted.

One of the first mental health professionals consulted to help Ashley was hired by her parents in 2002. This psychiatrist "ruled out the presence of mental health issues" (Ombudsman and Child Youth Advocate, 2008, p. 15). Later that year, Ashley was assessed at the Pierre Caissie Centre for youth treatment, where a psychiatrist's notes revealed the following "diagnostic impression" of Ashley: learning disorder, ADHD, borderline personality disorder, not depressed but narcissistic tendencies (p. 16). There were two different assessments, one day after the other, at the Nova Institution for Women in Truro, Nova Scotia (Vincent, 2013a). Dr. Jeffrey Penn (a psychiatrist) reported that Ashley experienced very little remorse and often enjoyed hurting others and herself. Further, she was described as getting bored by prolonged good behaviour and consistent positive reinforcement. She was, he said, a "fearful tyrannical child" with a high risk of suicide (Vincent, 2013a). He said she was deteriorating. He also said that her behaviour was affecting the other prisoners. He diagnosed her with a personality disorder with borderline paranoid characteristics and recommended that she be transferred to a secure facility with a twenty-four-hour behaviour modification program. The day before the above assessment, a psychologist, Dr. Alistair Webster, thought Ashley could be "effectively managed and assisted toward the adoption of pro-social behaviour" (Vincent, 2013a) where she was currently placed. Later, another psychologist said her self-harming actions constituted a bid for stimulation or experience. There is no evidence that she received individual supportive counselling while in custody, although she did in the early days of her acting out.

After her death, the forensic psychiatrist looking back at all the earlier reports described her behaviours retrospectively and said that "she had severe maladaptive personality traits with unremitting aggression, impulsivity, chronic suicidality, sadistic and masochistic needs, emotional lability and manipulative behaviour" ("Health board," 2011). This assessment reads as a descriptor of Ashley's behaviour through a backward glance. It does not, however, even retrospectively, provide a useful diagnosis, which might have led to a definitive treatment plan.

The two health professionals who were responsible for Ashley while she was at the Grand Valley Institution for Women, the federal institution for adults where she died, were brought before their professional association to account for their decisions regarding Ashley. Although Ashley had been increasing her self-harming behaviours and repeatedly tying ligatures around her neck, her treating psychologist at the time said that she was not suicidal but that "her tendencies were so high it was like playing Russian roulette" ("Health board," 2011). Someone had overheard Ashley saying that she knew the guards would come to her rescue before she died. The staff and mental health practitioners decided that, since none of her previous trips to hospital in search of a diagnosis and treatment had been fruitful, she might as well stay in a situation where the guards were used to her and knew how to manage her ("Health board," 2011).

In the following sections, I ask about the possible effects of a number of the policies that altered the life of Ashley Smith and most likely increased the likelihood of her continual incarceration and finally her death. I question the practices of solitary confinement, tasering, wrapping, and pepper spraying, as well as the changing diagnoses she received over time.

## Solitary Confinement

Solitary confinement was first introduced into the prison system as a positive improvement from the crowded and noisy prison experience. It was offered as a chance for prisoners to have time to themselves to think about the mistakes they had made and to plan how they might make changes in their lives. It was to be a peaceful respite. Over time though, it has often come to be used as a punishment for bad behaviour. Sometimes it is used for the protection of either the prisoner in custody or others who might otherwise be endangered. Ashley was almost always kept in solitary confinement over her four years of incarceration, from her first placement as a young teen until her death at nineteen in custody as an adult (*Fifth Estate*, 2010a).

Ashley was held in solitary despite the formal and legal restrictions on the use of such confinement at all levels of her incarceration (Ombudsman and Child Youth Advocate, 2008, p. 41). The official requirement was that, after a short period of time in isolation, usually five days, the individual's case was to be investigated thoroughly and every effort made to move the person into the general prison population. Further, there was an absolute limit under Correctional Service of Canada (CSC) guidelines of a sixty-day maximum sentence of solitary confinement before there was to be a mandatory review of the situation (Office of the Correctional Investigator, 2014). CSC avoided this requirement during the last eleven months of Ashley's life when she was at the institution for adults by moving her repeatedly. She spent virtually the entirety of this time in solitary because of her many inter-institutional transfers. After each transfer, the clock regarding the limitations for solitary confinement went back to zero. In 2007 alone, during the last period of her life, Ashley was transferred seventeen times back and forth to and from eight institutions. Furthermore, during her many years in the youth system, she was transferred out and then often came back in to the NBYC after just a few days. She was also transferred to psychiatric institutions and alternative secure institutions during her time in youth custody. After every transfer, the timer regarding the limitations for solitary confinement went back to zero.

There is a great deal of research that documents many negative consequences of solitary confinement. The literature review by the Ontario Ministry of the Solicitor General on the topic of solitary confinement (Larocque, 2017) noted that the research-based consensus is that there are many harmful effects directly from solitary confinement. These effects include insomnia, lethargy, back and joint pain, aggravation of pre-existing medical issues, anxiety, fear of impending death, panic attacks, irritability, depression, mood swings, unprovoked anger leading to outbursts, cognitive disturbances, perceptual disorders, paranoia, and psychosis, among others. The importance of each one is confirmed by cited research. It is clear from this list that some of Ashley's troublesome behaviours might very well have been produced and certainly exacerbated by the treatment she received in isolation in youth custody. In fact, there is also evidence of an increased risk of the possibility of self-harming behavior and suicide (Larocque, 2017, pp. 15–16; Office of the Provincial Advocate for Children and Youth in Ontario, 2015, p. 11). Significant physical health concerns are also associated with the solitary confinement of juveniles, including the worsening of pre-existing medical conditions, palpitations, and anorexia

Various commentators liken solitary confinement to trauma. For instance, solitary confinement, regardless of whether it is used as a punishment or for the security of the inmate or his or her colleagues, is a form of torture according to the United Nations (Mendez, 2011). It is thought to be especially egregious when used with children and youth because their brains and minds are still developing. Solitary confinement is known to be particularly problematic for people with mental health issues, because it can exacerbate these issues and create new forms of mental, emotional, and social suffering.

A diagnosis with a mental health issue would have been a logical and predictable sequel to Ashley's years behind bars locked in a small, often filthy room and lacking human contact (Ombudsman and Child Youth Advocate, 2008, pp. 41–2). Ashley was often not even permitted a blanket to keep her warm while sleeping. At times, her clothing was taken away from her. Sometimes she can be seen in video recordings with only a smock on. She was refused shoes. Sometimes even tiles from the cell floor were taken away. She was denied sufficient toilet paper, soap, tampons, and even underwear (Razack, 2014). She was often without any stimulation such as books or writing, painting, or drawing materials. That we have evidence she liked to journal, write poetry, and read highlights what must have been an especial loss and punishment for the teenager trapped in a cell by herself with virtually no social interaction, books, or writing materials and with only a food slot as a link to the world outside of her cell. Guards were told not to show warmth to Ashley, as it was said to reward her attention-seeking behaviour (Perkel, 2013). Add to this the fact that Ashley's guards often wore combat gear (Razack, 2014). It is not hard to imagine how Ashley's life and her ability to cope in a constructive and positive way were continuously diminished and her negative coping and adjustment strategies were strengthened by the lengthy and repeated institutional sanctions and solitary confinement, in addition to the ineffective and inconsistent medical and psychiatric interventions. Identity formation, so crucial to a developing youth, is severely challenged by excessive time in solitude (Martel, 2006). Ashley's treatment while in custody would have been a clear threat to the development of a stable and healthy sense of self.

Solitary confinement even in adults leads to a number of terrible outcomes. These negative outcomes are exacerbated among growing children (Martel, 2006; Mendez, 2011). Furthermore, the placement of youth with severe mental health problems in solitary confinement is most likely particularly problematic for their well-being and ultimate adjustment back into society. Ashley endured solitary detention for most of her years in custody.

For our purposes, with our focus on the health care aspect of Ashley's incarceration and eventual death, it is important to note that none of the diagnoses mentioned by the various health care providers included a prohibition of solitary confinement or a suggestion that the prison system itself might be one of the causes of Ashley's deterioration over time. The social context of her mental health assessments seems to have been routinely overlooked. The dangerous practices used to confine Ashley were ignored. Mental health care often has a focus on the individual and his or her behaviour. This concentration locates the pathology in the individual person. It may tend to neglect the interactional, social, and cultural contributions to well-being and suffering. It appears to have done so in the case of Ashley Smith.

## Tasered, Wrapped, Pepper Sprayed, Duct Taped, and Forced to Take Anti-psychotic Drugs While in Custody

In addition to being confined, isolated, and deprived of stimulation or even the basic necessities for human hygiene, Ashley was frequently treated with unkindness, insensitivity, and even brutality during her incarceration. For instance, as guards entered her cell, they sometimes tasered her, ostensibly for preventative protection for themselves (Zlomislic & Vincent, 2013). Ashley had at times made weapons from bits and pieces of things and had attacked guards when they entered her cell. There were numerous examples of other questionable interventions, such as male guards observing while she was told to remove all her clothes. The guards failed to videotape their own "use of force" interventions (which they were supposed to have done), thus hiding what may have been even more outrageous behaviours in their actions towards

Ashley. Further, guards failed to follow health guidelines in inter-actions with Ashley (Seglins, 2011). Some videotapes, though, did show how unkindly Ashley was treated by guards at times. In one example, the videotape shows "eight men and women wearing protective suits and combat clothes tie her down and forcibly inject her five times with anti-psychotic medication. She could be heard asking in a small voice that the guards keep her dress down and not exhibit her body for all to see. She was then left on a stretcher in her own urine for nine hours" (Razack, 2014).

Ashley also, a number of times, endured the "wrap," also known as the body belt. This technology essentially restrained her whole body and thus restricted all movement. Wrapping was com-pleted with the attachment of a hockey helmet to her head (Razack, 2014). While she was at a psychiatric institution in Saskatchewan, a "supervisor grabbed her, lifted her off the ground and called her a cunt. The same person stepped on her head, called her a f*** animal and banged her head on the floor" (Razack, 2014). Ashley repeatedly tried to complain and to challenge the conditions of her custody. Although complaints are legally required to be read and answered, several months after her death a number of unopened complaints were found (Perkel, 2013). To add to the trauma, Ash-ley was often held in restraints, even in solitary (Razack, 2014). One video of her time in prison shows her duct taped to the seat of an airplane as she was transferred from institution to institution. In this case, she is seen at her final destination wearing leg irons, a spit mesh mask, and a lead chain. She is being treated as if she is a huge and dangerous animal and not a troubled teenage girl in need of help and care.

The guards did not model positive behaviour. Although Ashley was a child when she was first detained, the day-to-day life in cus-tody was not warm, supportive, or encouraging. The treatment she received was not appropriate to her age or developmental stage. In fact, the cultures of the various institutions within which Ashley lived were clearly oppressive, harsh, rule-bound, and punitive at times, perhaps especially so in the eyes of a young girl. The cul-ture of the federal prison was described as intimidating (Vincent, 2013b). One of the staff was charged with attacking Ashley. She herself reported that he put a foot on her head and called her "the c word" (Razack, 2014). Contradictory evidence was given, and the case was ultimately dropped. The medical and criminal justice authorities appeared to have given up on Ashley. Five months before she died, a staff psychiatrist said that Ashley had reached a point of no return (Vincent, 2013a).

## Ashley's Contradictory Diagnoses and Treatments for Mental Illness

Despite the lack of a clear and consistent diagnosis, Ashley was prescribed powerful, even potentially dangerous, drugs, including anti-psychotics and mood stabilizers, among others (Vincent, 2013b). She was "restrained and forcibly injected with unnecessary tranquilizers and anti-psychotic drugs" ("Ashley Smith's sedation," 2010). Many of these strong pharmaceuticals have negative side effects. A mood stabilizer is the medication of choice for someone suffering from bipolar disease. Among its side effects are weight gain, nausea and vomiting, confusion, blackout spells, drowsiness, trembling, and even hallucinations (Citizens Commission on Human Rights, 2010). These are potentially very dangerous side effects for an already troubled young girl. To feel dizzy and confused or to have blackouts and hallucinations, although caused by pharmaceuticals ostensibly aimed to be of benefit, could clearly have also added to the suffering Ashley underwent. Among the common side effects for anti-psychotics are dry mouth, blurred vision, weight gain, drowsiness, and muscle spasms. There have been warnings about anti-psychotics causing stroke, heart problems, convulsions, seizures, and death, among other serious side effects (Citizens Commission on Human Rights, n.d.). Again, some of these side effects may very well have exacerbated Ashley's suffering and contributed to her continual re-incarceration from the time she was fifteen until she died at nineteen. There is a certain sad and egregious irony to the fact that the medications given to Ashley can, at times, cause the very problem they are ostensibly prescribed to alleviate. These very powerful drugs can have strong and negative impacts on a child or youth (Whitaker, 2001, 2010).

The fact that the medications were, at least some of the time, given against her will is also a serious problem. Canadian legislation requires that medication only be given with the free and informed consent of the individual receiving it, unless consent is impossible for the individual because of disordered inability to understand or imminent danger of harming the self or others (Canadian Medical Protective Association, 2021). Although there were times when Ashley would have been acting in a way that indicated her life was in imminent danger, there were times when that was not true. Still, she was given the medications ("Ashley Smith's sedation," 2010). Furthermore, at one point the psychiatrist prescribed these medications without even directly assessing (seeing) Ashley. Instead, this health care practitioner relied on the second-hand reports of Ashley's behaviour by a staff member who was unable to manage her. In another instance, Ashley was apparently given five medications in seven hours while confined to a bed (Vincent, 2013c). There is evidence that pharmaceuticals were weaponized and used as punishment at times. For instance, in one tape Ashley is told to calm down or "we'll give you some more medications" (Vincent, 2013c). In reply, Ashley is heard saying "no, no, no." This instance is hardly indicative of informed consent, particularly as guards in riot gear surrounded Ashley while she was being medicated.

### Mental Illness Both Created and Treated through Incarceration and Punishment

Ashley Smith died after spending most of her time as a teenager under the jurisdiction of the combined forces of various mental health diagnosticians and caregivers, along with criminal justice staff. The health care and criminal justice systems failed to provide adequately for her. Over her teen years, Ashley's behaviour was clearly troubling. She behaved badly on many occasions. The school, criminal justice and mental health experts, and authorities all agreed that she was having difficulties, repeatedly breaking rules and, at times, laws. They were, however, incapable of managing her, either through punishing or supporting her in her suffering and continual acting out.

We do not know whether or not Ashley was mentally ill when she entered the youth justice system. There were numerous different and contradictory diagnoses and non-diagnoses, even when she was first assessed. There were many other different diagnoses afterwards. It is clear that her experiences in this system resulted in what is manifestly counted as evidence of a disordered state of mental health: attempted suicide. Ashley made 168 attempts at suicide at NBYC. "Whether it started as an attention seeking behaviour and ended up being desperate calls for help, one cannot help but feel that something more could have and should have been done to help her" (Ombudsman and Child Youth Advocate, 2008, p. 35).

The placement of children with behavioural problems in punitive custody is always problematic. Some advocates and organizations have taken up this issue. For example, the Ombudsman's report for the province of New Brunswick states: "The fundamental premise is that youths suffering from mental illness or struggling with a severe behavioural disorder should not be sent to a correctional facility" (Ombudsman and Child Youth Advocate, 2008, p. 4). Nevertheless, there is often a link between mental illness and criminal behaviour and punishment. For instance, Fazel and Danesh (2002) found, on the basis of a systematic review of sixty-two surveys encompassing 23,000 prisoners, that 3.7 per cent had psychosis, 10 per cent had depression, 65 per cent had personality disorders, and 47 per cent had anti-social personality disorders. James and Glaze (2006) found that between 61 and 75 per cent of females and between 44 and 65 per cent of males, depending on whether they were incarcerated in local jails, state, or federal prisons, had various mental disorders.

Furthermore, the rate of criminalization of children's deviant behaviours (especially externalizing violent or aggressive behaviours such as opposition defiant disorder or ODD) is growing. At the same time that significant numbers of children and youth who exhibit deviant behaviours and emotional expression are (eventually) medicalized and sometimes medicated, so too are many of them criminalized and dealt with through the criminal justice system (Stout & Holleran, 2012). One US national survey found that 36 per cent of families whose children had severe mental illnesses reported that their children were in the youth criminal justice system because of the lack of mental health services (Shelton, 2002).

The rate of incarceration of children in the developed world is high (Waddell et al., 2005). In Canada alone, as many as 125,000 children and youth are charged every year with criminal offences, and 25,000 were incarcerated every year before the passage of the Youth Criminal Justice Act in 2003 (Perreault, 2012). Since then, the rates of children and youth being charged and incarcerated for some offences such as property damage have declined, but rates have continued to increase for violent offences (Taylor-Butts & Bressan, 2008). A significant proportion of incarcerated youth and children have diagnosed and/or undiagnosed mental health disorders (Cocozza & Skowyra, 2000; Hirschfield et al., 2006). One investigation concluded that almost all youth and children who were in custody met the conditions for at least one mental health disorder (Templin et al., 2002). Many symptoms of mental illness, especially externalizing aggressive behaviours, easily result in law breaking and become subject to the involvement of the criminal justice system. Some mental health disorders increase the risk of arrest (Hirschfield et al., 2006). Thus, although there is not enough good research on the existence and characteristics of mental health disorders within the juvenile justice system (Cocozza & Skowyra, 2000), it is clear that there is considerable overlap between (bio) medicalization and criminalization and that the majority of children and youth in the juvenile justice system have a diagnosis (Stout & Holleran, 2012). In fact, children and youth are particularly vulnerable to criminalization, and the rates of disordered mental health symptoms are highest among this age group of twelve to twenty-four (Statistics Canada, 2013). This issue is highly significant and reverberates far beyond the case of Ashley Smith.

Despite the evidence of the inconsistent diagnoses of mental health professionals and of the powerful and even at times negative effects of "coupling" medical treatments with punishment, the Ashley Smith inquest's recommendations include increasing the medical and mental health services available to inmates through Correctional Service of Canada (Chief Coroner, Province of Ontario, 2013). The report recommends that there be "adequate staffing of qualified, mental health care providers with expertise and experience in treating a population with mental health issues, self-injurious behaviours, suicidality, and trauma, at every women's institution to provide services and supports to female inmates." This recommendation goes on to list the following providers as being included: psychiatrists, psychiatric nurses (or nurses), a chief psychologist, psychologists, social workers, behavioural and recreational counsellors, general practitioners, and other professional service providers as required.

I take issue with the logic of this recommendation. Hiring more mental health practitioners is premature in the absence of evidence of the ability to develop valid and reliable diagnoses. The lack of robust diagnoses in the presence of both an intimidating punishment culture and the use of powerful symptom-causing medications does not make good sense. In fact, such a recommendation may very well lead to the suffering of others in a way that is similar to the suffering endured by Ashley Smith. In the concluding section, I will revisit the issues and questions raised by this in-depth look at the trajectory of one young person who suffered such an ignominious end.

## Discussion: How Did Medicine Go Awry in the Case of Ashley Smith?

That Ashley Smith was a troubled young teenager who regularly acted out is not disputed. Her parents had a difficult time managing her at home as she became a young teen. She rebelled at school. She was aggressive, crude, and even cruel with teachers and sometimes other students. She did not fit well into her local community. Many people tried to help her learn to contain her acting out before she was institutionalized for the first time for an assessment. That her incarceration continued for four years reflects on the system wherein Ashley was housed. The first institutional placement was cut short because staff could not handle her. Then, from the time she was fifteen, she was repeatedly re-institution-alized for longer and longer periods of time. Each time she was re-institutionalized, she amassed more and more "time," requiring further incarceration because of her (mis)behaviour. She received numerous conflicting mental illness diagnoses, along with asso-ciated pharmaceutical treatments, over her time in custody. She was mostly held in solitary confinement. She received aggressive, even violent, discipline. Her guards assaulted her physically and verbally. Eventually, Ashley was murdered when she tied a liga-ture around her neck under the watch of her guards who did not intervene. There are many lessons to be drawn from the egregious story of the life and death of Ashley Smith.

Medicalization played an essential role in the death of Ashley Smith. She was held in youth correctional institutions from the time she was sentenced to a thirty-four-day assessment at about fifteen years of age until she died at nineteen. In each youth cor-rectional centre, the rehabilitation of the distressed incarcerated youngster was based on custodial care under the auspices of men-tal health practitioners and their therapeutic and pharmaceutical-ized culture. It was the advice of mental health practitioners that was theoretically used for managing, treating, and shepherding to well-being the troubled young people in custody. It was the medi-cal model that guided practice and policy. The power of the medi-cal model, including mental health diagnoses and treatments, was undergirded and exacerbated in the residential settings. In such institutions, mental health advice and treatments become inextri-cably linked to all aspects of daily living from sleeping, to eat-ing, exercising, socializing, and recreating. Goffman (1961) wrote about how institutions become total and in doing so endeavour to execute near absolute control over the life of inhabitants. The total way of life for people within institutions is monitored and surveilled, even as it is separated from the life of the commu-nity. When this happens to people, young people most especially, and occurs over many years, they become institutionalized and increasingly unable to behave as independent actors. This was to be Ashley's fate.

In this context of great vulnerability, Ashley was subject to the powerful effects of numerous different interventions. She was aggressively pepper sprayed, tasered, and wrapped. She, as a young girl, was the recipient of contradictory, confusing, and ultimately ineffective mental health practices, which even included the forced administration of strong medications known to have strong and harmful side effects. That she was repeatedly and almost continually placed in solitary confinement during her years of incarceration increased the damage to her developing personality and her ability to be an independent actor.

Medicalization was powerful in this context, but it was not the result of a reliable or valid diagnosis or consistent treatments. The incoherence in the way that Ashley was seen and treated by those who held sway over her was ultimately lethal. The failure of a robust diagnosis linked to effective treatments made the power of medicine dangerous. Because she was also incarcerated, the medical care was forced upon her, which points to the putative dangers of coupling invalid and unreliable medical care in a punitive organization with a vulnerable, confused, and complex person.

In addition, for reasons emanating from her incarceration, Ashley spent most of her tenure in the system in solitary confinement. Although there were policies prohibiting ongoing solitary confinement and although the research literature was full of evidence documenting the negative side effects, the criminal justice personnel associated with her incarceration proceeded with solitary, and the medical professionals did not stop it. The specific practices of the guards, such as tasering, wrapping, and pepper spraying, would have been inconsistent with the psychiatric and psychological care and diagnoses, but they were allowed. Ashley could have benefitted from the presence of a caring individual who was neither medically trained nor an agent of the correctional system. She needed at least one adult who was able to stand outside the system and monitor how the system was interacting with her. The absence of a single individual (with authority) to oversee the well-being of each individual under the care of the state can mean that no one in particular cares about any individual, leaving them completely at the mercy of the state for medical and other care.

The role of social determinants of health is less obvious in the reports of how Ashley Smith quickly ended up in confinement. It is possible that the relative paucity of excellent services for distressed and acting out teens in the rural area of a small province may have played a role. Had an effective counsellor or program been available early on when Ashley was first running into problems at home, in school, and in her neighbourhood, she might have been able to avoid incarceration. Her aggressive and even violent acting out clearly violated gender norms of good female behaviour and might have been especially difficult to manage within a small community. Her sexual acting out may have been particularly troublesome because she was female. Being female definitely influenced her well-being once she was in custody. The fact that she was assaulted could have, independent of any of the other harms she experienced at the hands of the guards and the mental health professionals, led to her continued distress. We know that many people experience post-traumatic stress as an aftermath of assault (Ullman, 2016). Further, the experience of being held in solitary confinement, on its own, can cause symptoms of mental distress and a significantly greater tendency to self-harming behaviour (Kaba et al., 2014). Ashley was especially vulnerable because she was female in a sexist and punitive prison culture in which she was forced into solitary confinement for the majority of her time in custody, called names, and objectified by her guards. There were numerous examples of other questionable interventions, such as male guards observing while she was told to remove all her clothes.

Mental health care often has a focus on the individual and his or her behaviour. This concentration locates the pathology in the individual person. It has a tendency to neglect the interactional, social, and cultural contributions to well-being. This myopic focus on the individual in this case meant that the mental health professionals ignored the circumstances of Ashley's life while pathologizing her.

## Conclusion

The story culminating in Ashley Smith's murder at the hands of her prison guards is one that implicates the dangers of the powerful effects of medicalization within a punitive environment. In this case, medicalization's focus on individual bodies and minds obviates its potential to change the policies of confinement or the brutal, sexist treatment Ashley endured at the hands of prison personnel and also highlights the limits of mental health research and practice. That Ashley was diagnosed with a variety of different conditions and treated with various strong medications, despite the lack of evidence of a valid and reliable single diagnosis, became a powerful weapon at times. Ashley's gender was implicated in her repeated confinement because she was a victim of sexual assault and subject to brutalization and sexist denigration and name-calling by male prison guards.

Ironically, two of the recommendations from the inquest investigating Ashley Smith's murder recommend that "there be adequate staffing of mental health care providers with expertise and experience at every women's institution" and "that all female inmates be assessed by a psychologist within 72 hours of admission to any penitentiary or treatment facility to determine whether any mental health issues or self-injurious behavior exists" ("Ashley Smith inquest," 2013b). The irony here is twofold: First, the mental health professionals were not able to help Ashley Smith, even though they offered many different diagnoses, sometimes within hours of each other. Second, it is very likely that her mental health issues changed over time or perhaps began as a result of the sexism, assaults, and other cruelties she experienced while incarcerated. As medicalization theory would predict, the answer to problems such as Ashley Smith experienced is assumed to be more medical and likely pharmaceutical intervention, even though it has not worked adequately in this case.

# chapter three

# Vanessa Young and Marit McKenzie: The Potential Harm of Prescribed Drugs

## Vanessa Young and Prepulsid

This chapter discusses the pharmaceutical errors that led to the sudden deaths of two young women, Vanessa Young and Marit McKenzie. Both of these young women died after ingesting legally prescribed, if off-label, medications. In each case, the medication use may have been related to the beauty aspirations of the young women, as well as to the careless prescription and irresponsible availability of specific drugs. Issues in pharmaceuticalization, in the context of medicalization, are at the heart of these two tragic deaths. I question post-market monitoring practices. I look at conflicts of interest between Health Canada and the pharmaceutical industry. I ask how these deadly errors could be the result of normal pharmaceutical use, coupled with medical practice norms. These deaths, too, were the result of one of the social determinants of health, sexism, as manifest in gender beauty norms for women and girls.

Vanessa Young was a healthy and active fifteen-year-old girl living with her family in Oakville, Ontario, when she died suddenly of a cardiac arrest.[1] She had asked her father for permission to go out on a Saturday evening in April 2000. He responded that he was too busy to talk about it just then. He asked her to seek permission a bit later. As she turned to leave the room, she fell backwards and hit her head. Her father jumped up and ran to help her. She was already limp and pale. She did not seem to be breathing.

He screamed for his wife and son to call an ambulance, called his brother who was a doctor and a neighbour who was a nurse, and immediately began CPR and mouth-to-mouth artificial respiration.

A few days later, Vanessa died in hospital having never regained consciousness. She had had no obvious symptoms of illness before this catastrophic event. Otherwise a healthy young teenage girl, she had spent the afternoon of the day on which she collapsed making cookies and planning her evening of fun. Instead, she was in the hospital in a deep coma. As her father stood with her in the emergency room (ER) and talked with the accompanying paramedics and police, he heard discussion of the medication she had been on. It was Prepulsid, the brand name for cisapride. The ER doctors asked who had prescribed it. He overheard one doctor say: "They dish it out like water." He also heard talk of "long QT." He did not understand these conversations. But his curiosity and fear were raised. He promised himself and his daughter to find out what had harmed her and to warn others about it.

The first thing he did after Vanessa died, to fulfil this promise to himself and his daughter, was put in a phone call to the manufacturer of the medication Vanessa had been using. He called Johnson and Johnson's Canadian drug division Janssen-Ortho (now Janssen Canada) to warn them of his daughter's death from one of their medications. At the time, he thought they would respond immediately to this, to his mind, clearly urgent situation, remove the drug from the market, and warn others who might also be using it of the potentially deadly problem. Instead, they responded that they knew there were issues with the drug. They had already done what they were legally required to do to warn others of the potential danger.

There was a history of problems with Prepulsid, which were already well documented. The drug was sold worldwide in 119 countries. There had been many other reports of death and serious side effects, even though the drug was used mostly for the minor problem of heartburn. In July 1996, the *Canadian Adverse Drug Reaction Newsletter* reported that Prepulsid could be dangerous for patients with pre-existing heart problems and could cause serious arrhythmias (Health Canada, 2000). As of 1999, Health

Canada had received 127 reports of adverse events, 44 of which were related to heart arrhythmias and heart rate disorders. There had also been 12 reports of death from the drug in Canada. Janssen-Ortho had responded. They had done what they were obliged to do. They had faxed four advisory letters to Canadian doctors. Two warnings of adverse effects had been printed in the journal of the Canadian Medical Association. Clearly, the pharmaceutical company already knew of the problem and had acted as Health Canada required.

The problem was not Prepulsid per se, the company spokesperson said to Vanessa's father. It was that the drug had been prescribed by a doctor contrary to the warnings of the drug company and prescribed incorrectly to a child, a young girl with mild bulimia who was throwing up after meals and sometimes felt bloated. Neither the drug nor the pharmaceutical company was at fault. Prepulsid was specifically contraindicated for children, and it was not to be given in the case of bulimia or vomiting. Vanessa had all of the contraindications for use of this pharmaceutical treatment. This information was accessible to doctors and to patients if they would read the information sheet available with the prescription. However, apparently no one on Vanessa's medical care "team" knew of the contraindications. Vanessa had seen four doctors, including specialists, who had been treating her for her condition during the year or so that she was taking Prepulsid. Not one of them had ever asked questions about the medication or advised against it. The Youngs were a family that was very careful about any drug consumption. At least one of Vanessa's parents had always attended doctor appointments with her to ensure that information about her treatment was clear and remembered with precision. There had never been any warnings or mention of risks associated with Prepulsid. Nor did the pharmacists ask questions or advise against this prescription.

On the phone that day after Vanessa's death, the drug company representative claimed that he was very sorry for Young's loss but the company had done its part in ensuring drug safety. The situation was different in the United States at the time. In 1999, the U.S. Food and Drug Administration (FDA), as a result of a growing awareness of adverse events related to prior heart problems, had advised doctors to ensure that an electrocardiogram was undertaken prior to prescribing Prepulsid. This policy change and information bulletin was for a US audience only. A similar requirement was not put in place in Canada. Although Health Canada receives notice when any drug is removed from the list of acceptable drugs in other countries and responds by re-evaluating the position of the drug in their formulary, they had not yet acted on the US report when Vanessa died suddenly of heart-related problems. Prepulsid was withdrawn from the US market weeks before Vanessa's death on 23 March 2000. It was not removed from Canadian markets until August, months after Vanessa's sudden death.

The more Vanessa's father, Terence Young, discovered about Prepulsid – that the drug company had known about previous serious and even fatal problems associated with it and that Health Canada had also known about the danger – the more determined he became to fulfil his promise to Vanessa's memory and to work hard so this tragedy did not happen again to anyone else. Terence Young was particularly well placed to do this investigation and advocacy. He had already been a member of the provincial Parliament (MPP) for the province of Ontario, and he knew some of the players and lobbyists in political and decision-making circles. He was educated, healthy, hardworking, and intelligent. He had family members in medicine, including a brother and a cousin who were doctors. He wanted to know why Canadians had to experience serious side effects and to die before a drug, known to have potentially fatal side effects, was removed from the market. He wanted to determine Health Canada's role in this tragedy. To do that, he spent hours and hours online, in meetings, and conducting interviews, trying to understand the drug safety process in Canada. He wanted and finally, with the help of lawyers, secured an inquest into Vanessa's death to bring to light the causes so that the system could be changed. Ultimately, he sued the drug company and won the suit for an undisclosed amount of money. He established an organization called Drug Safety Canada. He spoke to hundreds of experts (McIver & Wyndam, 2013) and eventually spoke at conferences and wrote and published a book, *Death by*

*Prescription*, detailing all he had learned regarding why his daughter died of a prescribed medication while being seen by four different doctors (Young, 2012).

As a testament to Young's hard work, an inquest took place in 2001, the year following Vanessa's death. The inquest resulted in fifty-nine recommendations (McIver & Wyndam, 2013). Later, Young ran for federal office to work to enhance drug regulation and safety. He was successful in his pursuit of becoming a member of the federal Parliament of Canada (MP) in both 2008 and again in 2011. He initiated a class action suit soon after Vanessa's death against the pharmaceutical company. The suit was finally certified and ready to go to court as of 2007. In 2014, fourteen years after his daughter's death, a bill (Vanessa's Law) was finally passed. In summary, it provides for (1) strengthened oversight of therapeutic products through their life cycle, (2) improved reporting by certain health care institutions of serious adverse drug reactions and medical device incidents that involve therapeutic products, and (3) the promotion of greater confidence in the oversight of therapeutic products by increasing transparency (Parliament of Canada, 2014). Whether or not these changes would have been sufficient to prevent Vanessa's death is not clear. Furthermore, there are problems with the execution of the bill, according to Vanessa's father. Health Canada is still not requiring that serious adverse drug reactions be reported by doctors (Minksy, 2017).

## Marit McKenzie and Diane-35

There is another story of sudden death in a young girl still living at home that underscores the problems of Vanessa's death and adds more insight to the role played by the pharmaceutical industry and its relationship with Health Canada. This incident happened in 2013. It is the story of a medication, Diane-35, licensed by Health Canada in 1998 (Mintzes, 2004), which was designed for short-term use for severe acne only, and only when the acne is accompanied by signs of excess androgen. Diane-35 was only to be prescribed after other options had been tried unsuccessfully. Yet it became widely prescribed off-label for mild acne and was often prescribed over a lengthy period of time. It also became a popular (off-label) long-term birth control pill. The issues with the medication Diane-35 came to light in Canada largely because of the media attention garnered after another catastrophic, sudden death of a young woman. In this case, eighteen-year-old Marit McKenzie died of a massive pulmonary embolism followed by four cardiac arrests the next day. This outcome was related to use of the medication Diane-35 in 2013 in Calgary, Alberta. Marit was the thirteenth recorded death in Canada linked to Diane-35 according to the Canada Vigilance Adverse Reaction Online Database, a Health Canada voluntary reporting system tracking adverse effects of medication (https:// www.canada.ca/en/health-canada/services/drugs-health-prod ucts/medeffect-canada/adverse-reaction-database.html).

According to coverage in the *Toronto Star*, Marit, a first-year University of Calgary student, had been on this pill for her mild acne for almost one year when she woke up in the middle of the night at her parent's home so weak that she could not climb the stairs to their bedroom. She was too exhausted to go up to the second floor to say that she felt very ill and needed help. Instead, sounding afraid, she called upstairs to their bedroom on the telephone. She had been complaining of increasing tiredness in the weeks leading up to this evening, and friends and family were already concerned about her. A week before this night, Marit's mother had taken her to their family doctor who had originally prescribed Diane-35. The doctor had ordered a blood test to try to diagnose Marit's exhaustion. The results of the blood work indicated that there was no obvious blood-related reason for Marit's fatigue. She was said to be healthy. The doctor failed to question Marit's medication use and thus did not think to alert anyone of the possibility that the exhaustion might be a side effect of the drug that had been prescribed (Zlomislic, 2013a).

Marit's symptoms had been increasingly disabling and had led to dramatic changes in her behaviour in the previous months. Her boyfriend said that "they stopped rollerblading, going to the movies, hanging out with other friends and spent a lot more time just sitting quietly and trying to relax" (Zlomislic, 2013a). Still, no one in her world had any idea that her body "was shutting down" as the result of the acne medication. But on the night that she collapsed, she had severe chest pains, a racing heart, and trouble breathing. Rushing downstairs after the phone call, her father lifted up his daughter and carried her to the car, and he and her mother rushed Marit to the hospital. Marit suffered four cardiac arrests in the next forty-eight hours before she was pronounced dead. The cause of this devastation was a pulmonary embolism, which blocked the flow of blood to both of her lungs (Zlomislic, 2013a).

Introduced into the Canadian market in 1998, over time Diane-35 became associated with a number of deaths and at least 200 complaints of negative side effects to Health Canada, recorded in the Canada Vigilance Adverse Reaction Online Database. Since post-market surveillance and monitoring are voluntary, these numbers, in all likelihood, represent under-reporting (Mintzes, 2004). All hormone-based medications have some risk of minor and more serious side effects, including the blood clotting that led to Marit's cardiac arrests and death. However, Diane-35 has been shown in various studies to have a higher risk of blood clots, perhaps four times higher (Zlomislic, 2013b; Mintzes, 2004), than other oral contraceptives. Furthermore, it had not been officially approved in Canada as an oral contraceptive. Rather, it was officially to be used only as a last resort in the case of severe acne and for a short period of time. Nevertheless, it appears that many doctors were prescribing Diane-35 as a sort of two for one: acne medication and/or contraceptive. Health Canada's summary review of Diane-35 from April 2014 estimated that there had been about 450,000 prescriptions written per year since 2009. It also projected that approximately 35 to 40 per cent of the prescriptions were for the unapproved and long-term purpose of contraception (Health Canada, 2014).

## The Normal Functioning of the Pharmaceutical Industry

How could these sudden, tragic, and preventable deaths of young women in the prime of their lives have happened in Canada in the twenty-first century? There are a number of factors contributing to this egregious outcome. The first is the normal functioning of the pharmaceutical industry in Canada and around the globe. Because of its size and net worth, the pharmaceutical industry has more power than a number of nation states. This industry is one of the lowest risk and highest profit industries in the world. It operates globally and moves its operations and parts of its operations from jurisdiction to jurisdiction to increase viability, growth, and profits. Sovereign nations negotiate the terms under which they regulate the products of this industry with a balance between the economic benefits of hosting a pharmaceutical company, including tax and employment, and the costs of potential adverse events for citizens. Although its mandate is to develop products of benefit to the health of individuals, the pharmaceutical industry is directly beholden to shareholders and not to patients or consumers. Thus, its lines of accountability favour profit and the management of the risks of harm or death in the interests of profit. The industry must balance long-term harm or safety risks and concerns with the chance to generate substantial earnings quickly. There is an emphasis on speed and the speedy introduction of new discoveries to the market over the precautionary principle, which would assert the value of safety first.

Pharmaceuticals are an increasingly large part of medical treatment today. The reach of the pharmaceutical industry has been expanding in Canada as elsewhere. Drugs currently comprise a larger share of our health care dollar than any other sector except hospitals. Furthermore, the industry's segment of these expenditures has been growing in the past decades. In 1983, spending for pharmaceuticals was 9.8 per cent of the health care budget. In 1990, it comprised 12.6 per cent, and the estimated costs for 2010 and 2011 were 16.3 per cent and 16.5 per cent of the total health care budget, respectively. By 2018, Canada spent 16.8 per cent of its health care budget on pharmaceuticals (OECD, 2020). This growth pattern has also occurred in the context of a parallel expansion of the amount of the gross national product (GNP) that has been devoted to health care overall during the same period. Thus, a substantial and growing proportion of this money is for prescribed drugs (Government of Canada, 2018). Because of both the overall increase in the use of prescription drugs and the use of newer and more expensive drugs, Canada spends the third highest proportion of its budget on medications, about 22 per cent above the median for Organisation for Economic Co-operation and Development (OECD) countries. The majority of this cost, about 60 per cent, is covered by medicare (Clarke, 2016), and the rest is comprised of out-of-pocket and private insurance coverage.

Drug companies make most of their profits from medications that are under patent. A patent "protects" a new drug from being copied by rival companies for a fixed period of time. Newly patented drugs are much more profitable for companies. A new patent allows the establishment of a new price. Prices generally have little to do with the ingredients used and more to do with the ability of the company to charge what it estimates the market will allow. This price setting is regulated by the Patented Medicine Prices Review Board (2020) in Canada. The pharmaceutical companies negotiate with governments regarding the cost of drugs using the argument that they need to set prices that will enable them to finance ongoing research and new drug development.

A significant amount of the growth in the pharmaceutical industry and of its profit margins results from the manufacture and sales of what are colloquially referred to as "me too" patent drugs. "Me too" drugs are those that are developed through tweaking the active or inactive molecules in an already patented drug in order to maintain patent. This activity occurs as the patent protection is about to expire and the manufacturing drug company is about to lose the higher profits of patented drugs. When the patent expires, generic drugs that are considerably less expensive can be produced and sold. Thus, the production of similar or "me too" drugs obstructs the development and sale of cheaper generic drugs based on the ingredients of the drug whose patent is about to expire.

The standards for new drug approval in Canada are not high. For both new patents or slight tweaking to a drug to maintain a patent, a drug need only be as good as one previously developed and on the market for the same condition (Canadian Foundation for Healthcare Improvement, 2013). This "improved" drug for which a new patent is sought may simply involve some small degree of alteration of the medication. Of course, once the "new and improved" drug is developed and receives an additional extended or new patent, the company can begin to aggressively advertise, and the higher profits associated with patented drugs can continue.

There is also a great deal of evidence that drugs are frequently overprescribed in Canada. At times, the use of medications is as problematic as, or even more problematic than, the condition they are meant to treat. All drugs have side effects. Only a proportion of drugs on the market actually offer any benefit. For example, apparently about half of the antidepressants only work as a placebo on those who use them (Smith, 2012). As well as not having any effect, many drugs are also known to have deleterious, even if minor, side effects at times (such as a dry mouth or sleepiness). Users may be willing to put up with such seemingly minor side effects for the supposed benefit of the drug. However, less than minor side effects or serious adverse reactions also occur routinely. A sizeable proportion of hospital admissions result from drug misuse (either by incorrect prescribing, incorrect in-home utilization, or interaction effects of several drugs taken at the same time). About one-third of the visits made to the emergency room by the elderly are due to medication mishaps (Budnitz et al., 2011). Adverse drug reactions are one of the top causes of death in Canada (Rosenbloom & Wyne, 1999). In 2010, there were approximately 30,000 reports of adverse drug and device reactions, and about three-quarters were reported by Health Canada to be serious (Weeks, 2010).

## Patient Use of Medications

There are various types of medication errors or problems with the use of pharmaceuticals. While some are related to normative working of the pharmaceutical industry, others are more closely related to the characteristics of the patients who use the medications. One of the most grievous of medication errors today results from prescribing a specific medication to a person who becomes addicted to the prescribed drug and then needs to continue using it, or something else, to get the same results. This medical care decision can lead to the need to increase the amount ingested to maintain equilibrium. If a doctor is no longer willing to prescribe the drug because the condition for which it was prescribed initially is gone, then subsequent addiction to street drugs may occur. One example of this problem can be found in the widespread addiction to opioids. Opioids are prescribed for severe and intractable pain, but some people become addicted and need increasing amounts, not for pain per se but just to feel "normal." Many in this situation have turned to street opioid drugs, which has become an epidemic and led to immense suffering across Canada (Shield et al., 2011). The overprescription of opioids as painkillers for chronic conditions has been so costly to the population that it has resulted in thousands of deaths through addiction and overdose. The numbers have been so dramatic as to result in a decline in life expectancy (Belzak & Halverson, 2018).

Polypharmacy, or the prescription of a number of different drugs to the same person by one or more doctors, may lead to dangerous drug interactions. While each drug singly may be safe, or accompanied usually by only minor and easily manageable side effects, when taken in tandem with other drugs, it may cause serious adverse effects. Sometimes people get advice and treatment from more than one doctor. Sometimes the person does not explain that he or she has already sought help and received a prescription for a particular condition. Hopefully, each doctor will investigate the medications already prescribed before adding to the mix. But that is not always done. In addition, patients may forget the names of all the medications they are on or fail to bring them all to each medical appointment. In an absence of a digitally available drug/person inventory, this problem is bound to continue. Some individual doctors at times may unknowingly prescribe two or more drugs that can have problematic interactions and cause deleterious effects. This practice leaves open the possibility of drug interactions and subsequent medical problems. Furthermore, many of us take over-the-counter medications, including those we consider to be utterly benign such as "natural" health products, along with prescribed medications. Any polypharmacy is potentially dangerous.

Often times, pharmaceutical problems result from the inability or unwillingness of the patient to follow a schedule of use such as before meals, with meals, or after meals. Yet the medical care system assumes that patients are able to read and to organize and schedule their lives adequately. A significant proportion of the population is illiterate as defined by their ability to read and understand the directions on a bottle of prescribed medicines (Jamieson, 2006). People can forget, take with meals or without meals incorrectly, accidently overdose, stop precipitously, and so on. Women are more likely to take prescription drugs than men. Women attend the doctor more often than men. This difference is partly because women get pregnant and give birth, and these processes are medicalized. It is also because women are more likely to be caregivers of their children and more likely to go to the doctor in this capacity. Such familiarity may lead to easier consultation with the doctor. Women are more likely to be diagnosed with various chronic conditions. The elderly are also more likely to attend the doctor. Both women and the elderly are more susceptible to problems with medications (Manteuffel et al., 2014; Rotermann et al., 2015).

## Governance and the Pharmaceutical Industry

In Canada, Health Canada has the ultimate legislative responsibility to determine whether or not new drugs are safe and of adequate benefit, and therefore ought to be introduced to the market. Health Canada is also responsible for the ongoing monitoring of drugs for safety and efficacy after they are on the shelves and being prescribed. The initial introduction of a new drug onto the market is the result of evidence collected through clinical trials. But there are serious limitations in this governance and practice that affect the quality, efficacy, and safety of drugs on the market in Canada (Lexchin, 2009).

One of the most important restrictions regarding safety arises from the relationship of the pharmaceutical industry to Health Canada. Health Canada is dependent on pharmaceutical companies for a significant portion of its funding. In 2006, Health Canada received 30 per cent of its funding from the pharmaceutical companies. This figure was down substantially from the 70 per cent that had previously been the amount that Health Canada was beholden to the pharmaceutical industry (Lexchin, 2006). On the face of it, even this level of funding for Health Canada could easily be seen as a sign of a conflict of interest. However, this percentage climbed to 50 per cent in subsequent years, and Health Canada recently announced that it was raising the fees it charges for the introduction of new drugs into the marketplace (DATAC, 2018). While this funding is justified as enabling Health Canada to increase the speed of the introduction of new drugs into the country's market, there is little evidence that the sped-up process actually helps a substantial number of medication users. It is estimated that only 10.6 per cent of the new drugs offered substantial benefit. Furthermore, this faster process poses challenges to the safety of new drugs.

The structure and fiscal priorities of Health Canada thus seem to be biased in favour of the interests of pharmaceutical companies. Rapid drug approval is institutionalized and encouraged. The resources of Health Canada are geared towards rapid approval rather than sober second and third thought. If Health Canada does not meet certain targets in the speed of adoption of new drugs, it must rebate the pharmaceutical company that has developed the drug being tested. Once a drug is on the market, it is very difficult to remove it, even in the face of repeated documentation of adverse side effects. Health Canada can publish and circulate safety advisories and warnings, and it can provide the latest information to doctors and pharmacies about newly documented dangers that have been discovered as the result of post-market monitoring. But it cannot force a pharmaceutical company to take the drug off the shelf. Once a drug is approved, the power essentially belongs to the company to remove or leave a drug in the market, even after serious side effects have been found (Lexchin, 2009). Although there are various initiatives designed to strengthen post-market surveillance by the government (Sawler, n.d.), the relative contribution of the pharmaceutical industry continues to make drug removal challenging.

That the system favours the pharmaceutical industry is also evident in the processes of post-market surveillance or monitoring. To the extent that Health Canada stipulates that monitoring be based on volunteer reports from community members such as patients, doctors, pharmacies, or family members of someone harmed, it will be an uncertain procedure. Monitoring is a time-consuming process. It is sometimes difficult for community members to recognize or prove the cause of death or harm and to differentiate it from the disease process without assiduous and lengthy study of the available evidence on the pharmaceutical. Proof of association between the medication and the harm is always a complex and difficult process. Proof of causality is even more demanding, as it involves four fundamental conditions: consistent association of cause and effect, no other possible explanation for the observed link between cause and effect, time priority of the presumed causal variable, and a coherent and logical theoretical explanation. The complexity of measuring all four conditions of causal association to decide on one possible causal chain exacerbates the difficulties of withdrawal of a medication from the market once it has been approved.

There are many other impediments to ensuring ongoing drug safety. It is notable that medication error acknowledgement is often the result of active and often lengthy advocacy by patients, the families of patients, or medical care personnel. The process involves filling out complex forms that requires knowledge and skill. Doctors may be reluctant to report medication side effects mentioned by their patients in case they are personally sued for prescribing it in the first place. Furthermore, doctors have busy days and may not have the time to pay attention to such problems or to fill out the necessary forms. Patients and family members may be too disabled by grief or the side effects themselves to spend the time necessary to determine the cause of death or suffering. They may be afraid of the repercussions of "blowing the whistle." Even from a sophisticated scientific perspective, the cause of death or suffering is usually complicated to determine absolutely. It involves a number of different factors. It may often take a considerable number of years before the impact of the drug becomes manifest in any individual. Thus, determining the prime cause or the contributing cause of a drug-based adverse event may be prohibitively challenging.

It is likely that only a fraction of the errors or side effects of new medications are ever reported (Coleman & Pontefract, 2016). It is estimated that eventually 3.9 to 4.4 per cent of drugs introduced to the Canadian market have had to be withdrawn within five-year periods (Lexchin, 2014). This figure is probably only a small fraction of drugs that are associated with some harm. Moreover, during the time the withdrawn drug is on the market and before the complaint is successfully laid, many people will potentially have been harmed or have died as a result of ingesting it. The two young women who are the focus of this chapter are cases in point. The vast majority of the adverse effects, approximately 95 per cent, are likely unreported (Hazel & Shakir, 2006). Thus, probably only about 5 per cent of adverse events are reported. One French study found that there was only one report of an adverse event for every 4,600 drug reactions (Moride et al., 1997). With the lack of systematic follow-up and post-market monitoring, and the complexities of determining causality, the actual number of side effects is essentially unknown.

## Clinical Trials: The Drug Approval Process

Drugs are approved in Canada after they have been tested in clinical trials. It is difficult to get information about these clinical trials, even though they provide the fundamental evidence upon which drug licensing is based. Health Canada considers the results of their pre-market studies to be confidential and private. In fact, such studies are considered the property of the pharmaceutical company. However, clinical trials used to evaluate new drugs just before they enter the market are necessarily potentially problematic. For example, the subjects in clinical trials may be unlike the ultimate users of the new drug in many and systematic ways, such as age, weight, gender, and non-diagnosed health conditions. Clinical trials usually exclude pregnant women, but there is always a period of time in which women may be pregnant and not be aware of it. This situation is true for the trials themselves and then ultimately for the regular use of the medication. Trials also frequently exclude children and the elderly, who may later be prescribed the medication. There are many possible ways to differ sharply biologically from the average trial volunteer used to establish the efficacy and safety of a given dosage of a new drug (Jureidini et al., 2004; Tan & Koelch, 2008). It is not surprising, then, that adverse drug effects are more common in the elderly. They are the most frequent users of pharmaceuticals (Morgan & Kennedy, 2010). Boy and girl children are also frequently prescribed medications that have not been tested on their sex, age, and size groups (Jureidini et al., 2004; Tan & Koelch, 2008). On the one hand, there are serious ethical issues in experimenting on children. On the other hand, without such tests, use of pharmaceuticals with children may be unethical and medically problematic. It is a conundrum.

Drugs are also tested on people in various stages of health and biological functioning. They may be used on people with several disease conditions, or just one, and on people with differently functioning biological systems (for example, hormone differences between men and women). The required size of the clinical trial test group is statistically always going to be too small to locate rare but sometimes serious and even fatal side effects. In addition, some adverse effects may take years to develop (Canadian Foundation for Healthcare Improvement, 2010). But clinical trials are time limited. Indeed, there is pressure by the industry to speed up clinical trials so new drugs can get onto the market. There are many different types and stages of clinical trials for the introduction of new drugs, as illustrated in Table 1.

Issues with the length of the clinical trial and the types of participants used are prominent within published results. However, many trials are not ever made public. Ben Goldacre, founder of the organization AllTrials – which advocates for more transparency and regulation within the pharmaceutical industry – argues that only a small portion of registered trials even submit final reports (AllTrials, n.d.; Prayle et al., 2012). Furthermore, trials with positive findings are twice as likely to be reported in comparison to

Table 1. Types and Stages of Drug Trials

| Types/Stages of Drug Trials | Description |
| --- | --- |
| Laboratory Studies | Examine the effects of drugs on various cells and tissues |
| Animal Studies | Specifically examine the short- and long-term toxicity, physiological effects, cancer causation, rates of birth defects, and impact on reproduction through the use of animals as subjects |
| Phase I | **Studies in a small group of healthy volunteers**: small and short-term studies of the effects of the drug on the human body (including safety and side effects) |
| Phase II | **Studies of larger groups of people**: studies with a focus on effectiveness, safety, and short-term side effects; preliminary data on whether drug works with different diseases and conditions |
| Phase III | **Studies of the impact on larger groups of people with the condition**: these studies test approved dosage and mirror clinical prescribing patterns such as potential interaction with other drugs that patients may be taking |
| Phase IV | **Follow-up**: at times, a regulatory agency will require the manufacturer to complete a follow-up study and to monitor the impacts of longer term use |

Source: Adapted from Mintzes, 2004; National Institute on Aging, 2020.

trials finding negative or undesirable results (AllTrials, n.d.; Song et al., 2010). Both of these fundamental ethical issues further obfuscate the "evidence" on drug efficacy cited by pharmaceutical companies.

## Off-Label Prescribing

Once a clinical trial has demonstrated the required level of the safety and efficacy of a new drug, the drug can be brought to market. It is at this point that the appropriate dosage and particulars of utilization are determined. The new drug can then be advertised and sold. Once a new drug is on the market, the potential problems with its use may expand as it is used over time. Nevertheless, doctors are allowed to prescribe drugs off-label or for a different purpose than that for which the drug was initially approved by Health Canada. This potentially serious problem was implicated in both of the deaths we are now discussing. Off-label prescribing includes prescribing to categories of people, including children and the elderly, drugs that have not been approved for those age groups. It also includes prescribing a greater or smaller dose or frequency than has been approved. It may include prescribing in combination with another incompatible drug. It may include prescribing in the absence of full awareness of side effects and contraindications.

Still, off-label prescribing is common and widely accepted. As many as one in five prescriptions (20 per cent) may be for off-label use (Radley et al., 2006). A somewhat higher percentage of off-label prescriptions occurs in specific situations, such as in the case of terminal illness, when there may be no other option available. Doctors may choose an off-label drug as a last resort when nothing else seems to be working and there is a possibility that this different medication might help. There appears to be a greater tendency to use drugs off-label in the case of psychiatric symptoms (Radley et al., 2006). It is not uncommon for children exhibiting behavioural and emotional struggles to be prescribed one drug after another in the hopes that one will eventually work as desired (Clarke, 2013). Some argue that this strategy of medical care may be considered a violation of the human rights of children (Whitaker, 2001, 2010). A similar argument could be made with respect to the use of drugs such as antipsychotics in situations in which people are not able to understand the costs and benefits, and thus not able to give informed consent. For example, warnings about increased mortality among the elderly who were prescribed antipsychotics were issued earlier than 2005 (Singh & Wooltorton, 2005), but prescription has continued, especially in nursing homes (Pimentel et al., 2015). Off-label use may be normative in particular situations and remains common practice in Canada.

At other times, doctors may decide to use medication off-label because of the messages of pharmaceutical representatives. Unfortunately, this information is based on an essential conflict of interest. Drug company representatives are hired to promote their company's drugs. Such representatives are chosen not because of their knowledge of pharmaceuticals but because of their sales and coaxing ability (Young, 2012). Prescribing as the result of a sales pitch has led to significant errors and resulted at times in suits against doctors under the legal theories of medical negligence, failure to acquire informed consent, and unregulated use of a research drug (Wittich et al., 2012).

In both of our cases in this chapter, the medication had been prescribed off-label and in a situation for which it was not indicated. In the case of Diane-35, the doctor was prescribing it for minor acne. It was not approved for that purpose. Yet it was being prescribed for much broader purposes and over a longer period of time, which is problematic. Moreover, the doctor may have failed to see the three safety advisories that Health Canada had posted on their website or to be familiar with the association between the signs and symptoms Marit was experiencing and her ongoing use of the drug. In other words, the doctor not only prescribed off-label but essentially against the labelling. Marit did not have any of the other particular risk factors to suggest that this medication should not be used or that its use could lead to her death. She was not overweight and did not smoke; nor did she have a history of blood clots in her family. She was not sedentary. The McKenzie family did not know of these risk factors or of the possible side effects of the medication. Neither the physician nor the drugstore from which Marit obtained Diane-35 provided her with the detailed information about possible adverse effects or warnings of potential risks.

The medication prescribed for Vanessa was not prescribed as it was supposed to be either. It was not to be given to children, and she was only fifteen years old. It was not to be prescribed in cases of vomiting or bulimia, and Vanessa had a mild case of bulimia. Vomiting after meals and feeling bloated were the two reasons for which she had initially gone to the doctor seeking help. There were several other contraindications that should have prevented this drug from being prescribed to Vanessa. It was prescribed off-label.

Off-label prescribing contradicts the basic principles of evidence-based medicine. Medical practice is virtually universally legitimated by the appeal that it is based on evidence from good medical science. Further, good medical science, it is claimed, is based on the "gold standard" of medical research, the blinded experimental design with at least two comparative groups, one using the new drug, device, or intervention and the other subject to a placebo. Evidence-based medicine is the formal bedrock of good medical practice today. When drugs are used off-label, they are not prescribed on the basis of peer-reviewed best practice guidelines. We are asked to put our trust in medical care because it is founded on the very best practices of science, including objectivity, precision, reliability, and generalizability, among other basic guiding principles. When doctors use drugs off-label, they are essentially ignoring these basic principles of medical science. They are disregarding the public trust under which the drugs are licensed and supported. Off-label use is not based on any science at all. It arises from ad hoc hypotheses, informal conversation, and even sales persuasion made by the drug detail men and women working for pharmaceutical companies. It must be admitted that sometimes off-label prescriptions have been beneficial to patients, but so too are placebos, and placebos do not come with the possibility of adverse events (Dresser & Frader, 2009). The problem is that the peculiar benefit of an off-label pharmaceutical may be idiosyncratic and thus unique to only one patient or one type of patient. It may be very harmful to a different type of patient. Without systematic record-keeping – including transparency – regarding ongoing evaluation, the value and the danger of off-label prescribing is unknown, and doctors are taking risks without adequate safety, efficacy, and knowledge.

## Drug Advertising: To Doctors or Direct to Consumer

Pharmaceutical companies are the major source of information about both new drugs and drugs already on the market. Although doctors say they are not influenced by drug detail men or drug company advertising, the evidence is clear that they are. Doctors have serious deficiencies in their education, both during school and continuing education, regarding the safety and efficacy of pharmaceutical products (Tannenbaum & Tsuyiki, 2013). Moreover, from medical school on, doctors are potentially influenced by the practices of the pharmaceutical industry through expensive material gifts, including holidays, meals, office furniture, and so on. They may also be employed and paid as "experts," and they may be financially rewarded for offering their own patients as subjects in clinical trials in return for generous payments. With growing awareness of these dangerous practices, medical schools are developing policies to educate doctors about these ethical conundrums and to prevent conflict of interest vis-à-vis doctors and pharmaceutical product prescription (Glauser, 2013).

Direct-to-consumer advertising (with limited exceptions) is not allowed in Canada. However, because Canadians consume media from the United States, where direct-to-consumer advertising is allowed, we are frequently exposed to drug advertisements. There is evidence that, when consumers/patients see drug advertisements, they are in general more likely to experience the symptoms described in the advertisements and to seek out the specific advertised treatment or medication by name. Doctors, in turn, are more likely to prescribe the exact named medication when asked by a patient for it, even in the absence of the condition for which the drug is indicated (Mintzes et al., 2002, 2003; Kravitz et al., 2005). Thus, advertising both to doctors and to consumers no doubt contributes to the overall rate of dependence on drugs.

Diane-35 was widely advertised for purposes for which it was not approved, that is, as a contraceptive. It was not legal in Canada to promote the drug to doctors or to the public for this use. Despite this legal restriction, it was "advertised" to doctors for birth control through the "back door" and via the circulation of a report resulting from an "unrestricted educational grant" (Mintzes, 2004). Furthermore, it became widely used and advertised to the public as a birth control method on billboards, in magazines, on television, and in movies. Health Canada did not take action against these violations, even though it received complaints from women's groups and health advocates. As we have indicated, once a drug is on the market, Health Canada has limited power. Prepulsid, too, was essentially being prescribed when it ought not to have been. It had been linked to deaths and pulled from the market elsewhere. It had been offered to Vanessa despite her youth and her possible symptoms of an eating disorder. This had happened under the guidance of four different physicians who were overseeing her case.

## Lack of Transparency Regarding Drug Safety and Efficacy Information

In addition to off-label prescribing and direct-to-consumer and other advertising, another serious problem is the lack of transparency concerning the reports of the research that lead up to the approval of drugs, as well as a lack of public information on the ongoing side effects. "Whereas the U.S. Food and Drug Administration and the European Medicines Agency routinely publish details of post-market safety reviews of drugs as a basic accountability measure, Canada refuses, citing 'confidential business information'" (Zlomislic, 2013b). For example, Health Canada did not require that Bayer/Berlex provide empirical evidence that Diane-35 was more effective than a placebo. In fact, according to a scholarly review of the available studies that tested the efficacy and safety of the medication when it was introduced to the Canadian market, there was no evidence that Diane-35 was effective for the specified use. Furthermore, it was three to twenty-nine times riskier than other available medications with respect to the incidence of venous thromboembolism (VTE) or blood clots (Mintzes, 2004). There were other worrying adverse effects described in the literature, including evidence of liver cell changes or hyperplasia in the liver. Furthermore, on the basis of summary reports of all Phase III trials accessed (after delays) through Access to Information legislation, Mintzes (2004) found that the clinical trials failed to provide evidence that this medication was better, either in its positive effects on the condition under treatment or in terms of having fewer adverse effects, than other previously developed and used medications for either acne or birth control. In addition, Diane-35 had been linked to liver cancer in a woman who had used it off-label as a birth control measure for fourteen years. It had also been linked with some cases of blood clots. Diane-35 had not been approved in the United States. Indeed, it was initially rejected by Health Canada because of connections to liver cancer.

As of 9 April 2014, Health Canada released a brief ten-paragraph synopsis to the public in which they concluded that the benefits of Diane-35 continue to outweigh the risks of using this medication for severe acne. Thus, Health Canada was not removing the medication from the market (Zlomislic, 2013b). This synopsis of a review was the result of months of "pushing" and battling by Marit's family and the *Toronto Star* newspaper against the standard secrecy regarding adverse effects by Health Canada. Bayer/Berlex, the company that manufactures Diane-35, claims Canadian health care providers have all the necessary information on the drug. The head of Health Canada's Marketed Pharmaceuticals and Medical Devices Bureau would not say whether this conclusion was arrived at on the basis of its approved use for severe acne for a short term or included its widespread use for birth control. Health Canada neither stopped these abuses from occurring nor invested in post-market surveillance of untoward advertising that would have observed encroachments on the law.

## The Role of the Pharmacist and the Pharmacy

Pharmacists do have some responsibilities regarding the provision of information about medications to consumers. These responsibilities are not monitored, however. Nor are dispensing errors systematically monitored or counted. Different pharmacies and pharmacists have varying norms regarding the extent of the information they provide. Pharmacists face many practical constraints in their ability to provide information, including pressures to perform and sell quickly, as pharmacies are for-profit entities. Thus, pharmacies provide different levels of service about side and long-term effects of medications. Some pharmacies spend time with patients explaining how drugs are to be consumed and for how long. They may also suggest potential problems of which the patient should be aware. Others do not have the knowledge or time, or do not take the time. At times, the printed inserts accompanying medications are clear and provide the necessary information about how to take a particular drug, what possible contraindications there may be, and what sorts of side effects may occur to which the patient should be alert in an accessible manner. Sometimes, the printed inserts are many, many pages long and may even leave important factors regarding contraindications to the very end. Moreover, the language used may be abstruse and easily understandable only to the medically trained. Some pharmacies gave information on the various adverse effects of Diane-35, including blood clots. The pharmacy from which Marit bought her pills did not. The warning she received only included minor side effects such as headaches, tender breasts, menstrual pain, swelling, and low sex drive.

## Gender and Body Image

We turn now to a different explanation for the deaths of these two young women. It addresses the role of the social determinants in health outcomes. We argue that the conditions for which the medications that caused their deaths were being prescribed were socially constructed conditions reflecting oppressive gender-based beauty norms. Rigid expectations of the behaviours, attitudes, and bodies of women and men characterize our society (see, for instance, Clarke & Miele, 2016; Clarke, 2009; Rice, 2014). These norms create demand for ideal bodily appearance and functioning. They reinforce ideas about sexuality. Great projects of medicine and consumption are enlisted to achieve these aims. Drugs, cosmetic surgeries, and medical interventions are marketed for body enhancement. Products, stories, and images are promoted and consumed (Hajli, 2014). The focus of self-improvement is often on skin, hair, weight, and breasts (Rice, 2013). Those with differences in bodies and bodily abilities do not fit in (Odette, 2013). Whiteness and beauty become conflated, and beauty becomes defined through the eyes of the colonizer (Donella, 2019).

Prevalent media images have powerful impacts on all young women. We live in a mediated world and are surrounded by mass images around the clock. Personal and ubiquitous items such as cell phones offer constant pictures through Instagram, Facebook, and other social media. Mass-produced entertainment, such as shown on Netflix, offers an endless stream of makeover series such as *100% Hotter*. Television, too, offers numerous makeover series such as *Extreme Makeover* and *Extreme Weight Loss*. Women tend to be seen as their bodies. Their bodies are objectified and understood as commodities – commodities that need to be constantly improved. This is an important part of sexist oppression. Social media is effective in many ways, such as encouraging consumerism (Hajli, 2014). The pressure felt by those who do not conform has even, at times, coalesced into social movements of resistance, such as the body positivity movement and the fat acceptance movements. The women whose stories are featured in this chapter were vulnerable, as are all young women, to the insecurities engendered by sexist body images. It led them to seek help for perceived body image problems. That they sought help from the medical care system rather than elsewhere and that they thought they needed to change themselves in the first place is what is at issue here.

In this context, it is important to understand that women are more likely both to go to the doctor and to use prescription drugs (Hunt et al., 2011). Women and their bodies are more likely to be medicalized than men and their bodies. In this case, these two young women may have been prescribed the drugs in part because of gender performance demands. Thus, Vanessa Young's problem of mild bulimia could have been related to her position as a young, modern woman. Eating disorders such as bulimia and anorexia nervosa reflect a concern with appearance and body image. Marit McKenzie's problem was similar in that the medication was being taken in response to a beauty norm, in this case for mild acne. Worry about mild acne reflects the internalization of the same gendered beauty demands. The same argument could be made about the medication in question, Diane-35, being taken for birth control. Women, as part of "doing gender," are more likely to be responsible for birth control than men. Indeed, being responsible for birth control is paradoxically said to empower women. In these cases, both women appear to be white and middle-class women from caring families who seem to be involved in their lives. The role of social class in body image is unclear (Kashubeck-West & Huang, 2013).

Body image is a significant concern for women, especially for young and adolescent women. Eating disorders are one result of this concern. Anorexia nervosa and bulimia are two of the most common eating disorders. Estimates of their incidence and prevalence are high and may even be growing in the presence of mass and social media. That these disorders are more common among women than men is documented both nationally and internationally. In the United States, 85 to 90 per cent of those with bulimia are female (Office on Women's Health, 2017). Vanessa was taking Prepulsid to help prevent her from vomiting after meals. We do not know for certain whether or not she was ever diagnosed with bulimia, but vomiting after meals is one of the most telling symptoms.

Young women are particularly vulnerable to eating disorders in a celebrity culture (Evans & Riley, 2013) dominated by a pervasive mass media. Bodily objectification and norms of thinness and dissatisfaction are endemic (Swami et al., 2010). Beauty norms are prescribed, but never achievable (Prieler & Choi, 2014). That they are not achievable may exacerbate the continuing power of these messages. Beauty norms may be even more problematic because they are coupled in a neoliberal regime with the notion that they are almost attainable through choice, unrelenting hard work, and the purchasing of appropriate products. Blum and Stracuzzi (2004) refer to this process of continual work as that of disciplining the body. This body discipline is one of the most essential and demanding jobs for young women in the new economy. Women are constantly bombarded with messages asking that they critically evaluate their bodies as objects of shame, pride, and embarrassment. Body image in turn reflects feelings of self-worth. These messages sexualize and subordinate women. They portray women as needing to be improved (Collins, 2011).

The rate of eating disorders varies cross-culturally. Eating disorders are also socially linked to particular activities and occupations where body size is an important component of success in areas such as dancing, gymnastics, and modelling. Eating disorders appear to have been growing in North America since about the 1950s. Some have argued that this growth mirrors the expansion of mass media such as television, which underscore the normative emphasis on thinness and beauty for women, in particular, and men as well. Others argue that it reflects a "hunger strike" and an attempt at empowerment against rising and contradictory expectations of females in the workplace (Orbach, 1986). The global gender gap between men and women in education, earnings, political power, engagement, and health reinforces women's need to compete harder for scarce resources and for male attention. The World Economic Forum (2017) continues to document the significant gender-based inequality wherein women have fewer of the primary determinants of life chances, including health, education, occupation, and political empowerment. In its 2017 report comparing 144 countries, Canada ranked sixteenth in its gender gap in a global context. Thus, in 15 countries around the world, women are more equal to men than women are here in Canada. Such inequality about all aspects of their life chances feeds into the insecurity that women may feel about the importance of their appearance.

As stated, Marit was taking medication for mild acne. Diane-35 was also taken by 35 to 40 per cent of users (off-label) as a birth control method (Office on Women's Health, 2017). In a sense, taking this drug fulfilled a double promise. A young or adolescent woman could take this drug ostensibly for acne but actually use it as a birth control method. Acne, too, is a condition that violates beauty norms for young and adolescent women. Appearance is correlated with achievement in school and in work (Talamas et al., 2016). It is also valued as a characteristic to attract heterosexual partners by young women. The beauty myth has influenced women's identities for many decades (Wolf, 1990).

The issues regarding body image have resulted in enormous profits for the cosmetic surgery, beauty products, and diet industries. Turning to medicine is just one of several options in the demand created for improvement. In fact, Canada ranks number one globally in proportionate spending on prestige beauty products. This spending amounted to 2.5 billion dollars in 2019, and the rate of spending is growing at 3 per cent per year (NPD Group, 2019).

One billion of this spending came from skin care, the largest category of consumer spending in this sector (NPD Group, 2019). This figure would suggest that including the general (not prestige) cosmetics market in Canada would increase the amount of monies dedicated to cosmetics. Suffice it to say that the market for cosmetic products alone is large and most likely falls somewhere above 2.5 billion dollars per year in Canada.

The diet industry is also significant and appears to be expanding (Ellis, 2013). This industry is worth approximately 7 billion dollars per year in Canada and has been on an upward curve since the 1980s (Ellis, 2013). The Canadian fitness industry amassed 3 billion dollars in 2017, employs 54,731 people, and includes 6,325 businesses (Review Chatter, 2017). On the one hand, you might counter, this fitness craze is all to the good. There are health benefits of fitness. On the other hand, perhaps ironically, the industry growth is mirrored by the growth in the percentage of Canadians considered obese or overweight. About one in four Canadians is considered either overweight or obese (Government of Canada, 2011).

The cosmetic surgery industry is another profit-making but medical enterprise that extracts huge benefits from oppressive gender beauty norms. Nose, hip, facelift, and breast are among the most popular surgeries (Solomon Facial Plastic, n.d.). The top three cosmetic surgery procedures worldwide are breast augmentation, liposuction, and eyelid surgery (International Society of Aesthetic Plastic Surgery, 2019). They are all related to female beauty expectations about breast size, slimness, facial symmetry, and youthful appearance. Worldwide, almost 2 million people have breast augmentation annually. More than 1.7 million people have liposuction, and approximately 1 million undergo eyelid surgery. Americans spend 16 billion per year on cosmetic surgery. While it is very difficult to compare this figure to Canada because of our national medicare system, it does speak to the size of the industry (American Society of Plastic Surgeons, 2019).

Another growing medical intervention that reflects the demands for body slimness is bariatric surgery. It is major surgery and associated with serious negative side effects and after effects (National

Institute of Diabetes and Kidney and Digestive Diseases, 2020). Nevertheless, in 2012–13, there were about 6,000 bariatric surgeries in Canada, reflecting a fourfold increase over six years (Canadian Institute for Health Information, 2014).

There are numerous social changes necessary to eliminate the oppression of women in many areas of life, including education, occupation, political power, parenting, sexuality, and appearance. These two case studies reflect the medicalization of women's identity struggles in an oppressive social and cultural environment. The social determinants of health lens, emphasizing gender inequities, understands how one of the results of gender oppression is a turning to medicine for an answer.

## Discussion: How Did Medicine Go Awry in the Cases of Vanessa Young and Marit McKenzie?

A number of different threads need to be unravelled to thoroughly understand the problems that led to the deaths of these two young women. First of all, they died because of pharmaceuticalization in the context of a continually medicalizing society. Their deaths are largely due to the functioning of the pharmaceutical industry within the medical and social system that is uncritical of the possible problems of medicalization. The immediate cause of sudden death in both cases was that the medicine each young woman was taking was being prescribed incorrectly and/or off-label. In both cases, the medicine was contraindicated (not prescribed in the manner in which it was supposed to have been prescribed). In neither case did a pharmacist or a physician notice, acknowledge, or act on this known violation of the conditions under which the medication was to be used. In both cases, in a medicalized culture, the parents and/or child accepted the authority of the doctors that the medicine would be of help and was safe and appropriate. Vanessa Young was under the care of four different doctors. Apparently, according to the drug manufacturer Janssen-Ortho, these doctors should have each received four different letters warning them of the dangers of the medication being used by Vanessa. Had even one of these doctors intervened to prevent Vanessa's continued use of a medication that she should not have been taking for several simple and obvious reasons, such as her age, she would not have died. The problem with Marit's medication was that it was being prescribed over a long period of time and not for the condition for which it had been approved. It had been approved for short-term use only and just for severe acne. Marit had mild acne and had been continuously prescribed the medication over a long period of time. In this off-label use, presumably the doctor had not seen the advisories on the website of the pharmaceutical company. The dispensing pharmacists did not warn Vanessa or Marit about the advisories or the side effects associated with these potentially lethal drugs.

A basic problem of pharmaceuticalization is the relative power of the for-profit pharmaceutical industry as compared to the Canadian state. Health Canada is even more dependent on the pharmaceutical industry for funding today than it was at the time that either young woman died. Other root causes for these deaths have not changed. Medicalization and its unquestioning stance towards the use of medical products and services endure. Even today, for example, despite years of work by Terence Young as a federal legislator, the bill that was unanimously passed under his tutelage is already being rolled back. The interests of pharmaceutical companies continue to hold sway over those of the consumers of drugs and their prescribers. Off-label prescription is accepted and considered normative. The lack of post-market surveillance is assumed to be relatively unproblematic and still reliant on voluntary reporting.

In both cases, the social determinants of health played a role in the initial request for a prescription, as both pharmaceuticals were linked to aspirational health and gender performance. Gender beauty norms persevere in a mediated culture dominated by inequality between men and women in all walks of life and by the powerful effects of idealized images and of celebrity within the media. These cases demonstrate the way that medicalization prevails through gender performance in the context of pharmaceuticalization.

## Conclusion

These two cases illustrate the particular dangers of pharmaceuti-calization under medicalization. The deaths of Vanessa and Marit are the tragic, tangible results of turning to medicine for discretionary issues rooted in gendered beauty norms and receiving a deadly pharmaceutical "solution." They also represent the power of the pharmaceutical industry to override the Canadian federal government, to advertise drugs inappropriately, and to keep medications on pharmacy shelves in Canada even after repeated findings and warnings about dangerous side effects in other countries.

Adverse drug reactions continue to be lethal and are a significant cause of death in the developed world today. They are thought to be the fourth to sixth cause of death in the United States, leading, it is estimated, to 100,000 deaths and 2 million adverse events annually (FDA, 2018). Still, these are only the most obvious cases, because about half of all error impacts take many years to reveal themselves. In Canada, drug adverse effects were already, in 1998, one of the top ten leading causes of death (Rosenbloom & Wyne, 1999). With the expansion of both the use of drugs and the spread of health care use itself, drug-related adverse events are likely to be higher up this potential ranking than they were at the time of this study. The case of opioid drugs, discussed above, illustrates the continuing problem. Furthermore, the body image issues detailed in this chapter continue today and are even growing in an increasingly mediated culture.

# chapter four

# Amy Tan: Lyme Disease and the Battle for Legitimacy

## The Issue

"Nearly everything about the disease is disputed," Michael Specter reported in 2015. He had followed the story of the diagnosis of and treatment for Lyme disease for the *New Yorker* magazine. Virtually all aspects have been the subject of controversy and contradictions in what Specter calls the "Lyme Wars" (Specter, 2015). The disease and the ensuing conflicts about its very definition and process of diagnosis have become embroiled in politics. The associated economic issues are enormous. The Lyme Wars include opposing sides on an extensive list of issues, including the very reality of the disease as a chronic condition, its case definition, its incidence and prevalence, its location, and its treatment. It has turned doctor against doctor, patient against doctor, and doctor against patient. It has led to the suspension of doctors from practice and lawsuits against other doctors for the way they practise. Some insurance companies or governments will support one treatment as legitimate, and others will reject the same treatment. Testing for Lyme disease seems to result in many false negatives as well as false positives. The interests of for-profit labs for Lyme disease testing have been questioned. Different lab tests and clinical assessments lead to markedly different results and diagnoses. Tests done at the same lab with the same sample at different times have resulted in varying outcomes. Early government denial of the possibility of the disease existing in Canada has slowed research and testing.

I am going to begin this chapter with the typical – in many ways – story of the Lyme career via the tale of the highly successful and well-known writer Amy Tan. I have selected her story because it illustrates many of the characteristics of the archetypal Lyme trajectory and the many controversies that swirl around it. Amy Tan is not a Canadian, but nevertheless she is a part of the argument of this book, because the inclusion of Lyme as a possible disease category has only been recognized very recently in Canada. Before about ten years ago, Canadians who felt they might have Lyme disease had to travel to the United States for diagnosis and treatment. It only became nationally reportable in 2009 (Hatchette et al., 2014). There were merely 315 cases reported in 2012. Thus, information about Canada is and has been much more difficult to acquire (Ogden et al., 2019). The disease has a much longer history in the United States. Moreover, Amy Tan, a writer, has documented her many different experiences over time, which allows me to discuss some of the crucial issues raised by diseases such as Lyme. These issues include the inevitable medical system, practice, and research problems associated with new diseases, particularly those with multiple organ and system involvement. The role of the social determinants of health in the diagnosis of new diseases is also discussed. I return to a brief discussion of the situation in Canada at the end of the chapter, just before the discussion section.

## Amy Tan's Battle with Lyme Disease

Amy Tan is a celebrated American writer, perhaps best known for her book *The Joy Luck Club*, published in 1989. For more than twenty years, since 1999, she has been living with an illness that many doctors and governments, including the Centers for Disease Control and Prevention (CDC) in the United States, do not think exists. According to her website, she continues to suffer from chronic Lyme disease, or late-stage neuroborreliosis as it is also called by some supporters (Tan, n.d.). Amy Tan lives in California but had spent a great deal of time on the East coast in the woods, on hiking trails, and sitting in tall grasses during her many trips back and forth across the United States. She travelled across the country with book promotions because of her enormous success as an author. She chalked up the first symptoms of which she became aware to tiredness resulting from the time changes and the long flights. Maybe it was stress that caused her sore back, frozen shoulder, stiff neck, constant headaches, and insomnia. Her jitteriness she attributed to coffee. Mostly her life was, she says, great. She had a happy marriage, a satisfying career, plenty of money, great friends, and dogs she loved. She was never sick and basically only went to the doctor for an annual check-up until these shifting, varied, and increasingly debilitating symptoms began (Tan, n.d.).

In the summer of 1999, Amy says, she had "the flu" but was better soon enough and pleased with her great immune system (Tan, n.d.). After the summer, more symptoms developed, including unusual things such as tingling and then numbness in her feet. She'd had a funny rash surrounding a pinprick of red. Then she noticed more odd symptoms that seemed to come and go. She had hearing sensitivity, a sore jaw, and pain like a shock in her legs. She awoke startled, as if injected with caffeine, at 3:00 a.m. every night. Sometimes she felt her heart racing. She continued on living her more restricted life, day by day, all the while normalizing the many changes to which she was adjusting.

After her next novel was published, she went on a four-month promotional book tour, still suffering bizarre, recurrent, and changing symptoms but carrying on nevertheless. But at the end of this tour, while she was in New Zealand, she collapsed dramatically, she says, as if something in her had broken (Tan, n.d.). This episode was followed by terrible anxiety, which was so incapacitating that, among other things, she was afraid to use a public washroom unless her husband waited outside. She had to have her dog with her at all times. She decided to go to her doctor, who discovered she had low blood sugar. Her father and her brother had died years before within months of one another of brain tumours. In consequence, the doctor tested her for brain and pancreatic cancer. Although she had thirteen lesions in her brain, the doctor felt they were benign and that this number could be normal at her age. The MRI and other tests ruled out either of these two cancers. There was one small adrenal tumour. It was described as incidental and benign. After treatment for this tumour, she was prescribed corti-sol. Her energy seemed to pick up, and she felt somewhat better. Then, when she stopped taking the cortisol, the health problems returned.

Finally, in response to her increasing anxiety, she went to a psy-chiatrist. She was diagnosed with post-traumatic stress disorder (PTSD) and major anxiety disorder. The psychiatrist suggested that she should go back to a "medical" doctor to have a complete work-up. She experienced other "bizarre" symptoms. She was referred to ten different specialists and underwent copious lab tests. Her cognitive difficulties increased. She had a terrible time concentrat-ing and couldn't read because she could not follow a story from page to page. She gave up writing her next novel. Once someone asked her what she was writing about, and she could not even remember the subject matter of her book, certainly not the nar-rative line. Something was definitely wrong. She withdrew from public, was unable to drive, and seemed to "space out" at times. She had recurrent visual hallucinations that, she said, "looked like they were made for B movies" (Tan, n.d.). She was prescribed the antidepressant Prozac in case the problem was actually based on the possibility that she was depressed. The antidepressant seemed to cause terrifying nightmares.

She visited many doctors and underwent numerous lab tests. One doctor, in trying to rule out multiple sclerosis (MS) and, unbe-knownst to Tan, syphilis too, had an ELISA (enzyme-linked immu-nosorbent assay) test done. The results were negative. However, in the meantime, after learning about the name of the test from her doctor, Tan looked it up on the internet and found that it was also a test for Lyme disease. Intrigued, she began to read about Lyme. She recognized that her changing and manifold symptoms fit the Lyme diagnosis. She also found out that the results of the ELISA test were not always accurate and told her doctor that her own bizarre and changing symptoms matched with those of Lyme. The doctor said it couldn't be Lyme because the disease was too rare and did not occur in California, and in any case, he had been test-ing her for syphilis, not Lyme. Because of her growing confidence that Lyme was the right diagnosis, Tan looked for a doctor who "believed in" and was knowledgeable about Lyme disease and practiced in California where she was living (Tan, n.d.).

By this time, Tan had sixteen lesions on her brain according to a new MRI, plus her other, seemingly spreading and growing, neurological symptoms. She was convinced that Lyme disease could no longer be ruled out. She finally found a doctor who was willing to consider Lyme as a diagnosis, and Tan was tested for it and other tick-borne illnesses. Within two weeks, the doctor confirmed the Lyme diagnosis. She was, she says, lucky to get the confirmation, because 50 per cent of those who later turn out to have Lyme disease do not test positive on the test that had given her the positive diagnosis (Tan, n.d.). Lyme testing is often unreliable (Wilske, 2005; Halperin et al., 2013). As a measure and illustration of the unreliability of the tests, Tan later, as part of a small study, sent her blood to five different labs; they all came back with different readings and diagnoses (Tan, n.d.).

The day after the diagnosis, Tan began to receive antibiotic treatment. Initially, she responded, as is typical in the case of Lyme disease, with fever and sickness, classic signs of a Jarisch-Herxheimer reaction indicating an immune system response to the treatment. After a few months, with the pain somewhat abated and the cognitive problems on the wane, she began to write again. After six months, she began to get her strength and energy back but still could not overdo it without getting feverish and ill all over again. She continued to take antibiotics for seven years. Whenever she tried to stop the antibiotics, her symptoms resurfaced (Tan, n.d.).

Tan now is able to keep the disease at bay with the daily ingestion of a Chinese medical treatment, an antimicrobial mushroom that she takes six times a day. Because of the brain lesions, she has to continue to take anti-seizure medications. She has her life back now, she says, and knows she is lucky because she had the money and the support to keep on looking until she found an answer (Tan, n.d.). But, as she says, Lyme disease is a stigmatized and controversial diagnosis, and many people have lost their health, jobs, houses, and marriages as a result of suffering from Lyme. Some have even lost their lives.

There are many reasons why I have chosen Amy Tan's narrative to illustrate the story of Lyme disease. Typically, Amy Tan did not realize that there was anything seriously or unusually wrong with her for a long while after her first symptoms. She normalized her exhaustion and strange signs of illness. She explained them away as resulting from stress and too much travelling and caffeine. When she realized that something was seriously amiss and continuing, she went to her doctor. He did not even consider that Lyme was a possibility because she lived in California, where the offending tick was very rare. It took a while, and numerous different doctors, before she was able to get a diagnosis. At least one test, the ELISA, intended to rule out syphilis, came back from the lab with a negative reading for Lyme. It turned out to be a false negative after later and different tests were done. As is typical, it was the Lyme patient, Amy Tan, who was the first person to think that the diagnosis might be Lyme disease because many of her symptoms matched the numerous and changing indications that she found describing Lyme on the internet. Eventually, she found a doctor in California who was what the support group community call "Lyme literate" (Tan, n.d.). As many others experienced, Tan's search for answers included seeing a psychiatrist, not only because her "foggy brain," cognitive difficulties, and disabling anxiety suggested the relevance of a psychiatrist but also because her symptoms did not seem to match any conventional physical diagnosis based on biological measurements, according to her regular allopathic doctors. Ultimately, Amy Tan learned how to manage her varied but chronic and frequently gravely debilitating symptoms using antibiotics, along with symptom specific medications and complementary care.

## The History of Lyme Disease in North America

It was not until the middle of the 1970s that Lyme disease was first noticed and identified in the United States. It happened when doctors in Connecticut started to see an unusual pattern of disease in children in and around the town of Lyme (Ballantyne,

2008). Groups of children who seemed to have juvenile rheumatoid arthritis were appearing in doctor's offices and hospitals. But
a clustering of juvenile rheumatoid arthritis did not seem likely.
Such a pattern would normally be the result of a contagious process. There were, however, other things the children had in common. They tended to live near densely wooded areas populated
by deer and field mice, both of which were known to carry black-
legged ticks. The potential relevance of the ticks arose because the
recurrent disease outbreaks seemed to be patterned on the feeding
cycles of the ticks. Some of the children had strange rashes on their
bodies before they developed the symptoms of arthritis. By 1981,
researchers and doctors had isolated the cause as a corkscrew bac-
terium soon named *Borrelia burgdorferi* in honour of its discoverer,
Willy Burgdorfer. It has been colloquially called "Lyme's disease"
because of its early appearance in and around the town of Lyme
(Ballantyne, 2008).

Lyme disease has since become the most widespread tick-
borne infection in America, although it has been known in
Europe for a longer time (Ballantyne, 2008). The deer ticks are
very small and difficult to see, about the size of a poppy seed.
Some people have a rash, and others don't. Sometimes the bite
is on the scalp, where it can be almost impossible to find and
observe. It does not cause pain or itching, which may make its
early signs invisible. The early noticeable symptoms often mimic
the frequent illnesses of influenza or a cold. The symptoms can
soon spread and become multisystemic. They may include neurological, heart, joint, and muscle involvement. Some people suffer with changing and more or less serious symptoms for many
years, and for some, serious symptoms seem to appear a length
of time after the initial symptoms. There are even cases of whole
families being diagnosed with Lyme disease. This finding has
led to speculation that it can be passed in utero to a new baby
and to a spouse via sexual intercourse, according to a report in
*Hospital News* and other anecdotal evidence ("Unravelling the
mystery," n.d.). However, there is no scientific documentation of
any means of acquiring the condition other than through a tick
bite (Auwaerter et al., 2011).

Lyme's early appearance was said to be due to changes in land use (Haines et al., 2006; Patz et al., 2008). Land that had previously been utilized for farming was reforested. It was then developed as housing for suburban residences. Lyme disease has since spread across the United States into Canada (Ogden et al., 2019). Some attribute its spread to the climate change that has occurred during that time (Haines et al., 2006; Patz et al., 2008). It is also known in Europe and in temperate Asia (European Centre for Disease Prevention and Control, n.d.). Acute Lyme disease is now recognized as a real disease in the United States and Canada, and is being diagnosed in more and more geographic areas across North America, Europe, and parts of the rest of the world. Chronic Lyme disease is not universally recognized.

## Lyme Disease: Prevalence and Incidence Disputes and Estimates

Lyme disease is the most prevalent tick-borne illness in the world (Stricker & Johnson, 2014). It is an urgent health issue. In a 2014 article, Stricker and Johnson called for a Manhattan Project similar to that established at the beginning of the Second World War, whose goal was to develop nuclear weapons to end the war and route out Hitler and his supporters. Stricker and Johnson argued that similar expense and effort would be required to address the problem of Lyme disease. Some have likened the crisis to that of AIDS in the very early days of its sudden frightening emergence, its ambiguous and changing symptoms, and its rapid spread (Connor, 2015). In fact, it is still difficult to be sure of the actual counts of Lyme disease (Centers for Disease Control and Prevention [CDC], 2021) A Manhattan Project for Lyme would be very costly in both money and effort. It would require the same concerted, almost single-minded, determination as that which led to understanding the causes of, prevention strategies for, and finally treatment that enables people to live with HIV/AIDS as a chronic condition.

The Centers for Disease Control and Prevention (CDC) estimate that about 35,000 cases of Lyme disease are reported and confirmed each year in the United States alone (CDC, 2021; Schwartz et al., 2021). They also acknowledge that this number represents an under-reporting. It is likely only a fraction of the true number or incidence rate of cases that begin, and go undiagnosed, each year. The CDC postulates that the number of cases is probably closer to 476,000 if approximations are not based on reported cases but on studies of the incidence of positive lab reports plus insurance claims (CDC, 2021; Schwartz et al., 2021; Kugeler et al., 2021). Alix Mayer, a former corporate researcher, interpreted statistics extrapolated from a national self-report study in the United States that asked a random national sample of people if they had ever been diagnosed with Lyme disease in the previous year. Based on the responses to this survey, Mayer (2014) arrived at different guesstimates of the annual incidence. Results showed that about 3 million respondents said they had been diagnosed with Lyme disease in the previous year, and about 1.5 million said they were currently suffering from Lyme.

It is probable that all figures and estimates of Lyme disease are in error to a degree. Self-reports can be biased when respondents do not understand the question or have some reason to provide a false answer. Sometimes self-reports are in error if the respondent does not have a diagnosis yet or does not have a correct diagnosis. Official statistics, too, can be in error when they rely on the reports of doctors to the CDC, as these reports may depend on unreliable tests. Further, potential patients often do not know that their flu-like symptoms may be masquerading Lyme. Other different errors result from alternative means of estimating incidence, such as lab and insurance company numbers. Taking all of this ambiguity into account, the CDC guesstimate that the annual rate of diagnosis in the United States might be as high as almost half a million cases (CDC, 2021) may be within range.

As early as 2006, Ogden and colleagues documented the not as yet officially acknowledged but nevertheless wide range of Lyme-bearing ticks in Canada (Ogden et al., 2006). Further ongoing research and mapping estimates suggest that, as the climate continues to change and warm, the spread of infected ticks into Canada is very likely to grow (Ogden et al., 2014). The official

Canadian figures for the incidence of Lyme disease are likely underestimates. Until recently, it has been impossible to be tested or treated for Lyme in Canada because the disease was said to be non-existent. Thus, people who felt that they had the signature symptoms or experienced unexplained multisystem issues had to send their biological samples to labs in the United States for testing. If the results were positive, finding a doctor who was willing and able to treat Lyme became a huge problem. For a long while in Canada, there was only one "Lyme-literate" naturopathic doctor in Richmond Hill, Ontario, and one "Lyme literate" allopathic doctor in Montreal (Kingston, 2014; Zarzour, 2015). Since it was not possible to treat formally or bill for Lyme disease in Canada, this doctor was only able to treat patients in Plattsburgh, New York, where they had to pay the medical fees from their own pockets (Zarzour, 2015).

Thus, the incidence of reported and confirmed acute Lyme disease cases is much smaller in Canada, not only due to population size but also because of climatic and geographic differences. Complicating this picture, the disease was not officially reportable until 2009 when there were 144 cases (Government of Canada, 2021b). The colder climate is not as hospitable to Lyme-bearing ticks. In 2012, there were 338 cases diagnosed in eight provinces, according to Canadian governmental statistics (Government of Canada, 2015). By 2016, there were 992 confirmed cases of Lyme (Government of Canada, 2021b), which represented an increase from 0.4 to 2.7 per 100,000 population from the initial date at which it was acknowledged that Lyme disease was occurring in Canada and was thus reportable. The Canadian government, however, realizes that not all cases of Lyme are being or have been reported. Estimates as of 2019 were that there were 2,636 cases in Canada (Government of Canada, 2021b).

Official statistics and self-report data, whether in Canada, the United States, or elsewhere, are clearly problematic for a variety of reasons. Another, unofficial yet commonsensical, way of considering the incidence of Lyme and the needs of people suffering from it (whether because they have a diagnosis or because they are searching for an explanation and treatment for one or more of their baffling symptoms) is to look at the results of various internet-based searches. In the summer of 2017, I searched Lyme disease on YouTube and in .46 seconds found 945,000 YouTube postings on the topic. In 2020, possibly reflecting the decrease in the need to search for answers because of the increase in capacity to diagnose Lyme across the country, there were 139,000 postings. I then searched Lyme disease blogs, and within .24 seconds there were 1,010,000 results. I searched Lyme disease alone, and within .31 seconds there were 24,200,000 results. There are many other searches that could be easily done, such as Lyme disease symptoms, but these three basic searches suggest something about the importance of Lyme disease in public discourse and most likely in the spread of suffering. By comparison, when I searched two other diseases with disputed but still more widespread historical and present legitimacy, along with multisystem involvements – chronic fatigue and fibromyalgia – I came up with 2,330,000 hits and 16,000,000 hits in fractions of a second. If we added Facebook, Instagram, and other social media to this populist method of estimating the problem of the incidence of new and questionably legitimate diseases such as Lyme, the figures representing talk and concern about Lyme would likely be much higher.

Lyme disease seems to be more common in women and children, although gender and age differences are difficult to determine with confidence for several reasons. In the first place, the lack of reliable testing methods makes gender comparisons problematic. In addition, there are extensive differences between men and women in health care utilization and attention to their bodies and thus willingness to be tested (Stricker & Johnson, 2014; Clarke & Miele, 2016). At every stage of life, women are more likely to be diagnosed with various chronic diseases than are men (Turcotte, 2015). On the other hand, men are less likely to frequent doctor's offices, but they may be taken more seriously and may have developed a more serious condition when they do finally attend to the doctor. Measuring and estimating Lyme incidence within socio-demographic conditions such as educational level and social class is impossible because of the absence of relevant data.

## Lyme Disease: Changing and Overlapping Biological Symptoms

There are over one hundred known symptoms of Lyme according to the Canadian Lyme Disease Foundation (CanLyme, n.d.-a, n.d.-b). Many individual symptoms overlap with other discrete and complex diagnoses. This factor in itself makes distinguishing Lyme from other diseases and syndromes very challenging. Moreover, the symptoms are found in a wide variety of systems and organs, including the head, face, and neck; the musculoskeletal, gastrointestinal, genitourinary, psychological, neurological, respiratory, circulatory, and nervous systems; eyes/vision; ears/ hearing; mental capability; and so on (Maloney, 2009). Symptoms range in severity from mild to extremely debilitating. They vary in types from seizures and tremors, to difficulty walking and balancing, to nausea and fever, to arthritis, to headache, and Bell's palsy. They may change over time and even from day to day. They often differ from person to person. The symptoms associated with Lyme can be overwhelming and serious, and impede the ability of a person to live a meaningful life. Sometimes they are minor. Later stage Lyme may include memory loss, fatigue, headache, spinal and radicular pain, depression, sleep disturbances, irritability, difficulty finding words, fibromyalgia, hearing loss, and distal paraesthesia (Maloney, 2009).

There may be many cases of misdiagnosis or underdiagnosis in the case of Lyme disease. There are undoubtedly both false positives and false negatives. Among the common misdiagnoses, according to the Canadian Lyme Disease Foundation, an advocacy group for Lyme sufferers and supporters, are chronic fatigue syndrome, colitis, early ALS (amyotrophic lateral sclerosis), early Alzheimer's, encephalitis, fibromyalgia, infectious arthritis, and MS (CanLyme, n.d.-a), as well as other symptoms associated with neurological disorders (Kingston, 2014). On the other hand, there may, at times, be a tendency to overdiagnose Lyme. For example, influenza and cold symptoms are extremely common, and there may, in some places, be a tendency to overzealously diagnose Lyme disease when a lengthy flu diagnosis might have been more appropriate.

## Further Suffering with Lyme: Socio-Psychological Symptoms

The risks and suffering from the disputed condition of chronic symptoms associated with Lyme disease are also vast. They go way beyond the physical suffering noted above (Ali et al., 2014). There are grave socio-economic and emotional costs (Ogden et al., 2019). Depending on the seriousness of the symptoms, people may need but not be eligible for sick leave or disability benefits, may not have health insurance, and may in the end become unemployed and lose their income. There are also costs associated with alternative treatments, to which many people may want to turn in their desperation to feel better. Even those who, like Amy Tan, do not suffer financially from the lengthy symptomatic suffering may fear the future and even fear death in the absence of a clear diagnosis. People with Lyme disease often feel stigmatized because their disability is undiagnosed and usually invisible. In fact, they commonly say that some people have a hard time believing they are sick because they look well. Others may marginalize them as malingerers or accuse them of pretending to be sick. Many people with Lyme experience a profound uncertainty about themselves and their future. Because of the diametrically opposing medical views about the reality of the disease and the difficulties of getting a diagnosis, patients cannot predict whether they will be seen as hypochondriacs or worse, on the one hand, or be taken seriously and treated with compassion, on the other. While the sample size in the research done by Ali and colleagues (2014) among Lyme patients is much too tiny for generalization, the many blogs hosted by people with Lyme disease and other anecdotal data document a widespread repetition of these same sorts of problems.

## Diagnoses and Diagnostic Disputes

The wide variety of multisystem and frequently fluctuating symptoms makes the diagnosis of Lyme disease even more difficult, because most of the symptoms, aside from the signature bull's-eye rash, may be part of other minor and/or serious diseases. Furthermore, even what might be considered typical symptoms differ at different stages of the disease trajectory. Further, testing results can vary as a result of changes in the character of the disease-bearing organisms themselves. Increasingly complicating diagnosis and treatment is the fact that symptoms sometimes do not appear for months. Even when people are tested for Lyme, false negatives as well as false positives are common at all stages of the disease. The development of reliable and valid testing for Lyme has been challenging because of the disputes about where it occurs and the denial that it could possibly occur in certain places at all.

Theoretically, the first stage of the disease is a bull's-eye rash located at the place of the Lyme-infected tick bite. I use the word "theoretically" here because many people either do not observe or may not have (had) a rash. After the tick bite, the initial signs of Lyme infection, usually occurring up to a month after the tick bite, are typified by flu- or cold-like symptoms. But as you know, flu and cold symptoms are endemic in the population and are not usually a cause for alarm or even for a doctor visit. Moreover, without the presence of the bull's-eye rash, or without observing the tick on the body prior to the rash, there is no way of knowing one should think about the possibility of Lyme disease. Furthermore, even when present, identifying the bull's-eye rash is not always simple. For example, it may be on the back or under the hair of a person. Since there is no pain or itchiness as a result of the tick bite, it can easily go unnoticed. It would be unlikely that anyone would reasonably think to test for Lyme in the early stages when the only symptoms are similar to influenza. Even if testing occurs in these early days, it may result in a false negative because it takes a while for the antibodies to appear in reaction to the bacterial infection (Glauser et al., 2016). Still, however, early treatment is critical. Guidelines from the CDC (used at times now in Canada too) therefore suggest that early treatment may begin if a person has been in a known Lyme-infected area and has a rash. Otherwise, doctors are to assume that the symptoms will clear up on their own or may reflect one of many alternative diagnoses.

Early testing is problematic, therefore. Once the disease is at its next stage or disseminated, testing can be useful. With disseminated disease, the common test ELISA will pick up antibodies 98 per cent of the time (Glauser et al., 2016). However, there is still a high rate of false positives of between 4 to 11 per cent. Some people therefore recommend a two-stage approach to testing, involving the ELISA test first and then a confirmatory immunoblot IgG test. Still others recommend the testing developed by the CDC. Some advocates who feel that none of these tests are sensitive enough may send samples to private for-profit labs that have higher rates of positive Lyme results. Clearly, single reliable and valid tests of Lyme, and of Lyme at various putative stages, still need to be developed.

## Treatment and Treatment Disputes: Acute vs. Chronic Lyme

Some people are diagnosed accurately and early enough that they are treated successfully with the basic level of treatment – two to four weeks of antibiotics. At the end of this time, no more antibiotics need to be given. If the antibiotics are started early enough, this limited treatment is often adequate for a long-term cure. There may be some residual fatigue or other relatively minor symptoms for a while during the time the person recuperates completely. In many cases, though, this length of treatment does not result in a cure. Many people with Lyme report a resurgence of symptoms once they end their prescribed period of antibiotics (Cameron, 2009). If symptoms of the disease reoccur after the intensive antibiotic use, many people consider that they have chronic Lyme disease, even though the bacteria is not observable by available Lyme tests. One of the most disputed issues is that, after this initial period of treatment, many doctors and insurance companies refuse to continue or to reinstate antibiotic treatment and deny that Lyme is or can be a chronic condition.

The issue of the legitimacy of continued treatment has divided many in the health care field. There are disputes among doctors, medical organizations, governments, and insurance companies. However, none of the highly respected and mainstream health care organizations in the field thinks that continuing symptoms should be treated with antibiotics; this list includes the CDC and the Infectious Diseases Society of America (IDSA). The CDC (2015) acknowledges the ongoing chronic suffering after the acute stage but call it by a different name, one that distinguishes it from "chronic Lyme." The term used by the CDC is "post-treatment Lyme disease syndrome (PTLDS)." The ongoing symptoms from Lyme are merely residual, according to this view, and take a while before they are completely eliminated. In making this distinction, the CDC is warning against the long-term prescription of antibiotics (CDC, 2015).

Thus, the chronic manifestation of Lyme remains a particularly disputed condition. The CDC (2015) admits that some people continue to feel poorly for months after treatment, but they explain this problem as the period of time it sometimes takes for the immune system to recover from a serious infection. To support this view, the CDC notes that a long period of recovery is also characteristic of other infectious diseases. They say that the ongoing symptoms may be the result of lingering damage to the nervous and immune systems, which would be better treated in a different way.

There are three (at least) alternate theories to explain the experience of chronic symptoms associated with acute Lyme disease. They include autoimmune syndrome, which essentially means that, after the course of antibiotics, the immune system continues to react as if it still has the infection (Rebman & Aucott, 2020; Singh & Girschick, 2004). In other words, it is the ongoing immune system response that continues to cause the symptoms. A second theory is the novel pathogen theory, which posits that the ongoing symptoms are not due to Lyme but to another pathogen that the offending tick was carrying (Rebman & Aucott, 20207). While the antibiotics may eliminate the Lyme bacteria, they do not eliminate the other pathogen(s) that may be causing the ongoing problems. The third theory suggests that the ongoing symptoms are due to bacterial persistence of Lyme itself in the body (Rebman & Aucott, 2020), which is thought to be the reason that some people do respond to long-term antibiotics and contend that they have chronic Lyme disease. Furthermore, despite acknowledging the potential dangers of lengthy antibiotic use, certain medical practitioners and researchers point out that some infectious diseases, such as tuberculosis, are associated with ongoing symptoms and are known to require long-term antibiotic use (Connolly et al., 2007). In the absence of good, reliable, and sensitive tests for acute and chronic Lyme, it is impossible to determine the indisputable answer to the question of veracity of Lyme as a chronic condition or to determine the best and safest treatment protocols.

Research is ongoing to investigate the chronic Lyme and/or PTLDS (post-treatment Lyme disease syndrome) debate. However, in the meantime, mainstream medical professionals advise that the continued use of antibiotics is dangerous. They also point out that repeated studies have shown there is no difference in outcome between patients treated with antibiotics over a long time and those treated with placebo. This research has determined that long-term antibiotic treatment is essentially ineffective and may be dangerous (see, for instance, Berende et al., 2016). There are many documented problems associated with long-term antibiotic treatment (Feder et al., 2007). One issue is that continued treatment may mask or obviate the need to explore the possibility of other potentially treatable diseases consistent with the symptoms. Another is that there may be substantial associated side effects, after effects, and various health risks and little or no benefit to ongoing antibiotic treatment. The spread of antibiotic resistance around the globe is another reason to be wary of overuse and to avoid antibiotics whenever possible.

## The Context of Political and Economic Chaos and Controversy

The context of ambiguity in the definition, measurement, and treatment of Lyme disease has led to the growth and development of many different opposing factions and interest groups. Because Lyme disease is still without a reliable definition, diagnostic tests, or treatments, the controversy over Lyme has become very political. There are a variety of players with some similar, some overlapping, and some competing interests. There are significant economic consequences for the national health care system in Canada and also for the various labs that test for the presence of Lyme, as well as for health maintenance organizations (HMOs) and other medical care insurance companies in the United States. This area of medical practice is so fraught that "sides" have become entrenched and serious conflicts have ensued.

The language of disputation in the following quotation from the very popular citizen-led blog called The Lyme Maze gives a glimpse into the desperation and dramatic extremes of the different perspectives on science, doctors' authority and autonomy, and conflicts of interest in medical practice: "In the U.S., like in Canada, most family doctors and infectious disease specialists side with the IDSA (Infectious Diseases Society of America), and stick with the extremely flawed and outdated guidelines set out by this organization" (Lyme Maze, n.d.). This patient advocacy blog goes on to list a number of places where readers may be able to find a doctor who "believes" the patient and is willing to do what the patient wants regarding Lyme diagnosis and treatments. It usually involves a willingness to send a biological sample for testing to a lab of the patient's choice, often a for-profit lab with a high rate of positive Lyme diagnoses. Such sites also recommend "Lyme-literate" doctors who are willing to prescribe and even administer antibiotics over the long term. Critics accuse these Lyme-literate medical doctors (LLMDs) of conflict of interest. In fact, they may benefit from the costs of the care they provide (Auwaerter et al., 2011). Some may have investments in Lyme-friendly labs or with antibiotic-producing pharmaceutical companies. Antibiotic-producing pharmaceutical companies stand to profit from long-term use of this drug. Heroes and villains are made in this contentious field of play.

Most doctors side with the conventional CDC-approved standard of care, including the 9,000 physician members of the IDSA (Auwaerter et al., 2011). They are a group of mainstream specialist doctors who refuse to provide ongoing antibiotic treatment because of the risks of side effects and because they do not think that the ongoing symptoms are directly susceptible to the antibiotics. They abide by the results of the published peer-reviewed research and the decision-making of the CDC. This stance reflects a strong belief in the gold standard of conventional medical practice, evidence-based medicine (EBM).

This cohort is the larger, mainstream group of doctors with conventional science on their side. However, many patients and some other doctors and alternative health care specialists excoriate the conventional practitioners and the standards of treatment they prescribe. These are patients and their affiliated health care providers who believe in chronic Lyme and in the prescription of antibiotics for the long term. They are represented by another group of Lyme activists and advocates, including some doctors and the alternative medical association, the International Lyme and Associated Disease Society (ILADS). Within this group are doctors who believe in chronic Lyme and the efficacy of long-term antibiotic prescription. They have issued their own treatment guidelines and, in turn, severely criticize doctors who do not prescribe long-term antibiotics. As Auwaerter and colleagues (2011) say, there are parallel medical and patient universes in the contentious area of Lyme.

The controversy has been, at times, equally political and disputatious in Canada. At a national conference on Lyme disease in 2016, one Canadian doctor charged that much of the conventional and widely acceptable peer-reviewed treatment for Lyme disease contravenes the Canadian Medical Association ethical code (Payne, 2016). Dr. Hawkins, a Calgary physician, stated that the current treatment "reflected dismissiveness, clinical arrogance, condescending patient contact, prejudicial treatment and humiliation" (Payne, 2016). He added that the patient stories he heard at the conference brought him "to tears." In Canada, the national health care system decides, along with medical associations, which diseases exist and are legitimate and which are not. This assessment may change over time. It may be more or less understood by doctors practising across the country. Health ministries may not fund the ongoing work of a doctor for diagnosing a disease that the government, the payer for the national health insurance scheme, does not consider a real or legitimate disease. In just one example, Dr. Ernie Murakami from British Columbia allegedly lost his licence to practise from the College of Physicians and Surgeons in British Columbia because he prescribed ongoing antibiotic treatment for a case of what he termed chronic Lyme (Lyme Maze, n.d.).

According to the Canadian Lyme Disease Foundation, the majority of Canadian doctors have historically dismissed the Lyme-related experiences of patients because it is so newly recognized as occurring in Canada. The available tests for Lyme in Canada may be inadequate (CanLyme, n.d.-b). They may only be able to effectively and reliably test for one strain of the disease. Over the years, many patients have gone to the United States and paid for-profit labs from their own funds for tests in order to get a positive diagnosis. Critics of this practice say that the majority of the US tests that Canadian patients pay for are false positives and thus both a waste of money and unhelpful for patient health (Gregson et al., 2015).

In response, Canadian Lyme activists claim that Lyme is spreading quickly through migratory birds and climate change, and that the Canadian health care system has not kept up with the reality of this new disease (Green Party of Canada, 2014). The (former) leader of the Green Party in Canada, Elizabeth May, took up this cause. May is a supporter of activist Lyme disease patients and introduced a private members bill, Bill C-4. This bill, called the Federal Framework on Lyme Disease, was passed through the senate in December 2014. Responding to the news that the bill had successfully passed through its third and final stage, May said: "This victory belongs to all Canadians coping with Lyme disease and their loved ones. This bill would never have been passed into law without their advocacy and willingness to tell their stories" (Green Party of Canada, 2014). The results of this new bill have led to the development of increasingly reliable and valid measures for Lyme, surveillance of Lyme across the country, the introduction of national treatment standards, and other innovations for prevention and treatment across the country (Government of Canada, 2021a).

There are continuing disputes in Canada and the United States between governments and doctors over the right to diagnose and treat as they see fit. As the result of strong advocacy by Lyme patients, for example, the governor of the state of New York signed a law in December 2014 that is colloquially called the Lyme Doctor Protection Act. This law forbids the board of medicine in the state of New York from investigating complaints about doctors "based solely on their recommendation or provision of a treatment modality that is currently not universally accepted by the medical profession" (Specter, 2015). The argument is that doctors should not have to use the standard guidelines based on the best published scientific evidence but should be able to try to help their patients by providing what the patients ask for and/or what they, on the basis of clinical experience, may think they should do. This law also values the patient's subjective experience and even subjective self-diagnosis (in this case of chronic Lyme) over that of the established mainstream medical practitioners and researchers, and indeed over evidence-based medicine (EBM).

Doctors who believe in chronic Lyme disease can become heroes to sufferers and their supporters. Charles Ray Jones was one doctor who believed in chronic Lyme (Ballantyne, 2008). He treated about 12,000 children for Lyme and other tick-borne diseases. They came from all over, including every state in the United States, Canada, South America, and overseas, to his clinic in Connecticut. But eventually Dr. Jones was fined and placed on probation for violating the standards of treatment for Lyme disease. He had to hire lawyers and spent many thousands of dollars fighting to continue his practice. His patient supporters raised hundreds of thousands of dollars to back his fight. Dr. Jones's story is just one example of the history of conflict between the patient advocacy organization ILADS and the medical association IDSA about whether or not chronic Lyme exists and whether or not it is safe to treat people long term with antibiotics.

There are also government entities at various levels that prosecute doctors for providing continued antibiotics and diagnosing chronic Lyme. At other times, states have legislated that insurance companies must pay for long-term antibiotic treatment, even though the major organization of mainstream doctors (IDSA), along with the CDC, opposes this treatment. Connecticut conducted an antitrust investigation of the IDSA, arguing that the organization was influenced by the insurance industry (Feder et al., 2007). The insurance industry did not want to pay for ongoing antibiotics until the science was absolutely clear that antibiotics would be safe and efficacious for long-term treatment. Canadian doctors who have given antibiotic treatment for longer than the recommended thirty days have also faced serious repercussions, including being investigated by their regulatory bodies, and have lost their licenses as a result (Frketich, 2013).

## Modern Medical Science and the Diagnosis of New Multi-organ, Multisystem Diseases

Modern medical science and practice are not well suited to the incorporation of new diseases into research and the discovery of treatments. The problems associated with the care of people with Lyme disease arise from the fact that it is a fairly new condition that has spread rapidly across North America. It is also a disease that sufferers recognize and have experienced longer and more often than the medical system of research and practice have been able to keep up with. That the burden is on patients to find a name and a treatment for their unusual way of feeling is characteristic of multisystem diseases in the early days of their emergence into a population. Lyme disease is emblematic of a problem in the health care system with the identification of new diseases, particularly diseases that involve multiple systems and a changing variety of symptoms, which initially cannot be measured objectively but only, by and large, presented subjectively through oral reports.

Medical practice is structured in ways that make the early iden-tification of patient-defined problems difficult. In the first place, doctors tend to have a lot more power, prestige, and income than the average member of society. Those higher up in the social pres-tige hierarchy are less likely to listen to those below them than the reverse. Doctors are typically engaged in a busy, stressful, and even high-risk job, and diagnosing a complicated disease takes time. Doctors learn to trust themselves and what they have learned as relevant to a diagnosis more than they trust patients and their subjective expressions of distress, pain, and suffering. Most doctors are paid by the fee-for-service model. They are accountable to their payers, whether insurance companies or governments, for spending time efficiently. A quick diagnosis is a desired efficiency in this paradigm. Relying on evidence-based medicine is the safest strategy.

Medical practice is also divided into specialties, and many of these specialties are based on organs. Urologists focus on the urinary track, neurologists on the brain, obstetricians and gynaecologists on women and their reproductive systems, dermatologists on the skin, and otolaryngologists on the ear, nose, and throat. The job of the general practitioner is often to see the patient, make a preliminary assessment, and then refer him or her to an appropriate specialist. In the case of multisystem, multi-symptom, and frequently changing diseases, there may be no obvious specialist to whom to refer a suffering person. Further, modern medicine is based, as we have said earlier, on positivistic empirical science and evidence-based medicine, which means that doctors are to make decisions based on evidence. The whole thrust of the diagnostic endeavour is to use the best information available from scientific or "gold standard" research. Lyme disease is an example of a new disease that stands outside of the fundamental medical value of practice based on published and peer-reviewed research. In other words, at the outset, in the case of a new disease, there is no generalized EBM upon which to base treatment.

Not only will there be no evidence base in the case of a new multisystem, multi- symptom disease, but oftentimes there is no objective measurement that would indicate the nature of the problem or even the dominant system involved. This circumstance, then, is one where doctors, who are increasingly being encouraged to use evidence and not clinical experience, will be asked to trust the subjective views of their patients rather than their textbooks, peer-reviewed research published in top and recognized medical journal articles, pharmaceutical reps, and medical colleagues. Given the social distance between doctors and patients (Malat, 2001; Oxtoby, 2013), it is likely that doctors will have an increasingly difficult time going against their training and norms, which encourage relying on the results of published research, to listen to the words of suffering from patients. Indeed, over time and over the duration of their careers, doctors may have to distance themselves increasingly from an empathetic stance towards suffering patients to prevent burnout and stress. Scepticism and doubt about the veracity of patient experience can easily become normative whenever a diagnosis is difficult, particularly when the complaints are diffuse. Almost by definition, then, it will be hard to get diagnoses in cases of new diseases that are multifaceted, such as AIDS was and as chronic fatigue, fibromyalgia, and Lyme are.

Medical practice is also located in a political and economic world. There are power and money interests at play in the training and work of scientists and doctors. Science depends for the most part on grants from the government and medical device or pharmaceutical companies.

There has been a decline in the willingness of both the US and the Canadian governments to fund basic research (Mervis, 2017; Marshall McNagny, 2017). Basic research is designed for the furtherance of knowledge and is not driven by practical outcomes. But under neoliberal governance, grant allocation is increasingly based on the assessment of the granting committee that there will be direct practical and financial benefits from the research. The faster these benefits result in marketization, the better for the granting groups. This pressure becomes part of the values of the scientists or a burden that they have to withstand if they want to continue to do basic research (research for its own sake and with no immediate time line for practical implications).

Good positivistic research is characterized by such values as objectivity, reproducibility, and parsimonious explanations. All of these features are more difficult goals to attain in a disease with changing and multisystem symptoms. Consequently, it seems reasonable to suggest that studying complex multisystem diseases tends to take a longer time than studying those that seem to be limited to one organ or another. Thus, there will be much less incentive for scientists to write research grant proposals for this type of study. Practising physicians are expected to rely increasingly on scientific findings, which will be slower to achieve in subjectively described multisystem and multi-symptom situations. Clinical insights are increasingly considered to be of secondary value as compared to scientific and lab results (Maloney, 2009).

## A Few Cases of Lyme in Canada

In Canada, Lyme disease has been diagnosed in thousands of people since 2009. Each year following 2009, the number of cases increased except in 2017–18, when it decreased from 2,025 to 1,487 (Government of Canada, 2021b). Among these numbers are some well-known Canadians, including music stars such as Avril Lavigne, Justin Bieber, and Shania Twain (Telling, 2015; Radcliffe, 2020; Adams, 2017). It is likely that all of these people would have had access to the best possible medical care. Nevertheless, in each case there were difficulties of diagnosis, the long-term symptoms, and/or after effects, as well as confusion and fear in the face of changing and multisystem symptoms. What we are told of their experiences reflects the findings discussed below. Avril Lavigne went to numerous doctors until she finally got a diagnosis. She felt exhausted and light-headed for months. She said that she thought she might die and was fully bedridden for five months. Justin Bieber's Lyme disease caused him depression that lasted, undiagnosed, for about one year. At the same time, he reported that he had a case of mononucleosis. Because Lyme disease affected her vocal cords, Shania Twain's symptoms led her to think that she would never sing again. The time to diagnosis was shorter for Shania Twain, however, because she saw the tick fall off her and then subsequently got so tired that she almost fell off the stage while singing. She took her experiences to her doctor and was soon given a diagnosis. These stories remind us that Lyme disease can have severe consequences, the symptoms are varied and can be confusing and frightening, and the disease and its after effects can last a lengthy period of time.

## Discussion: How Did Medicine Go Awry in the Case of Amy Tan?

At first, the case of Amy Tan seems to illustrate the effects of non-medicalization. After all, it took years and years of assiduous searching as Tan travelled from doctor to doctor until she was finally able to get a diagnosis. She included alternative health care providers in her search, as the allopathic or conventional medical doctors could not offer an explanation for her symptoms. As is often typical of multisystem diseases involving changing symptomatology, Amy Tan did not realize that there was anything seriously or unusually wrong with her for a long while after her first symptoms. She never observed a rash. She normalized her exhaustion and strange signs of illness. She explained them away as resulting from stress, too much travelling, and caffeine. When she finally realized that something was seriously amiss and continuing, she went to her doctor. He did not even consider that Lyme disease was a possibility because she (and he) lived in California, where the offending tick was very rare. It took time and numerous different doctors before she was able to get a diagnosis.

As is typical with many "new" diseases, it was the Lyme patient, Amy Tan, who was the first person to identify Lyme disease. But, I argue, this case does illustrate medicalization. In the first place, the process of identifying new diseases frequently begins with the patient identifying a patterning of symptoms. This trend is because it is a logical outcome of the modern medical system's emphasis on evidence-based medicine. Such a strong but limiting focus on basing diagnosis only on the results of already published work means that new diseases are invisible and non-existent. The power of the EBM ideology means that, if a symptom pattern is not part of a known, identifiable configuration or diagnosis, it does not medically exist.

An additional problem in this case is that not only is Lyme a new disease but it has symptoms that change over time and involve multiple systems of the body at one time and over time. These characteristics conflict with medicalization's association with increased specialization. New diseases and multisystem diseases may incorporate symptoms that would be relevant to a neurologist, an internal medicine specialist, a cardiologist, a rheumatologist, a pulmonary specialist, an immunologist, a psychiatrist, and so on at any one time and over time. In the absence of a specialization in such new diseases, they can become orphans of the medical system.

Furthermore, those suffering the changing and often vague and difficult-to-describe symptoms can easily be dismissed as malingering or psychiatrically ill and may experience symptoms of mental distress (Loevinger et al., 2012). In addition, as is the case with Lyme, such new and patient-identified symptom patterns may lead to disputes among various medical specialties, governmental bodies, health insurance companies, and nation states about the reality of these diseases as well as about their chronic manifestations and corresponding treatments (Kumbhare et al., 2018).

There were medical errors in Amy Tan's case in the medical system, medical science, and medical practice. Tan had to spend years and try multiple doctors of different specialties. She was referred to a psychiatrist in case the symptoms were fabricated. Finally, she herself found the diagnosis online and then found a doctor who was willing to listen to her and to test for the self-diagnosed disease. By that time, she had been to see at least ten different allopathic doctors and had begun to seek complementary health care. She had been tested for different cancers and given MRIs for brain lesion investigations. Finally, a doctor ordered an ELISA test, ostensibly to rule out MS but also, unbeknownst to Tan, for syphilis. Although the results of this particular testing were negative, she decided to read about the ELISA test and found references to Lyme disease. The symptoms described matched hers. Then she looked for a doctor based in California, where she lived, who believed in Lyme. She found one who believed her, and he ordered other relevant tests, confirmed her diagnosis, and began treating her with antibiotics. Although initially she felt worse, after about six months, she finally began to be well again.

## Conclusion

The Amy Tan case illustrates the medical system issues that arise when a patient is experiencing a new disease, particularly a disease with multiple and changing symptoms. As such, the patient who is suffering is essentially powerless. She experiences her symptoms, but she cannot get help. The power of EBM, coupled with the assurance of doctors in their own correctness, means that the patient's reality is, in a way, denied. The patient is told that he or she is not sick, even as the patient's knowledge of his or her own bodily experience is negated. New diseases, by definition, lack published research and are thus not susceptible to knowledge based on EBM. The case also illustrates the fallibility of lab tests. The socio-political nature of medicine is also evident in the conflicts of interest among doctors, patients, different medical organizations, and insurance companies. These conflicts suggest something of the complexity of the medical system issues at the heart of this story. Medical practice and research issues are implicated in the debates about whether or not Lyme can become a chronic disease and/or should be treated with antibiotics over the long term. Finally, it is possible that the social determinants of health played a role here too, as there is evidence that physicians tend to take the symptoms of men more seriously than those of women.

# CASE STUDIES, PART 2

## Focusing on the Health Care Provider Causing Medical Error

# Dr. Charles Smith: The Case against Blaming the Individual Doctor for Medical Error

## The Issue

There were twelve documented cases of wrongful convictions for crimes against children and babies that occurred between 1981 and 2005 in the province of Ontario. These convictions were for infanticide, murder, sexual abuse, and abuse. As a result of these convictions, a dozen people were erroneously imprisoned. Those who were incarcerated lost friends, families, and employment. Children were removed from their families. One innocent man spent twelve years in prison for the rape and murder of his niece. A circle of suffering much larger than that of the wrongfully convicted resulted. One individual was responsible for testifying and providing evidence in all of these situations. He was acting as a paediatric forensic pathologist. His name was Dr. Charles Smith.

The usually temperate and influential *Globe and Mail* newspaper summarized the results of the Goudge Inquiry (2007–08) into the work of Dr. Charles Smith at the Hospital for Sick Children (Sick-Kids) in Toronto as follows: "In 2008, Mr. Justice Stephen Goudge concluded that Charles Smith was an arrogant, unqualified pathologist whose biased, inconsistent and unprofessional testimony precipitated a string of wrongful murder charges and convictions" (Mahoney & Bonoguore, 2010). This view was repeated in a number of other mass media, including the national broadcaster, *CBC*, and the high circulating and prominent *Toronto Star*. The public perception was that Dr. Charles Smith was essentially solely responsible for this series of egregious outcomes for a number of parents and other caregivers of children and infants. It was Smith's mistaken and misleading reports and testimony as a paediatric forensic pathologist that had led to devastating results for many families over several years.

This chapter will explain how features of the medical care system, including, among others, labour force issues, the development of a new specialty without adequately trained personnel, and the colleague-dependent relationships in the pathology department, contributed to Dr. Smith's ongoing behaviour and to years of suffering for innocent people, their families, and friends. The fact that the structure of accountability within the pathology department unit was not enforced is another important contributor to the many errors in interpretation that Dr. Smith made. The interaction of the medical system with the judicial system is a concern that will be discussed. The lack of training regarding the role of the doctor as an expert witness is another issue. The chapter will also look at how aspects of the social world related to the social determinants of health likely infused the observations and decisions of Dr. Smith and contributed to his faulty and biased diagnoses. The chapter ends with a brief description of two cases of wrongful conviction, those of William Mullins-Johnson and Richard Brant, both of whom were Indigenous men.

## Dr. Smith's Early Life and Medical Training

This story, thought of as the Dr. Charles Smith case, highlights a variety of issues that may be at play when health care goes awry. We don't know very much about Dr. Charles Randal Smith's personal life or even his early personality. We know that he was born in a Salvation Army Hospital in Toronto and was adopted as a three-month-old baby. His adoptive family moved a lot, including, for a while, to Germany. Apparently, he had searched for his biological mother during his life. When he found her, she refused to see or talk to him. Many people who are adopted feel that they fit so well into their adoptive families that they never want to look for their biological parents. Others search for biological parents because they want to know about their own genetic histories. They want to be forewarned of what sorts of diseases they might need to be on guard for. Charles Smith was one of those people who wanted more information and maybe even a relationship. That was not to be ("Dr. Charles Smith," 2009).

Charles Smith graduated medical school from the University of Saskatchewan in 1975. He moved to Toronto and took a job in surgery at the Hospital for Sick Children (SickKids) in 1979. After a year, he began training in pathology. At this point, he was learning clinical pathology, which involves helping in the determination of medical diagnoses. It focuses on the examination of cells, tissues, organs, and fluids in a laboratory. This training was directed towards assisting other doctors working in the hospital to make good decisions about the underlying pathology of presenting medical problems. By 1980, he was certified as an anatomical pathologist and soon joined SickKids as one of several rotating pathologists. Despite his lack of specific training, he began to practise paediatric forensic pathology by doing autopsies on infants and children whose death had been surprising or suspicious. This type of investigation is required by the state when a person has died suddenly or without known cause. The results may become part of a criminal trial or an inquest. Thus, this job encompasses both medical and legal components, both of which ideally require highly specialized education and experience.

## Dr. Smith at the Hospital for Sick Children

In 1992, Charles Smith, despite his lack of training or certification in the field of forensic pathology, was appointed director of the newly created Ontario Paediatric Forensic Pathology Unit (OPFPU) at the Hospital for Sick Children (SickKids) in Toronto. He became responsible for investigating suspicious child deaths in Ontario. He "soon came to dominate pediatric forensic pathology in Ontario" (Goudge, 2008, vol. 1, p. 6) and eventually in Canada. He was quickly perceived to be the expert in the specialty, due in part to the position that he held and in part, as the Goudge Inquiry noted, because "his experience seemed unequalled, and his manner brooked no disagreement" (vol. 1, p. 6). He trained lawyers and "expert" witnesses in how to give opinions in court. He saw and gave testimony on more cases of suspicious deaths in children than anyone else in Canada during this time. In many ways, he acted as if he were an advocate for the "innocent" dead. He was even known to use arrest warrants to have bodies exhumed when he thought there might be a reason to be suspicious ("Dr. Charles Smith," 2009).

Even prior to Dr. Smith's 1992 appointment as the director of the OPFPU, concerns about his work had arisen. In 1991, for example, a judge had overturned a conviction in the case of a babysitter who had been charged with the death of an infant ("Dr. Charles Smith," 2009). The ruling determined that the conviction had been based on error-ridden methods and faulty conclusions made by Dr. Smith. In 2002, Dr. Smith received a caution from the College of Physicians and Surgeons of Ontario, stating that he was being "overly dogmatic" and had a "tendency towards overstatement." Nevertheless, he continued to hold his position as the head of the OPFPU until 2005. Finally, on the basis of many more complaints about the work of Dr. Smith, the new Coroner for the Province of Ontario asked for a full review of all Dr. Smith's decisions involving "suspicious cases and homicides" (Goudge, 2008, vol. 1, p. 7). The purpose of the review was to evaluate and compare the evidence that Dr. Smith used against the conclusions that he drew. The chief coroner engaged five reviewers with training in forensic pathology to evaluate forty-five "criminally suspicious" cases.

The findings of the coroner's review were mixed (Goudge, 2008, vol. 1, p. 7). In all but one instance, Dr. Smith had apparently carried out all the appropriate tests. However, in 20 per cent of the cases, the expert panel did not agree with significant findings or facts. In addition, in twenty of the forty-five cases, the experts disagreed with either or both Dr. Smith's verbal testimony and/or his written report. Twelve of these twenty cases had resulted in findings of guilt in criminal cases. The finding of so many errors under the jurisdiction of one doctor led to the establishment of the Goudge

Inquiry. The Goudge Inquiry was intended as a "systemic review and assessment of the way that pediatric forensic pathology was practised and overseen in Ontario, particularly as it relates to the criminal justice system from 1981 to 2001, the years in which Dr. Smith was involved" (vol. 1, p. 7).

## The Goudge Inquiry

The Goudge Inquiry found there were a number of serious problems in the work of Dr. Smith. Some of these were his responsibility alone, and some were the responsibility of others in the Coroner's Office in the sense that his superiors had not intervened to stop Dr. Smith, even as evidence of his faulty practice came to light. Some of Dr. Smith's mistakes were common to the field of pathology or paediatric forensic pathology at the time and reflected the state of the field at SickKids and in Canada more generally. The whole department of paediatric pathology lacked a focus on excellent practices (Eggertson, 2008). Dr. Smith had been asked to do a job for which he did not have appropriate training at the time. Nor, however, did most of the other pathologists working in Ontario have this formal training (Goudge, 2008, vol. 1, pp. 11–12). Indeed, the field itself was still being developed.

It was routine for doctors in Ontario to do coroner's autopsies on a fee-for-service basis, even though they did not have the requisite knowledge base for this activity (Goudge, 2008, vol. 1, pp. 11–12). Furthermore, the training for the job of a doctor focuses on learning to diagnose in order to treat the patient appropriately. By contrast, a doctor whose work involves forensic pathology practice is not working for the patient but rather for the state, for the criminal justice system, and possibly for the family of the deceased. This different perspective is assumed to be self-evident and non-problematic. It is not taught in medical school except to a few in the subspecialty of forensics. However, the fact that autopsies were fee-for-service work likely incentivized practitioners (some of whom had no training at all in pathology, let alone forensic pathology) who wanted to make a bit of extra money to do the autopsies. This method of payment may even have encouraged fast and sloppy techniques and reporting.

Still, Dr. Smith had a growing reputation and influence, largely based, according to the Goudge Inquiry, on his speaking engagements (Goudge, 2008, vol. 1, p. 13). Many, including the police and Crown counsels, positioned him as the reigning expert. He was willing to get involved in criminally suspicious cases, whereas a number of other people were not prepared to take on that particular challenge. Others were not willing to testify in court. Dr. Smith was. He became the point person in cases of accidental, sudden, or suspicious death in children and youth in Ontario. Dr. Smith was not adequately prepared for this task. Moreover, he essentially did not know what he did not know (vol. 1, pp. 13–14).

Dr. Smith was not a careful and precise practitioner. Instead, he was described as "sloppy and inconsistent" (Goudge, 2008, vol. 1, p. 14). He failed to account for contradictory evidence. He did not explain his thinking or conclusions with reference to existing literature or reasoning. He was often late in providing findings. He ignored requests for urgent reports. In three cases, a subpoena had been required before he brought his report to court (vol. 1, p. 15).

Dr. Smith was poorly prepared for his court appearances. Nevertheless, he testified frequently. He offered unscientific and biased opinions (Goudge, 2008, vol. 1, p. 16). He was described as inflexible about his views. There was a culture of advocacy in regard to the abuse of children at the OPFPU at the time. The implicit bias was towards finding an accused person guilty. There was a widespread belief that child abuse had been under-reported. Dr. Smith said that he did not see his task as one that required neutrality. Instead, he thought of it as supporting the Crown in getting a conviction (vol. 1, pp. 16–17). Dr. Smith did not see and did not acknowledge the limitations of either his own knowledge or that of the field of paediatric forensic pathology. He gave no evidence of understanding the importance of validity and reliability in observations. In fact, "rather than acknowledging the limits to his expertise, Dr. Smith sometimes misled the court by overstating his knowledge in a particular area" (vol. 1, p. 17). At times, he used casual, personal experience instead of scientific judgment to determine his testimony on a case. For example, he explained that a certain injury could not have happened the way some accused parents had described it as happening because it had never happened that way with his own children (vol. 1, p. 17). He disparaged other experts in court. When confronted about the fact that he had used speculation, he responded to the inquiry that he did not realize that speculation was out of bounds in court proceedings (vol. 1, p. 18). At times he made "false and misleading statements to the court" (vol. 1, p. 18) and spoke about matters authoritatively that he had no expertise in, even though he was under oath. In sum, there was a long history of Dr. Smith behaving improperly in court. He presented biased findings and conclusions. Even when he was being investigated, he was "not above using deception" (vol. 1, p. 20).

Clearly, there is a great deal of evidence that the quality of the Dr. Smith's work as a forensic paediatric pathologist was lacking. He had joined the pathology department at SickKids quite soon after he graduated from medical school. He was willing to take cases that others were unwilling to take. He was catapulted to the position as the head of the OPFPU, even though he lacked training in forensic pathology. Looking back, it appears that he was ill prepared for the responsibility he had been charged with. With his decisions and courtroom style characterized as prejudiced and opinionated, many questions arose about his personality, his intelligence, and even his moral compass. He had a history of sloppy work practices, and yet he was allowed to continue his work. How can this be explained?

In the next sections, I ask questions about how the Dr. Smith saga could have happened and how the very nature of medical practice, medical science, and the medical labour force structure tolerated such problematic work. In doing so, I will discuss the following topics: institutional culture and monitoring practices; medical and social knowledge; variability in medical practice, regulation, and oversight; and specialty practice; as well as the social construction of child abuse. I end with a brief discussion of two cases. Findings in each of these areas will help us understand the reasons that the innocent were found guilty through the work of the pathologist at

SickKids. I will point to the ways that the outcome of the inquiry largely took an individual blame and shame approach rather than a medical systems error approach as described in previous chapters.

## Institutional Culture and Monitoring Practices

To understand the Dr. Charles Smith case, it helps to examine the institutional culture of the Ontario Paediatric Forensic Pathology Unit (OPFPU) at SickKids. It is useful to look at the processes of the evaluation and monitoring of the work of individual doctors. The OPFPU was a very small unit in which there was no clear hierarchy defining responsibility. There were two colleagues whose positions led them to have authority over Dr. Smith: Dr. James Young, the chief coroner for the province, and his assistant, Dr. James Cairns, the deputy chief coroner. These two men were at least aware of some of Dr. Smith's problematic behaviours and errors. They had received complaints and been witness to appeals of his decisions. They failed to confront or stop him (Eggertson, 2008).

Furthermore, while Drs. Young and Cairns held positions to which Dr. Smith was accountable, there was no clarity about channels of responsibility or authority. Nor were there policies in place to enable a regular review of his work or that of anyone else in the unit. There were very few quality control standards, monitoring strategies, or compliance actions documented for any of the staff in the field of paediatric forensic pathology in Ontario at the time. There was "no legislative framework ... to ensure proper oversight and accountability of forensic pathology in general, or pediatric forensic pathology in particular" (Goudge, 2008, vol. 2, p. 206). Dr. Smith was not the only practitioner who lacked appropriate training. Throughout the 1990s, local coroners were usually family practitioners (vol. 1, p. 22). There were therefore no colleagues who had the expertise to monitor Dr. Smith's work, which was not unusual at the time. For example, there were only seven paediatric pathologists working in the United States, and the number around the world was likely "vanishingly small," according to the report commissioned by the Goudge Inquiry (Cordner et al., 2008).

The responsibilities of various new specialties such as paediatric forensic pathology were essentially under construction. They were being clarified and institutionalized. Peer-reviewed research and training were relatively unavailable.

Numerous alarms were raised about Dr. Smith's work during the 1990s by police officers, Crown counsels, and others. These concerns were taken to the Office of the Chief Coroner of Ontario (OCCO). They were responded to informally. There was no institutional direction for complaint handling. Dr. Cairns and Dr. Young did far too little and did not hold Dr. Smith accountable (Eggertson, 2008). Evidently, this strategy was ineffectual. In the final analysis, Drs. Young and Cairns "had a kind of symbiotic relationship with Dr. Smith" (Goudge, 2008, vol. 1, p. 32). They actively supported and protected him to their own benefit, because his increasing prestige, based on his talks at conferences and meetings, enhanced the prestige of the OCCO (vol. 1, p. 32). Moreover, Drs. Young and Cairns recognized that "without Dr. Smith there would be nobody to do the work in criminally suspicious pediatric cases" (vol. 1, p. 32).

Furthermore, Drs. Smith, Young, and Cairns shared a culture in which there was a tendency to consider the deaths of children that came before them as suspicious. They assumed that the children's deaths were likely the result of child abuse. As the inquiry states, the pathologists shared the same commitment to "think dirty" (Goudge, 2008, vol. 2, pp. 111–13) in their approach to paediatric forensic pathology. This bias was not unusual at the time. The notion of the existence and prevalence of child abuse was newly emphasized in the surrounding culture. In fact, this philosophy of advocacy for children seemed to have prevailed elsewhere at the time. For example, a peer-reviewed paper in a relevant medical journal published at the time promoted the role of the paediatrician as a child advocate (McRae et al., 1984).

The Goudge Inquiry (2008) concluded that there were numerous systems level problems that contributed to the dreadful malfeasance in the work of Dr. Smith. In fact, the inquiry resulted in a number of different questions related to medical system issues, including the professional, jurisdictional, organizational, and inter-organizational systems within which Dr. Smith had worked as a paediatric forensic pathologist and as a court witness. The questions highlighted the ad hoc nature of these fundamental processes in the Office of the Coroner. Justice Goudge advised that basic questions of policy had not been considered. Prudent rules and regulations had not been established. As a result, Dr. Young, the chief coroner, and Dr. Cairns, his assistant, were asked to, and did, resign rather than face the sort of detailed investigation experienced by Dr. Smith (Boyle, 2015).

There were inadequate or missing procedures in regard to virtually all the relevant aspects of the decisions made about "suspicious" child deaths. The following is a shortlist of a few of the places where adequate social, criminal justice, and medical policies were missing: the police work related to forensic pathology, the responsibilities of the Crown, the role of child protective services, the basic education and training requirements for entry into the profession of paediatric forensic pathology, the role of colleagues and peer review in decisions made by pathologists, the role of the family in a dispute, and the maintaining of scientific objectivity in autopsy work and in providing evidence (Goudge, 2008, vol. 1, pp. 3–52). All of these multilevel issues played a role in Dr. Smith's testimony and court reports, and in the ultimate decisions made in each case. The lack of formulated policy in all of these areas contributed to the dreadful outcomes for individuals and families documented by the Goudge Inquiry.

## Medical Knowledge Is Social Knowledge

In the case of Dr. Smith, and his medical practice in general, it is useful to understand the potential influence of social forces, such as the media, family and personal experiences, friendship networks, and contemporary values, on medical practice and knowledge. The primary legitimacy and basis for the power of the traditional or allopathic medical system is that its knowledge and therefore practice are based on science. A consequence of this underlying premise is the assumption that findings are generalizable. Behind this avowal is the idea that science is above the vagaries of everyday common sense. It is said to be objective. However, that is not the case. Neither medical science nor medical knowledge stands above the world of everyday reality. Instead, there is considerable evidence that preconception is normative in medical decision-making (see Eddy, 1984; Singh et al., 2014). All knowledge is subjective in certain ways. In other words, what we know as citizens, as family members, as teachers, as workers, as commuters, and in any other aspects of our lives derives from the social context in which we engage. Knowledge is essentially a product of language. It is built and maintained by groups of people sharing observations, reflections, and explanations of the surrounding world at a particular time and in a unique place.

Knowledge is dependent on the tools and technologies available for seeing the world. Without a magnifying glass, you might not be able to find or remove the sliver in your finger. Without the thermometer, you might not know whether you have a fever. Mirrors permit us to see the reflection we offer the world. Medical technologies such as X-rays allow access to a viewpoint under the skin. Microscopes facilitate access to viewing the cellular level of the body. Electrophoresis enables speedy gene sequencing. Cars, planes, and trains provide opportunities for us to move and thus to see and then describe different parts of the world. Until the Roman Catholic Church distinguished the body from the soul, autopsies were not allowed. Autopsies provide a particular vantage point for knowledge. The artistic and anatomical knowledge of both Michelangelo and Leonardo Da Vinci depended on illegal autopsies and grave robbing. It was the eventual acceptance of the autopsy because of changes in church doctrine that provided the groundwork for empirically based biological and medical sciences as we understand them today.

Knowledge is based on community engagement and points of agreement, as well as, at times, conflict and disagreement. Thus, we have agreed to call the sky blue on particular days when it looks a certain way, and we have agreed to consider an upturned mouth a signifier of happiness, or something else, depending on the cultural context. Medical knowledge is similar in many ways to what we might call common sense knowledge in that it is socially located and perpetuated. However, medical knowledge is also different, because it is knowledge that is created, known, spread, and transformed among an elite of highly and specifically educated scientists and medical practitioners. Its language is often esoteric, specialized, and may even be based on the "dead" language Latin.

Medical knowledge is considered to be prestigious. The power of medicine is based on this status. It is also said to be unbiased and universal in application. It is based on the principles of positivistic science. Positivistic science is reflective of probabilistic logic and statistics, not determinative knowledge. Consequently, at its best, all scientific findings or truths are only ever probably true or probably not true with a known and estimated degree of error. All diagnoses and all treatments, then, are only probably correct and will only probably work. Diagnosis operates through a process of hypothesis formulation and testing until the clinician decides what seems to best fit the evidence. In fact, a substantial portion of diagnoses made in everyday medical practice is wrong. According to a review of research on diagnostic error, a substantial number of diagnoses are incorrect, and of these incorrect diagnoses, many are life threatening (Newman-Toker et al., 2021). It is very likely that these figures represent underestimates, because most misdiagnoses are unreported and many are unrecognized, either by the patient or the health care provider (Singh et al., 2014). One study published in the *BMJ Quality and Safety Journal* estimated that approximately twelve million Americans are misdiagnosed each year (Singh et al., 2014).

Medical science and practice are based on the empirical reality of probability. Thus, there is always a margin of error. Furthermore, scientists and medical practitioners are fallible, just like humans in other fields. Medical science requires safeguards for ensuring the validity and reliability of its findings. Uncertainty is endemic in all medical decision-making. Further questions can always be asked and answered. There is uncertainty about what is known in medical science at any one point in time and place, and there is also the personal uncertainty of the practitioner, who undoubtedly does not have total recall of what he or she has learned in medical school or in continuing education since. "Uncertainty, biases, errors and differences of opinions, motives, and values weaken every link in the chain that connects a patient's actual condition to the selection of a diagnostic test or treatment" (Eddy, 1984).

Central to medical knowledge and practice is the ability to distinguish between diseased and healthy. This distinction is not necessarily a categorical or binary one. There is often a continuous fluctuation between what is considered health and what is considered ill health. The line distinguishing one from the other is changeable, depending on a variety of factors such as, for example, the willingness and ability of the sufferer to experience and report pain or discomfort. Those noticing and reporting pain may fall into the category of "the ill." Those with the same biological situation who do not feel pain may be placed in the category of "the well." Furthermore, sometimes disease can appear and then disappear spontaneously. Some "diseases" may be outside the awareness of the patient and may not necessarily cause harm. Other times, the patient may claim a disease that medical science and practice have not observed, studied, or diagnosed.

There are deeply contradictory views on the scientific nature of medical practice. On the one hand, there are those who argue that medicine is based on science. Others maintain that clinical experience and art or creativity are inherent in a good diagnosis, hypothesis, and treatment. "Medicine is an art whose magic and creative ability have long been recognized as residing in the interpersonal aspects of patient-physician relationships" (Hall et al., 1981). Clinical experience involves a knowledge base plus pattern recognition. Intuition and diagnosis often arrive almost instantly. The busyness of modern practice requires quick work. This rapidity is generally satisfactory, as most patient needs are common and easily identified. However, there are important and even life-threatening exceptions.

To improve the practice of medicine, there is a current thrust towards founding medical decisions on the best available science published in peer-reviewed medical journals around the world. For example, the Cochrane Collaboration is a British non-profit organization with an independent network of people around the globe. Its mandate is to review, summarize, and systemize published medical research to make it useful for practitioners and other interested parties (see https://canada.cochrane.org/). As a contributor to this initiative, Canada is one of 130 countries working towards evidence-based medical care through excellent scientific reviews (Cochrane Canada, n.d.). This drive for evidence-based medicine (EBM) promotes the idea that all medical decisions should be based on the best scientifically based research currently available. Inherent in the idea of EBM is the basic proposition that research itself needs to be evaluated and its quality ranked and assessed along a number of different criteria, such as research design, validity, and reliability.

The first level of scientific knowledge is based on informal discussions and sharing experiences with patients and others in conversations at conferences or in peer-reviewed journals. This type of knowledge might be called anecdotal. Some common medical practice is based on such informal processes of repeated seemingly similar experiences. Knowledge with a somewhat stronger foundation is based on reports in peer-reviewed journals of individual cases or small groups of cases. This type of knowledge is merely descriptive and cannot be generalized. It does not allow for causal analysis. It should not be the basis of widespread treatment decisions. At the next level is the cohort study. It is the basis of epidemiology and rests on following large numbers of people over time to observe changes in health and correlates of changes such as, for example, smoking incidence or sugar consumption. An advantage of this research design is that it can include a number of different variables. It might include a wide range of diverse life styles and their impact on health outcomes. Statistical reasoning in such a study allows for comparisons. For example, this type of study may link smoking and lung cancer incidence. Causality can be inferred, but only statistically, with this type of design. It can be suggestive for further research. A more robust research design is the randomized controlled trial. It is often called the gold standard of medical science. It involves one or several experimental groups who receive an intervention and comparison or control groups who do not. This classic experimental design is devised to observe the effects of an independent variable (a specific treatment) on a dependent variable and to therefore determine any causal connections. It is the only research designed explicitly to measure causality. Once a number of studies have been completed on a given topic using a wide variety of different research designs, it is possible to summarize the findings and draw probable conclusions. The most valid and reliable research involves a systematic review of all the studies on a particular topic. It is based on consistent comparators using standardized and systematic evaluative criteria (such as sample size) to establish conclusions regarding the best evidence related to the topic (for example, diagnosis and treatment of cystic fibrosis). The most robust design for evaluating the quality of research is the meta-analysis. This type of study is a systematic review of a number of peer-reviewed and published research studies. It provides a comparison based on statistical analysis.

The anecdotal research allows for the weakest evidence, and the meta-analysis is the strongest source. Thus, the best evidence is that which has been repeated from study to study over time and found to be consistent and statistically powerful. This level of evidence is still incredibly rare. Therefore, many medical decisions are inevitably based on incomplete, inadequate, or faulty knowledge. A number of studies critiquing peer-reviewed medical research have been published (see, for instance, Smith, 2014). The majority of evidence used for medical decision-making is not complete. Evidence is always changing as new studies are undertaken and their results published. New questions arise as newer models, theories, and findings occur. Thus, medical or scientific evidence is always open to further assessment. Paediatric forensic pathology is medical knowledge based on very small samples and relatively few published clinical research studies (Cordner et al., 2008). The very knowledge base of the discipline and practice requires further development. This problem is much bigger than Dr. Charles Smith's failings or those of the OFPFU.

## Variability in Medical Practice

There are wide variations in the ways that individual doctors and scientists practise from day to day, week to week, and year to year. Medical doctors and scientists are also subject to the same fallibility as other human beings. They get tired. They get bored. They become weary of their work or "burn out." All doctors were not at the head of their class. Some almost failed one course or another, or even the whole degree, the first time through. Over time, some doctors keep up and others tend not to. Some trust the drug detail personnel for information about pharmaceuticals and use this information in the treatment plans they offer their patients. Others strongly reject information provided by those with corporate interests. Some doctors take perks from pharmaceutical and medical device companies to lend their names and reputations to research studies and speaking engagements promoting products. Some doctors prescribe the drugs in which they have invested financially, or for other reasons have a conflict of interest. Doctors suffer from the same mental and physical illnesses and addictions as other people do. For instance, according to one study, approximately 50 per cent of male medical students and 43 per cent of female medical students drank alcohol in excess of low-risk guidelines (Newbury-Birch et al., 2000). There is no reason to think that the rates of illness and addictions for doctors are any different from those among the general population. Some of these issues may affect their judgment at work. Some doctors go through divorce or other marriage and relationship challenges. Patients sometimes abuse doctors at work (Elston & Gabe, 2016). These situations too can cause stress. They can affect the doctor's quality of work.

Medical practice is also guided by cultural and social norms. There are different medical cultures. Lynn Payer (1992) documented medical cultures in a comparison of nation states. She went from country to country to visit doctors. Each time, she presented the same medical "complaints." She found that doctors in different countries tended to attribute different diagnoses to the same symptoms. Countries could be characterized by the emphasis they placed on one set of health problems or another. Payer also examined morbidity and mortality tables, and read medical journals in each country. She found that the trends in diagnostic patterns reflected the history and culture of each country. For example, she noted that the Germans, building on their emphasis on the arts, particularly music and literature, focused problems on the heart.

German people were more likely to be given heart-related diagnoses and treatments than those in the other countries studied. She found that the French, by contrast, focused their medical diagnoses on the digestive system, which, she thought, was a reflection of their emphasis on the pleasures of eating and drinking. The British tended to stress the "stiff upper lip." They were less likely to offer diagnoses and were parsimonious in offering treatment. People had to be sicker to get treatment or a diagnosis in Britain. In comparison, the tendency in America was to take aggressive action with less serious symptom presentation and to get things done. This study is an impressionistic one done by a journalist. However, epidemiologists have consistently confirmed the presence of differences in rates of varying medical diagnoses and practices, depending on such variables as geographic area, gender, race, and class of the patient; the number of different kinds of specialists; and so on. John Wennberg is a leader in this area. He has spent his career examining socially patterned differences in rates of different diagnoses and treatments across a wide variety of social conditions. He established the Dartmouth Atlas of Health Care to examine the social patterning of health, morbidity, mortality, and care availability across the United States (see https://www.dartmouthatlas.org/). The Wennberg International Collaborative serves a similar function with global rather than national comparisons (see https://wennbergcollaborative.org/). Wennberg and his group have published numerous atlases of medical practice variation. You can see examples in the Dartmouth atlas website. Among other things, the group has repeatedly and across time and place documented how diagnoses and care vary substantially by geographic area where racialized people and various ethnic groups differ in population proportion.

There are similar efforts being made by epidemiologists across Canada. In Ontario, published accounts of research comparing different components of medical care and outcomes are completed by the Institute for Clinical Evaluative Sciences (ICES; https://www.ices.on.ca/). Payer's impressionistic study, Wennberg's atlases, and the comparisons published by ICES, along with the work of innumerable scientists studying variations in medical care, all reflect the fact that medicine is not practised in exactly the same way in different jurisdictions. It is not entirely based on principles of objectivity. Nor is it universally true. Instead, it is a field, like others, that is always in a state of flux. Its knowledge is always incomplete. Like other fields of medical research and practice, pathology is also subject to alteration in different circumstances. Forensic pathology as a field is built on medical science that demands perhaps even more subjectivity in the interpretation of the causes of the pathology. It may be more vulnerable to human error, as well as to the vagaries of science and practice discussed above. Furthermore, the requirement that the forensic pathologist testify in a court of law adds another dimension and an additional opportunity for error.

## Child Abuse

Child abuse is not necessarily an easily observable condition. It is always subject to social definition and construction (Gelles, 1975). It has a natural history of recognition and definition (Parton, 1979). What is defined as child abuse varies from time to time and place to place. For example, child labour was generally acceptable in the early days of industrialization in North America, particularly among some classes of children. Now, however, child labour is considered to be an abuse of the rights of children. Today, it is illegal in Canada and through much of the developed world (Library of Congress, 2007). Elsewhere, there are still approximately 215 million children working, part or full time, around the world (United Nations, 2017). Sometimes the work is very hazardous. It is often controversial. From the perspective of the developed world, this practice amounts to widespread yet accepted child abuse. From the viewpoint of the developing world, it is often necessary for family and child survival. At times, parents have been charged with infanticide as the result of what is termed "sudden infant death syndrome" (SIDS). At other times, the very same cause of death (SIDS) has been thought to result from "natural causes" such as sleeping position, biochemical or molecular abnormalities, various environmental risks, and so on (Kinney & Thach, 2009). In many ways, mothers and other caregivers may be particularly vulnerable to cultural anxieties about acceptable and unacceptable mothering behaviours. For example, mother-infant bonding may now be pathologized (Tuteur, 2016). That breast feeding has become mandated as the only acceptable way to feed a baby has led to a new concept, "lactavism" (Gottlieb, 2015).

As a consequence, parents may be especially susceptible to being labelled as deviant and criminalized. In another example, a series of unreliable test results from a laboratory at SickKids, taking place over a number of years, was recently discovered; these errors led to many children in Ontario being taken into state care erroneously over more than a decade. When the problem was noticed, a commission chaired by Justice Susan Lang (2015) was instituted. The commission found that the Motherisk Drug Testing Laboratory (MDTL) at the Hospital for Sick Children had tested approximately 24,000 hair samples from parents from the 1990s to 2015 (Lang, 2015). The Children's Aid Society (CAS) had ordered these tests because of its mandate to protect children from abusive or negligent parents. The hair analyses were focused on the detection of drug or alcohol abuse. As a result of the faulty investigations of parental hair, the CAS determined that a number of children should be taken into care, put up for adoption, or left with their parents.

The climate and culture of variability in the definition of child abuse, coupled with a tendency to be suspicious of parents but advocate for their children, undergirded the decisions made by Dr. Charles Smith and the unit within which he worked at SickKids.

## Regulation and Oversight

The uneven and changing regulation and monitoring of medical work also led to variations in practice. Both contributed to the fiasco perpetrated by Dr. Smith. Conventional allopathic doctors are essentially self-regulating through professional bodies; unless doctors break a law and are taken to court, their practices go largely unmonitored by outsiders. Regulating medical practice is mostly a provincial matter. It is managed under the authority of the College of Physicians and Surgeons of each province. Before 2014, the governance of the College of Physicians and Surgeons of Ontario (CPSO) was composed primarily of sixteen working physicians, plus three medical faculty. In this situation, the point of view of doctors would clearly have dominated policies and procedures. Now, however, thirteen to fifteen members of the public have been added. Still, the majority of the group is medical in orientation. According to the CPSO website, its purpose is to protect and serve the public interest by regulating the practice of medicine in Ontario (College of Physicians and Surgeons of Ontario [CPSO], n.d.). Doctors must be members of the college to practise in the province in which they are working. It is the college that provides certification to practise as well as some degree of oversight and regulation.

The CPSO assesses doctors infrequently. Practically speaking, the college has the goal of assessing all doctors every ten years. A lot can happen in a doctor's life that may jeopardize his or her ability to practise safely over that lengthy period. Thousands of patients could be seen, and a parallel number of treatment decisions could be made. In addition, the college continues to admit that it is not perfect but is working towards developing consistent (and high) standards across the province in all practice areas (CPSO, n.d.). Of course, this goal has not been reached. Thus, even today, more than a decade after the Charles Smith case, we cannot rely on adequate standards of practice in every jurisdiction or in every doctor's office across the province of Ontario or, in fact, anywhere else in the world. According to the CPSO *2014 Annual Report*, only 88 per cent of the 2,396 physicians who were evaluated in the ten-year cycle were found to be fit to practise, and only 94 per cent of Independent Health Facilities passed their assessment (CPSO, 2014). In other words, at any one time, patients face a one in ten chance of receiving inadequate health care or being the subject of a medical error in Ontario at the hands of their doctors. Patients may face a slightly better chance of valid and reliable medical tests. However, these figures, based on the self-reporting of the medical profession, should give us pause and a reason to think seriously before we subject ourselves to medical intervention. In addition, there are doctors who receive formal complaints, although there may or may not be overlap with the doctors found to be inadequate in the ten-year cycle. The average time before a decision was made as to whether or not these doctors (or health care sites, which may also receive complaints) were fit to practise was eight to eleven weeks. Consequently, even after complaints and concerns have been raised about the abilities and functioning of physicians or health care sites, they may very well be continuing to work and could possibly cause patient harm while doing so.

The College of Family Physicians regulates the practice of family doctors. It makes ongoing medical education mandatory. However, since some doctors do much of their work in their own private offices, in solo practice, they may be less likely than others to be informally monitored (Canadian Medical Association, 2019). They may work outside of a network of informal judgment and censure. Patients will not necessarily have any reason to doubt their technical medical care. Patients can evaluate the personal style or the bedside manner of doctors. However, the correlation between a good bedside manner and excellent technical skills is unknown. Specialists are more likely to experience informal reprimand because they depend on referral and often work, in part, out of a hospital where they can be observed and may be subject to informal checks or criticism.

The Canadian Medical Protective Association (CMPA), established in 1901, is another potential source of oversight for the medical profession in Canada. Supported by both taxpayers and doctors themselves, it operates as an insurance company for medical practitioners (see https://www.cmpa-acpm.ca/). Its website says that the CMPA provides "medical-legal protection [that] enables doctors to practice confidently and to make decisions that result in better patient care" (CMPA, n.d.). Although primarily an insurance provider, the CMPA offers a number of classes designed to reduce the risk of lawsuit and complaint in medical practice in order to minimize problems that require payouts, as well as in the interests of good care for patients. As such, it teaches practitioners techniques for minimizing mistakes and negligence.

There is a myriad of topics within courses designed for continuing education. I will list a few to give a sense of the complexity and breadth of medical responsibility above and beyond the medical and biological sciences that are the focus of medical school education. A shortlist shows courses on how to document each patient's visit, on meticulous notetaking, on responsibilities regarding the meaning of informed consent, on disclosure of medical mistakes or possible medical mistakes, on how to make apologies, on how to manage medication use for children and the elderly, and on how to prescribe opioids and anticoagulants. This list is a small fraction of the issues discussed. It suggests the complexity of the social, administrative, practical, and ethical work of the doctor. That there are courses relating to ethics, such as privacy and confidentiality, suggests the importance of personal qualities of character associated with integrity, conscience, and values in working as a doctor.

The fact that approximately one quarter of the doctors practising in Canada were trained internationally also speaks to the potential complexity of the (possible) retraining and oversight necessary because of the wide variety of values and basic ethical principles represented by doctors from other cultures upon entering practice (Canadian Institute for Health Information [CIHI], 2020, p. 20). Attention to issues such as confidentiality and privacy, which Canadian patients expect from their doctors (and yet are hard to monitor), speak to the fundamental assertion that medicine is more than technical and based on more than evidence. Its practice also depends on ethical awareness and attention to principled decision-making. All medical work is therefore personal as well as professional. Practice embodies ethical decision-making.

As well as problems related to appropriate or ethical practice norms, physicians also have different personalities, stresses, and psychological and health profiles. Sometimes these issues in the lives of individual doctors can cause problems with patients and with colleagues. The term used by the CMPA to describe this problem is "physician disruptive behaviour." According to the CMPA (2018), this term refers to unacceptable conduct that affects patient care and/or collegial relationships. It is not an insignificant problem. For example, approximately 5 per cent of physicians are repeat offenders who have come to the attention of regulatory authorities and medical care institutions, such as hospitals (CMPA, 2018). The examples offered of physician disruptive behaviour by the CMPA included abusive language, shaming, intimidation, angry outbursts, and threats or use of physical force by fellow physicians. The CMPA has an online article on the topic to help people cope with such difficulties (CMPA, 2018), which suggests that personality issues such as those described by the Goudge Inquiry as characterizing Dr. Charles Smith may not be isolated issues among health care providers (or indeed among any of us).

In spite of the efforts being made in continuing education, online support, and monitoring the work of physicians, there were 854 legal actions in 2019 and 732 in 2020 (CMPA, 2020). These figures may represent a small fraction of the total number of malpractice issues. Only one in ten medical malpractice cases makes it to trial (Milne et al., 2014). Approximately 35 to 40 per cent of cases generally lead to before suit settlement. The CMPA has a history of defending doctors, even at great cost. In fact, it is willing to spend more on the court case than it would have to spend on a settlement. Consequently, even in cases of clear liability, lawyers are often unwilling to take cases for patients because the chances of winning are so low and the cases can be dragged out over a lengthy time period. This situation arises partly because of the immense resources of the CMPA as compared to individual patients. The CMPA fights hard, spends money, and has the assets to continue the fight against any individual patient in order to defend its doctors. Thus, the system is heavily weighted against the patient ever winning a medical malpractice settlement, regardless of the facts of the case. Ironically, because taxpayers support the CMPA along with the fees that the doctors pay, the CMPA has money from patients to fight against the interests of patients.

## Specialty Practice

The next topic of discussion has to do with the particular characteristics of forensic pathology as a science and practice that may have contributed to the terrible outcomes for so many caregivers and finally for Dr. Charles Smith. During the time of Dr. Smith's wrongful convictions, forensic pathology was not a new field. There were, however, very few forensic pathologists in North America or elsewhere in the world. There were still fewer paediatric forensic pathologists. The specialty was very small. The science was constantly changing, and the whole area of pathology was being divided into smaller and smaller specialty areas. As in all medicine, knowledge and practice were constantly evolving. As we have seen, medical knowledge, by definition and method, is always a matter of probability and not certainty. Perhaps even more than some other specialties, the field of forensic pathology needs to be treated as one that is, in part, particularly subjective and vulnerable to interpretation. Different pathologists can see and notice different things. There may not be as many different sources of evidence upon which to base a decision. For example, there is no patient with whom to communicate who might be able to add information to enhance the probability of a valid diagnosis. Furthermore, there is a relatively small and preliminary knowledge base and science.

The field of general pathology has a long history, but the professional specialty in North America was not distinguished until the 1920s and 1930s. Under pathology, there are numerous emerging subspecialties with names such as digital pathology, clinical pathology, histopathology, neuropathology, pulmonary and renal pathology, and anatomical pathology, among others. However, specialty subdivisions differ from geographic area to geographic area, and there may be fewer subspecialties in one area than in another. According to the Royal College of Physicians and Surgeons of Canada, there are eight subspecialties in the field of pathology (Royal College of Physicians and Surgeons of Canada, n.d.). Wikipedia lists sixteen subspecialties (see https://en.wikipedia.org /wiki/Pathology). Regardless of the exact number in Canada today, it is clear there has been increasing specialization in the field of pathology. The division of labour and knowledge appropriate to each specialty is always in some mild state of flux and debate, rendering peer review imperative in the field.

## Case Discussions: William Mullins-Johnson and Richard Brant

Let us first look at one of Dr. Smith's cases in a little depth. It illustrates several features of the ongoing errors that Dr. Charles Smith committed in his medical practice as a paediatric forensic pathologist. William Mullins-Johnson, a twenty-two-year-old Indigenous man from Sault Ste. Marie, had been staying with his half-brother and sister-in-law for about two months in 1993 (Harland-Logan, n.d.). One evening, he was asked to babysit the three young children in the home who were three, four, and six years old. The four-year-old girl, Valin, watched television with her uncle and then put herself to bed. She wasn't feeling well and had had a fever during the day. Mullins-Johnson said he looked in on Valin at 8 p.m. and found that she was sleeping. Her mother came home shortly afterwards and did not check on her daughter. Her father came home still later. He apparently did not check on Valin either. In the morning, at about 7 a.m., Valin's mother went to say good morning to her daughter. She observed vomit on the bed and her daughter lying face down. When she turned the child over, she found Valin's face was purple and Valin was unresponsive. The mother called 911. Ambulance attendants arrived at the scene and concluded that Valin was already dead. Within twenty-four hours, the police arrested Mullins-Johnson and charged him with aggravated assault. A pathologist at a local Sault Ste. Marie hospital, Dr. Rasaiah, did the autopsy examination. Since he was worried that Valin might have been sexually abused, he asked Dr. Zehr, a colleague with training in child abuse, to examine her. Dr. Zehr concluded that there was evidence of chronic sexual abuse. At the trial, there were five expert witnesses. Four stated that, although it appeared that Valin had been sexually abused in the past, the abuse had not been recent nor had it contributed to her death. Dr. Charles Smith was the fifth expert witness at the trial. He did not directly observe Valin's body, but he stated, on the basis of postmortem slides he had observed, that Valin had suffered trauma to her rectum. He testified that the injury was most likely the result of penetration by a large, blunt object. Although there was no evidence of semen, Mullins-Johnson was charged with murder and rape, and found guilty. His guilt was determined, in part, by Dr. Smith's assurance that Valin had been sexually abused immediately prior to her death. The jury was faced with contradictory evidence, and although Mullins-Johnson asserted his innocence, he spent twelve years in jail for rape and murder.

The guilty verdict was appealed to both the Ontario Court of Appeal and the Supreme Court of Canada. Both were denied (Harland-Logan, n.d.). It was not until 2003 that a lawyer named James Lockyer, on behalf of the organization now known as Innocence Canada, asked for the slides and tissue samples that Dr. Charles Smith had used in his determination of guilt. Although he was asked repeatedly, Dr. Smith did not provide the slides and tissue samples, claiming he had returned them to Dr. Rasaiah. After a period of almost a year of Dr. Smith's avoidance and failure to send the evidence upon which he had made his determination, the slides and other evidence were eventually found on the shelves of his office (Goudge, 2008, vol. 2, pp. 28–9). In the end, this evidence was central to overturning Mullins-Johnson's conviction. What Dr. Smith had interpreted as signs of rape and murder, and therefore key to his determination of Mullins-Johnson's guilt, were actually post-mortem changes to Valin's body. They were not the result of intentional pre-mortem harm that amounted to murder and rape or sexual assault ("Wrongfully convicted," 2010).

Mullins-Johnson was finally released in 2005 after it became clear that Smith had misinterpreted and mislaid evidence that could have shown the four-year-old died of natural causes ("Mullins-Johnson happy," 2007). The Goudge Inquiry found that, along with poor and inadequate evidence managing and invalid autopsy conclusions, Smith – as well as his colleagues in the unit – also had the tendency to offer biased judgments about the families of the dead children. They spoke as if they knew and understood "social risk factors," and they felt that, although they were by no means experts in sociology, psychology, or any other relevant field, they ought to take such factors into account. Furthermore, the Goudge Inquiry observed that Dr. Smith presented himself as particularly capable. Dr. Smith emphasized that he was, in fact, especially qualified because he was director of the OPFPU, and it was a "unique" department, not only in Canada but in all of North America. He also asserted that he had probably performed more paediatric forensic autopsies than anyone else in the country. He positioned himself as having "vast experience with pediatric cases." He was repeatedly able to convince juries of his expertise (Goudge, 2008, vol. 2, p. 119).

Let us now look at a second of Dr. Smith's cases – the case of another Indigenous man, Richard Brant, who was wrongly convicted after his baby died. Again Dr. Charles Smith's sloppy and unethical work was responsible for this miscarriage of justice. Richard Brant was imprisoned for aggravated assault for a period of six months. His case, too, represents the tendency of Dr. Charles Smith to use tunnel vision in determining causes of death. The doctor who performed the original autopsy said that the causes of death were bronchopneumonia and subdural hematoma (Vijaykumar, 2018, pp. 178–9). A second opinion was sought from Dr. Smith. He based his conclusions on a deteriorating tissue sample. Later, a technician discovered that the baby's brain had been mistakenly stored in water instead of formaldehyde and was thus in the process of decomposition. It was therefore actually impossible to use it for assessment (p. 179). Despite the absence of adequate tissue samples or slides, Dr. Smith argued that the baby had been assaulted.

Years later, after Brant had been convicted and served his six-month prison sentence, the truth of the baby's death came out at the Goudge Inquiry. Dr. Smith was found to have determined that Brant was guilty because he had the "social risk factors" of a person prone to shaking his child. It was this bias that had led to Brant's wrongful conviction. One has to wonder about racism in this case, as in that of William Mullins-Johnson.

## Discussion: How Did Medicine Go Awry in the Case of Dr. Charles Smith?

The first and most obvious explanations of Dr. Charles Smith's medical errors were his personal but highly inappropriate argumentative style in court and his assertions regarding the significance of social factors in determining guilt and innocence. His contentions about social risk factors were not based on his area of expertise but rather on his social stereotypes. In regards to his pathology work, he exhibited sloppy practices and appeared to jump to conclusions affected by his biases. That he was asked to act as a forensic pathologist and not as a psychiatrist, psychologist, or social worker did not appear to occur to him, and he seemed to use personal biases and stigma in his deliberations. At least two of the twelve people (about 17 per cent) who were wrongfully convicted were Indigenous. This figure grossly over-represents the population of Indigenous people in Canada, which is less than 5 per cent. This over-representation may be related to Dr. Smith's biases and, indeed, racism.

The intermediate causes of ongoing medical error in this case were medical system organizational issues. Dr. Charles Smith was not stopped, despite many repeated complaints. There was a lack of an enforced accountability structure in the forensic pathology unit. There was no training or education for pathologists on how to interact with the court system and give evidence. Labour force issues played an important role in the egregious outcomes documented by the Goudge Inquiry. There were just not enough paediatric forensic pathologists from whom to choose. It was a new specialty, and few had yet been trained. The larger context of this case is one of a changing science, with shifts in the definitions of specialty practices. It is also a case in which the inevitable degree of subjectivity in all diagnoses played a role. The fact that, in the field of pathology, there is no patient to discuss and explain symptoms (for potentially corroborating a diagnosis) may make it a particularly difficult field of practice. Nor is peer review a built-in aspect of decision-making, although it has been recognized as an important intervention, especially given the many errors in pathology over the years (Chorneyko & Butany, 2008). As the work in the unit was fee-for-service, it may have been more vulnerable to personal exigencies such as the need or desire for money. This problem of subjectivity is even more significant when, as in forensic pathology, the science is supposed to not only investigate the causes of sudden, unnatural, or suspicious deaths but also liaise with the criminal justice system in order to help determine whether there was an intention behind the death. Thus, we have two inevitably complex and yet sometimes subjective interpretive systems working together to arrive at one conclusion that may have significant and powerful impacts on the lives of others. That Dr. Smith had not been trained for his role as a witness was another fundamental cause of his mistaken testimony to the court.

It also appears that the social determinants of health played a role in that the unit was highly sensitive to, and on the lookout for, the possibility of child abuse. This focus likely affected Smith's decisions. These medical errors may reflect the cultural emphasis on uncovering hidden child abuse that was evident during the time period in which the decisions were made. The influence of the mass media and the cultural ethos emphasizing the notion of a hidden epidemic of child abuse may have been an influence on Dr. Smith. Furthermore, Dr. Smith appeared to be influenced by discrimination and stigma against Indigenous people. He used what he called "social risk factors" to estimate the likelihood that a given injury was the result of intent or not.

## Conclusion

The immediate causes of these medical errors were the repeated and unchecked argumentative style and biased court appearances of Dr. Charles Smith. There were ongoing medical system issues, including the lack of an enforced accountability structure in the forensic pathology unit, the lack of training for pathologists about how to interact with the court system and give evidence, and the lack of personnel, including a peer-review system, to do the tasks required in the department. It also appears that the social determinants of health played a role in that the unit was highly sensitive to, and on the lookout for, the possibility of child abuse in the child deaths that they studied and upon which they decided cause of death. Dr. Smith's use of social risk factors in his determination of the causes of death was also both highly inappropriate and unchecked by the power and accountability structure of his unit. In fact, his social risk factors formulation may actually reflect his racism more clearly than anything else. His ongoing errors seem to also reflect the cultural emphasis on uncovering hidden child abuse that was evident during the time period in which the decisions were made.

# Elizabeth Wettlaufer: The Nurse Who Murdered Her Long-Term Care Patients While No One Noticed

## The Issue

Elizabeth Wettlaufer is a nurse who was convicted of killing eight elderly people while she was on duty in nursing homes in Southwestern Ontario. The circumstances described here and the factors that contributed to Wettlaufer's crimes were documented in a public inquiry launched in 2017 (Gillese, 2019). The murders occurred over the period from 2009 to 2016. She murdered her victims, who ranged in age from mid-seventies to mid-nineties in age, over a number of years. None of the deaths was considered suspicious at the time. The deaths were quiet and not entirely surprising to nursing home staff, family members, or friends. If there were questions asked about the suddenness of the deaths, they did not point to murder. The victims all had some degree of mental or physical frailty. They were all what is considered to be old. The deaths only came to light because Wettlaufer confessed. She admitted both to these murders and to a number of other attempts to kill or harm a nursing home resident in her care. In total, she confessed to and was charged with two counts of aggravated assault and four counts of attempted murder as well as the eight murders. Wettlaufer is now in prison and will be for a long time. She received a sentence of life imprisonment (times eight) with no chance of parole for twenty-five years.

Wettlaufer's crimes finally came to light when she herself sought treatment for drug addiction at the Centre for Addiction and Mental Health (CAMH) in Toronto. She disclosed her role in the murders to one of her therapists, who then reported Wettlaufer's actions to the police and to the College of Nurses of Ontario. Wettlaufer said that she had already admitted her crimes to a number of people, including her pastor and his wife. They may or may not have believed her but they prayed over her, and the pastor allegedly said that if she ever did it again, he would have to report her (McQuigge, 2017). Wettlaufer also said that she had told some of her friends, her Narcotics Anonymous Sponsor, and a lawyer (Fraser, 2017). The lawyer advised her to keep it a secret and told her not to do it again. Apparently, no one reported her to the police, to the nursing homes where she worked, or to the College of Nurses of Ontario, which is the regulating authority for nurses in the province. No one close to those who were killed was surprised or troubled enough by the deaths of these seniors to raise an alarm or to ask questions, demanding answers.

Wettlaufer said that she felt a compulsion to murder. She said that either God or the Devil wanted her to kill. She experienced what she called a "red surge" at each of the murders. Most of those whom she killed died peacefully after the injection of insulin, a drug chosen because it was not monitored by the nursing home (CBC News, 2017). Some of her victims had been experiencing symptoms of dementia, and all of them were vulnerable either physically or mentally and were in the long-term care home because they could no longer autonomously care for themselves. They were dependent for their well-being on their caregivers (Fitzpatrick, 2017b). In an explanation for her actions, Wettlaufer told police she picked some of her victims because they "were mean" and difficult to look after. She also said that she had a heavy workload (Fitzpatrick, 2017a).

Wettlaufer was a fully trained registered nurse (RN) who had been educated in Kitchener, Ontario, at the local community college, Conestoga College. Prior to her nursing education, she had attended a Baptist Bible college for a degree in religious education counselling. Despite her education, she had a troubled occupational history. Many years before Wettlaufer confessed to these nursing home murders, just after graduating from nursing, she had been fired from a hospital in 1995. She was fired because she was observed to be confused and disoriented at work, which was determined to be the result of ingesting lorazepam, a tranquillizer (Lupton, 2017). There were other indications from early in her career that Wettlaufer was a problematic employee and a troubled person. In another example related to work, restrictions were put on Wettlaufer's nursing licence due to overdosing on hospital medications while at work. Apparently, in consequence, she became a personal support worker (a job with less responsibility and lower pay) instead of a nurse for a period of time. However, details about those early days of her career are scarce (McQuigge, 2017).

Before the murders came to light, and after seven of the murders had occurred while she was practising as an RN, Wettlaufer was finally fired from the nursing home Caressant Care (see https:// caressantcare.com/long-term-care-homes.php), where most of the murders occurred. Despite having been fired, she was able to quickly find work again as a RN in another nearby nursing home, even though the nursing home that fired her did as they were required and reported the firing to the College of Nurses of Ontario. However, there is some difference of opinion about what was reported to the regulatory body. According to Caressant Care, they submitted a twenty-page chronological report on 17 April 2016, which documented the ten workplace violations that had caused multiple suspensions over the years. The college says that, when it received Caressant Care's notification about the firing of Wettlaufer, a college staff member called the home's director of nursing. According to the college's documentation, the nursing home spokesperson downplayed the reasons for the firing and emphasized that there was no "underlying issue or concern" because no resident had been seriously harmed. Furthermore, in support of their minimization of the issues precipitating the firing, the nursing home said that Wettlaufer had admitted to her mistakes. This reported acknowledgement of her errors was understood to imply that she had learned from them and would not repeat such behaviours. Thus, no action was taken to suspend or otherwise put limits

on Wettlaufer. In fact, soon after she was fired, she found employment at another nursing home where she killed her eighth victim
(Lupton, 2017).

In the meantime, and over the years, Wettlaufer had tried repeatedly to get help. She had admitted herself to a psychiatric hospital
and had gone to a psychiatrist for aid for her mental health issues.
Wettlaufer struggled with addiction to alcohol, opioids, and other
drugs and had sought help for these addictions over the years. She
had joined Narcotics Anonymous for a period of time. She tried
to get assistance by telling a number of people what she had been
doing. Apparently, she also tried immersing herself in religion to
cope with her life struggles, including her confusion about her sexual preferences. Wettlaufer told a student nurse about the murders
and how she had been involved. The student responded by saying
that she was going to report her to management. Wettlaufer per-
suaded her against this whistleblowing. How can we explain these
eight murders over time? Why were they not noted as suspicious
deaths at the time they occurred? How did Wettlaufer go unchecked
for such a long time? There are a number of threads of thought to be
understood and explored in this chapter. In the first place, we have
to consider how this case aligns with our critique of medicalization.
The route to the link between these murders and medicalization is
complex. It involves a consideration of the cultural attitudes and
behaviours, both at the individual and at the policy levels, towards
medicine. These cultural values place a high and unquestioned
value on conventional or allopathic medicine. They also embrace
the disproportionate investment in the aggressive heroic allopathic
medical care system. This investment covers research, practice,
and health systems. By contrast, the cultural emphasis on medicine exacerbates the tendency to under-support the caring functions of health care, especially for the complex chronic conditions
much more common among the elderly. The underlying problem is
that medicalization has both led to and underscored or supported
forceful high-tech medical intervention designed to save lives at
the expense of care. People who are ageing are inevitably nearer
the end of their lives than young people in general. In the final
analysis, they cannot be cured but only cared for. The dominance

of traditional medicine has led to the undervaluing of sustaining a comfortable life for those for whom cure is not likely and death is the logical outcome (Mezey & Fulmer, 2002).

That the murdered people were all elderly is also related to the outcome we are trying to understand. How might ageism play a part in these murders and in the fact that they were largely invisible until Wettlaufer admitted her crimes? At the broadest level, the demographic profile of Canada as an ageing nation also plays a part. Canada is characterized, in part, by discrimination and prejudice against its ageing population and thus fails to provide adequate resources, housing, staffing, and ongoing surveillance of care. Ageism may have played a role both at the systemic level and at the level of the perceptions of the people close to the victims of the murders. That no one apparently raised an alarm earlier might have been because of the stereotypes about the elderly. Had a younger person died unexpectedly and suddenly in hospital, an investigation would have likely been triggered. Instead, those close to the people who died suddenly did not ask questions about the sudden loss of the resident or loved one. What does the organization and state of nursing homes have to do with this situation? Nursing labour force issues, including the staffing levels of personnel representing various levels of training and compensation, must be considered. To some extent, Elizabeth Wettlaufer was an anomaly, a "bad apple." She was intermittently misusing various substances, and she had recurrent mental health issues. Furthermore, Wettlaufer was one of a category of health care serial killers (Gillese, 2019, vol. 1, p. 4). There was plenty of warning to the long-term care institutional sector that should have been acted upon. In this way, the continued murders are clearly a result of more than a single individual's malfeasance. These ideas are among those we will examine in the following discussion.

## The Ageing Population and Ageism

There is no doubt that Canada is an ageing nation. In fact, we comprise one of the "oldest" nations of the world. In 2014, the median age of Canadians was 40.4 years – in effect, half of all Canadians were older, and half were younger, than 40.4 years – compared to the rest of the world, where the median age was 29.7 years (MacDonald, 2015, p. 291). The Canadian census of 2016 showed that the one in six Canadians is over sixty-five years of age. These proportions of ageing people are historic and record breaking (MacDonald, 2015, p. 289). Statistics Canada's 2016 census data indicated that, for the first time in Canadian history, the number of persons sixty-five years of age or older outnumbered those under the age of fourteen (Canadian Association for Long Term Care, 2017). These figures reflect both increasing life expectancy and the baby boom following the Second World War. To add to this picture of an ageing nation, the elderly population is also getting older. An increasing number of people in the population are over eighty-five years of age.

These changes in the ageing of the population are associated with ageism. It has been argued that ageism is the most tolerated of the "isms" today (Revera Inc. & Sheridan Centre for Elder Research, 2016). It must be added to the list of other "isms" such as racism and sexism. Ageism can be defined as "an alteration in feeling, belief or behaviour in response to an individual's or group's chronological age" (Levy & Banaji, 2002, p. 50). Implicit in the notion of ageism is the idea that there is widespread acceptance of negative perceptions of the elderly, which is manifest in interpersonal and systemic interactions with the elderly. "This prejudice minimizes our expectations of older adults and influences how they are treated, their participation in society, and what steps are taken to enhance their engagement" (MacDonald, 2015, p. 309). According to reports from seniors themselves, the most commonly experienced characteristics of age discrimination include being treated as if invisible (41 per cent); perceived as if they have nothing to contribute (38 per cent); and assumed to be incompetent (27 per cent) (Revera Inc. & International Federation on Ageing, n.d). These values may relate to the fact that the deaths were neither observed nor questioned. The experience of ageism is especially true for women.

Ageism has been attributed to the decline in economic productivity in ageing people in a capitalist society. Thus, ageism is partly thought to be a reflection of the increasing proportions of people who are preparing for or have retired. There are, consequently, fewer people entering the labour force than leaving it, which represents a growth in the number of people who are, in economic terms, often called "dependent." Dependent people are considered as such because they are eligible to retire and live on old age security, governmental, and other privately held pensions. There is a perception that such people have a negative effect on society and are a drain on the economy. The reliance of the elderly on "non-productive" retirement income is one of the foundations of the resentment of the elderly, one part of ageism. As the population ages, more services and tax income are devoted to supportive housing, additional health care, and other such services that are needed by the elderly. At the same time, the proportion of the population that is younger is decreasing. Thus, fewer people are available to be responsible for the greater "burden" of taxes used to provide health and long-term care for the elderly. There is also relatively less tax money for services for the young and middle-aged populations. In one example, elementary and high schools and universities may receive decreased investment as tax dollars are funnelled into pensions.

Coupled with economic dependence, the elderly are often thought to experience both poor physical and mental health. Ageing is stereotypically associated with physical sickness, disabilities, dementia, and death. The elderly are thought to be a drain on the universal health care system. Ageing people do cost the health care system more per person than those under sixty-five (Canadian Foundation for Healthcare Improvement, 2011), but the reasons are complex. In part, they relate to the advance of certain expensive technological and pharmaceutical innovations that may be taken up by the elderly more than by the young. Hip and knee replacement, surgical advances in relation to chronic conditions such as diseases of the heart and cancer, and treatments for other chronic ailments such as steroids for arthritis and pain are among the developments that enable the elderly to maintain their health and mobility for longer periods of time. These medical interventions can, however, be costly and add to the bill for universal health care.

Another cost driver for the medical system is the lack of available beds in long-term care institutions. It leads to the elderly "using" expensive hospital beds when they could, if home care beds or assistance at home were available, be living in long-term care or in their own homes. Because of the irrational governmental policies, elderly people can become what is derogatorily called "bed blockers" at great expense. The health care system was designed for acute and not chronic care. Another reason the elderly consume disproportional health care dollars is that, lacking sufficient alternatives such as home care and hospices, the elderly are more likely to die in hospital. Dying could often be more compassionately managed much less expensively in hospices with palliative care (Canadian Foundation for Healthcare Improvement, 2011). Despite the higher cost of health care for Canadian seniors, they are less satisfied with the quality of the health care they receive than those aged sixty-five and older in ten similar developed countries according to an international survey (Canadian Institute for Health Information, 2017). This dissatisfaction may indirectly reflect the ageism they experience in a situation with an inadequate supply of either long-term care beds or home care dollars.

## Elder Abuse at Home, in Institutions, and in Public

There are times when the widely accepted prejudice and discrimination of ageism concentrates and results in elder abuse. This mistreatment arises out of the potential and real dependence of the elderly, especially the most vulnerable elderly, on others, particularly on those younger than themselves (Rzeszut, 2017). Elder abuse takes many different forms and occurs within families, within institutions, and in the public sphere. Such abuse can be financial, emotional, physical, sexual, and social (neglect) in expression (Department of Justice, 2015). Overall, about 4.5 per cent of seniors report experiencing some type of abuse every year. Financial and emotional abuse are the most common types. In addition, about 10 per cent of Canadian seniors are victims of crime, usually crimes of property, annually. There are numerous other crimes perpetrated against the vulnerable elderly. They include a variety of fraudulent schemes, including those related to duplicitous investments, false promises of reward prizes, pushy telemarketing, phony health products, and deceitful offers of home repairs. Approximately 1 per cent of Canadian seniors experience violent crimes or physical abuse yearly (Department of Justice, 2015). Seniors tend to know those who commit violence against them. All types of abuse and crime are known to occur in public and private institutions for the elderly. There have been a number of powerful media investigations of the dire situation in Canadian long-term care (Kelly, 2017; Mancini et al., 2018; Pedersen et al., 2018). A total of 2,198 cases of abuse by staff towards dependent residents were reported in homes across Canada in 2016 (Pedersen et al., 2018). This figure is likely an underestimate of the extent of the problem. Abuse is more common in institutions than it is in the community (National Research Council, 2003).

In addition to the varieties of abuse against an individual enumerated above, people in institutions are vulnerable to systemic institutional abuse. Systemic abuse is evident in deficiencies such as overcrowding, understaffing, poor meals, and failure to uphold the human rights and dignity of those housed in a particular institution. Caregivers working in institutions for the elderly report being troubled about the way that some staff treat their charges. Included among the types of abuse of concern are a culture that allows verbal abuse, swearing, and yelling, and various types of rough handling of patients. As women comprise the majority of nursing home residents, it is elderly women who are most susceptible and may be most subject to ageism. The most vulnerable residents may be those whose family live furthest away and are thus not available to monitor the care of their family member.

Furthermore, much of the abuse mentioned can be virtually invisible. For example, it may be very difficult for anyone but the personal care worker to see such signs of abuse as bruises because they may be hidden under clothes. Many rooms in long-term homes are private, and thus hostile actions of caregivers can easily be made invisible to other staff or residents. Residents may themselves be confused and unaware, unable, or afraid to report that they or others are being mistreated (National Research Council, 2003). In consequence, some family members have installed videocams in the rooms of their loved ones. Emotional abuse is essentially undetectable unless observed, and even then, is subjectively defined. The isolation of long-term care institutions from their local communities may also exacerbate the opportunities for those who work within their walls to behave badly towards the people in their care. Finally, the cultural and social denigration of the value of the elderly indiscernibly supports and underpins the normalization of serious and criminal mistreatment of the elderly.

It is important to note that all the numerical estimates of seniors who report they have experienced abuse or criminal victimization are undoubtedly an under-representation of the actual incidence. Many seniors likely fail to acknowledge or report being victimized at the hands of an intimate family member or caregiver upon whom they are dependent within or outside of an institution. They may not know their rights and may be ashamed and blame themselves. They may be fearful of retaliation if they complain about the way they are being treated. For a wide variety of complex reasons, seniors are not as likely as other age groups to formally report being victims of crime or spousal abuse. Instead, many crimes against seniors are not reported to police but only come to light when they are mentioned to or observed by informal caregivers, health professionals, or financial institutions and agencies.

## Institutional Care for the Elderly

The elderly in residential care homes are among the most vulnerable in society (Hawes, 2003). Close to 10 per cent of Canadian women and 5 per cent of Canadian men who are sixty-five years of age and over live in long-term care facilities, including personal care homes, nursing homes, and complex care facilities. In 2018–19, there were approximately 4,500 patients in hospital in Ontario waiting for nursing home placement or other non-hospitalized care service and accommodation (Health Quality Ontario, 2019). These people are sometimes negatively termed "bed blockers" because they may be housed in acute care hospitals over a long period of time while they wait for placement. This situation often occurs if a senior has no safe home to which to return. About 16 per cent of hospital beds are filled with people waiting for an alternate form of care. Most are waiting for long-term care in an institution. The illogic of this state of affairs is evident when we consider that long-term care is much less expensive than hospital-based care – approximately $175 per day as compared to $750 per day (Ontario Long Term Care Association, 2018, p. 8). There are 626 licensed and approved homes operating in Ontario. Still, many people who need such care languish in hospital or at home in expensive or unsafe, and in many other ways, undesirable circumstances. The wait list for long-stay beds, as of January 2020, was 35,308. Of the available homes, 58 per cent are privately owned, 24 per cent are non-profit/charitable, and 16 per cent are municipal (Ontario Long Term Care Association, n.d.). The long-term care homes are mostly for seniors but can be used for other purposes when there are no other options. Altogether, 77,563 long-stay beds are allocated to deliver care and housing to frail seniors who require permanent placement; 723 convalescent care beds are allocated to provide short-term care as a temporary placement between hospitalization and home; and 114 beds are allocated for respite to families who need a break from the exhaustion of caring for their loved ones while they wait for a bed or if they choose not to institutionalize their loved one (Ontario Long Term Care Association, n.d.). Many of the long-term care homes are in need of repairs and remodelling. But the money is tight. Long-term care is part of the province's health care system and partly publicly funded on a cost-shared basis with residents.

## Monitoring Long-Term Care Institutions

The lack of national standards, monitoring, or assessment may contribute to various types of elder abuse in long-term care institutions (Hawes & Kimbell, 2010). Provincial standards differ. The Canada Health Act does not cover home care and long-term care. Long-term care institutions in Ontario are, in principle, assessed annually. This frequency does suggest a degree of oversight. Although these inspections are legislated, the depth and breadth of these examinations may be somewhat curtailed and variable, depending on such things as political exigencies, time, and financial constraints. In an economic climate in which there are not enough long-term care beds and the political will to raise enough money is lacking, it is clear that less than ideal situations can and do exist. Families may feel deeply compromised when they allow their loved one to go into a home that they know to be somewhat inadequate but do so because they have no choice if they want to work and support themselves and other family members. Inspection is delegated to the provinces, and thus differences in standards and outcome occur (Norris, 2020). Across the country, both long-term care beds and home care service availability is insufficient.

## Staffing Long-Term Care Institutions

Staff at long-term care homes have numerous and diverse responsibilities. They have to care for people with a wide range of conditions varying in complexity, severity, and types of sickness and disability. Staff may be subject to being physically and verbally attacked by seniors and others in their care. The work is physically demanding at times. It involves lifting sometimes very heavy residents. It can include trying to convince people who don't want to go to bed, or eat their meals, or use the toilet to do so. Yet, many of those who are in residence are unable to look after themselves and must be helped with the basics of daily life. The vast majority of residents (97 per cent) need help with routine daily living activities such as getting out of bed, eating, or toileting (Ontario

Long Term Care Association, 2018, p. 3). Some degree of cognitive impairment is found in 90 per cent of residents. About one-third are severely disabled physically or cognitively. Almost half are sometimes aggressive, generally related to their cognitive impairment or mental health condition. About 61 per cent of residents take ten or more different prescription medications; 86 per cent need extensive help with performing daily activities; 80 per cent have neurological diseases; and 40 per cent need monitoring of an acute medical condition (Ontario Long Term Care Association, n.d.)

This high level of need, coupled with the lack of adequate staff numbers and training, means that accidents happen and problems arise on a routine basis. Some of the serious problems include the frequently observed and reported inappropriate use of anti-psychotics off-label (27 per cent); falls caused, at times, by inadequate supervision of the elderly residents (15 per cent); increasingly depressed mood over time in care (23 per cent); the use of restraints to manage aggression and uncontrolled behaviours (9 per cent); and inadequately managed pain (9 per cent) (Canadian Medical Association, 2016). These problems are well documented. A study of 4,500 registered nurses from 257 Canadian hospitals found that about 60 per cent felt there was not enough staff for them to do their jobs properly. Almost 12 per cent said that patient safety in their own hospital unit was compromised. About 25 per cent would not recommend the hospital in which they work to others (Hildebrandt, 2013). Although this study was a study of hospitals and not nursing homes, there is no reason to expect that the figures would be substantially different for nursing homes. As the level of staffing in nursing homes is minimal, there would not likely be sufficient staff to worry about patient safety on a daily basis. It is unfortunate that similar research does not appear to have been conducted on the perceptions of nursing home staff. The fact that Wettlaufer's murders went undetected and apparently unsuspected might suggest there are other relatively invisible problems that would become known were better monitoring and safer care the norm.

There are three levels and types of training among those who work in direct care with patients in nursing homes. First, at the top of the hierarchy of nursing caregivers, are registered nurses (RNs), who are licensed to medicate. However, there may be only one RN on duty in an entire nursing home; thus, there is essentially no peer or supervisor to monitor the work of the one RN who has access to many diverse medications for a wide variety of conditions. Increasingly, long-term care institutions are relying on caregivers with less education and training than RNs. Registered practical nurses (RPNs), who are diploma graduates of community colleges, are the second level of caregivers, while the third level are personal support workers (PSWs). PSWs are only required to have 600 hours of training, including 342 hours in the classroom and 10 hours of supervision plus 280 hours of practicum. They constitute a body of unregulated care providers whose job is to help a person manage daily activities such as dressing, toileting, eating, and the like. Registered nurses require more education including, increasingly, a university degree. Nurse practitioners (NPs) need more education than registered nurses, and their scope of practice is broader and can include diagnosing and prescribing medications. The proportion of RNs and NPs among regulated nurses has declined across multiple care settings since 2007 (Canadian Nurses Association, 2018). The average wages of the three major daily caregivers reflects the hierarchy of expertise of the service offered. The average salary of a nurse is $111,000 per annum across Canada. This figure includes nurses in highly specialized roles who earn well above this average. Nursing home workers are not at the top of the pay scale. The average wage for the other two nursing staff, the far more prevalent workers in long-term care homes, are hourly rates from $19.37 to $28.89 for RPNs (Payscale, 2018b) and $12.82 to $20.63 for PSWs (Payscale, 2018a).

It may be that the situation is somewhat poorer in Ontario nursing homes than elsewhere in the country. However, the only evidence of this claim is the assessment made by the Registered Nurses Association of Ontario's research designed to increase funding and support for such care within the province. The association argued that the long-term care facilities in Ontario have residents with higher care needs than a number of other jurisdictions, yet have fewer nurses per resident (Registered Nurses Association of Ontario, 2007).

An ideal scenario for care in nursing homes, based on research reported by the Registered Nurses Association of Ontario (2007), would include NPs, RNs, and RPNs, who would all be engaged in their complete and full "scope of practice." This ideal would provide the safest and healthiest outcomes for those who live out their lives in long-term care institutions. This team of regulated professional workers would be assisted by PSWs, who are not regulated as of yet. Ideally, the PSWs would work within the context of the regulated professionals. Added to these workers would be other health care providers such as physiotherapists, social workers, recreational therapists, and the like. Unfortunately, in order to save costs in these burgeoning institutions, there are virtually no NPs, a minimum number of RNs and RPNs, and a growth in the number of staff who do not have the training to work unsupervised or inadequately supervised, although they often do, that is, PSWs.

## Caregiving Stress and Burnout

Informal caregiving is ubiquitous among all ages of people, including elderly people, who, at times, care for one another and for those younger than they are. Elderly people care for spouses, friends, and their children, grandchildren, and others. Informal caregiving in the community can be more or less demanding of time and emotional, physical, and financial resources. It can be short lived, such as caring for someone with an acute illness, and it can take place over years when it is for a person with a serious chronic or a terminal illness. It can involve twenty-four-hour care or just a few hours per week. About 20 per cent of older people in Canada provide care to at least one other person at least once per week. About one-tenth of the population of elderly people provide more than ten hours of care to another. Often times, it is because there is no option available to support the elderly in caretaking. A sizeable number (34 per cent) of these caregivers report that they experience distress, anger, or depression while providing care (Canadian

Institute of Health Research, 2016). No matter the length or the demands of caregiving, it always disrupts the ongoing plans and activities of the caregiver and thus causes some stress. Caring for a person for twenty-four hours a day and caring over many years are especially taxing. Working to provide caregiving is also often stressful and unpredictable. Caregivers experience violence at the hands of those for whom they are caring (Sibbald, 2017). Without adequate levels of home care support, the stress and other negative consequences of informal home caregiving will continue, and people will be forced to place their elderly loved ones in long-term care institutions without being able to first demand higher standards and reliable monitoring across the country.

Caregiving in a long-term care institution with elderly residents who have complex needs and sometimes very difficult personalities, and where staffing levels may be less than ideal, can be particularly demanding for the mental health and well-being of caregivers. Nursing home workers and registered nurses in paediatric hospitals have been found to have poorer mental health than the average member of the Canadian population (Hoben et al., 2017). Mental health is especially problematic among nursing home workers who care for a very frail, vulnerable, and often medically complicated group of people. The increasing incidence of various dementias among the people to whom service is provided adds to the challenges of institutional caregiving (Berendonk et al., 2017; Tonelli et al., 2017). A review of the experiences of nurses in long-term care for the elderly documented negative experiences, including feeling devalued as professionals. This finding suggests that the prestige level of nurses working in this sector may not be as high as that of those in other sectors (Registered Nurses Association of Ontario, 2007).

## Addiction among Nurses

We know that Elizabeth Wettlaufer struggled with substance abuse over many years during the time that she was working as an RN and a PSW. We also know that this problem had been observed, and she had been reprimanded, suspended, and even fired. However, she was able to continue nursing and to change jobs in the nursing home field despite this record. She says that she was stressed, and stress can enhance the likelihood of abusing various substances. Neither stress nor substance abuse was unique to Wettlaufer among nursing home staff. In fact, a normal, if not higher than normal, level of addiction might be expected because of the nature and characteristics of the work. It is not only physically demanding; it also involves heavy emotional work. One consequence of stress is burnout, resulting in a caregiver who doesn't care for his or her patients and doesn't even want to be at work any longer. Burnout is especially endemic among front line workers, whose work often involves tedious, inauthentic, and personally costly emotional work (Hochschild, 1990) such as nursing home staff are required to do. Sometimes staff in hospitals and long-term care institutions deal with their stress and the demanding emotional work required, as well as the physical labour they endure daily, by abusing drugs the way Wettlaufer did. A wide variety of types of medications are easily accessible to RNs in long-term care. At times, access can lead to utilization of medications meant for others. Research on the topic of the link between health care work and addiction is scarce, and what is available is not based on large representative samples. Instead, it is often anecdotal. Some research documents that health care professionals have at least the same level of illicit drug use as the rest of the population (Kunyk, 2015). Anecdotally, many have suggested that the rate of drug addiction, partly due to the ease of access to a multitude of drugs, is much higher among those in health care professions. However, accurate and reliable empirical data on the relation between workplace access to substances and prescription-type drug misuse among nurses or other caregivers are limited. One study, using an anonymous mailed survey, collected data on three dimensions of access: perceived availability, frequency of administration, and degree of workplace control over storage and dispensing of substances. Each dimension was independently associated with increased use (Trinkoff et al., 1999). Based on this research, RNs appear to be more likely than RPNs and PSWs to abuse medications in use in nursing homes because they have direct access to such drugs. This observation may not generalize to the use of alcohol or other medications.

Even if the rates of substance abuse are merely at about the same level as in the general population, there is a safety problem for those who are cared for in hospital or in long-term care (Health Canada, 2014). Because the population-wide rate shows that about one in ten people face some sort of substance abuse problem, one in ten nurses is likely struggling with a substance use disorder. If we expand our concern to the occasional problem of alcohol or substance use at work, the reason for concern grows substantially. For example, more than 39 per cent of Canadians have used cannabis in their lifetimes, and almost 10 per cent used it last year. It would be very difficult to conduct reliable and valid research on the addiction rates of health care providers. It would also be virtually impossible to monitor casual (non-addicted) drug and alcohol use at work in long-term care homes. This type of deviant behaviour is often hidden, and respondents are unlikely to report their own transgressions or those of their co-workers. Regardless of the rates of substance abuse and dependence, only a very small percentage of health care providers is ever apprehended or disciplined. For instance, one study found that approximately one-half of the nurse respondents surveyed reported drug or alcohol use at work, while 40 per cent admitted that it likely had an effect on their ability to do their job competently. More than two-thirds of respondents thought their problem could have been recognized earlier (Cares et al., 2015). Alcohol addiction probably occurs at a comparable or higher rate than in the general population too. This higher rate is likely true in Canada, as in the United States and elsewhere in the developed world. For example, the American Nurses Association estimates that 6 to 8 per cent of nurses use alcohol or drugs to an extent that is sufficient to impair their professional performance (National Council of State Boards of Nursing, 2011). Although the available evidence does not offer a known degree of statistical probability, it suggests that substance use disorders exist at all levels of caregiving in nursing homes. In the absence of thorough and reliable oversight, this issue can amount to a significant problem regarding the safety and well-being of seniors in residence.

## Mental Illness in Staff

Elizabeth Wettlaufer was not alone as a Canadian or as a nurse in having a mental illness. According to statistics from the CAMH, one in five Canadians is diagnosed with mental illness each year (CAMH, n.d.). About 8 per cent of Canadians will experience a major depression at some point in their lives, and 1 per cent will develop bipolar disease during their life. Still, a substantial amount of stigma and discrimination surrounds those with mental health issues. Thus, for example, nearly half of those who say they have experienced depression have not gone to the doctor about it (Canadian Mental Health Association, 2021). Even if the rates of mental illness in long-term care institutions are merely the same as the rates in the population at large, there will inevitably be caregivers with various (treated and untreated) mental health challenges at work. However, due to the difficult work in long-term care with people who may be neglected by their families, demented, physically abusive, and violent, as well as other stressors, mental illness is inevitable and its probability likely enhanced. Again, in the absence of robust monitoring and excellent employee assistance programs designed to intervene and help a troubled caregiver, the actual incidence of mental illness is unknown and largely invisible.

## The Inquiry into Long-Term Care

An inquiry was called into the deaths caused by Elizabeth Wettlaufer in 2017, with Justice Eileen E. Gillese appointed as commissioner (Gillese, 2019). Commissioner Gillese delivered her report in 2019. The scope of the inquiry was the "circumstances and contributing factors allowing these events to occur, including the effect of relevant policies, procedures, practices and accountability and oversight mechanisms" (vol. 4, p. 3). Unfortunately, many of the issues that we have discussed as pertinent to the nursing home deaths were excluded from the report. These issues included staffing levels, funding, the handling of grievances and complaints, union/institution labour relations, the treatment of staff with mental health or addiction issues, and the number of staff in long-term care homes (vol. 3, p. 175).

The inquiry report does, however, point out that serial killing within health care is not unprecedented and "while rare, is longstanding and universal in its reach, with documented cases reaching back to the 1800s" (Gillese, 2019, vol. 1, p. 4). Furthermore, the report emphasized that, since 1970, there have been ninety serial killers within health care who have killed around 450 patients around the world, including in Canada. This figure, according to the report, is most likely an underestimate. According to experts, the real number of people killed is likely more than 2,600 (Pearson, 2021). My point, though, is that this particular serial killer ought to have been discovered long before she was. The reasons that she wasn't discovered are linked to medical systems and practice errors, along with the social determinants of health.

The inquiry report concluded that there were systemic problems that enabled Wettlaufer's murders to go unchecked but no one was to blame. The report argued that the long-term care sector is not broken but strained. It made a number of suggestions for increased support of the system and for prevention, awareness, deterrence, and detection enhancement. In conclusion, the report stated: "There is real significance to my finding that the long-term care system is not broken. Ontario has no need to jettison the existing regulatory system and start over. Instead, we need to identify and acknowledge the strengths of the existing system and build on them. Celebrating the existing areas of excellence in the long-term care system should inspire others in the system to follow suit" (Gillese, 2019, vol. 1, p. 16). The regulatory system may not be broken, but its functioning clearly is.

## Health and the Long-Term Care Sector

Early in 2020, Canada was hit by a pandemic virus called COVID-19. By 10 May, 82 per cent of all deaths in Ontario from COVID-19 were in long-term care (MacCharles, 2020) and possibly as many as 86 per cent in Canada (Loreto, 2020). Serious problems in all long-term care homes were brought to light during the COVID-19 crisis of 2020. The risk of dying from COVID-19 was significantly higher in for-profit homes (Ireton, 2020). In one such home, 37 per cent of the residents died. Only 13 per cent of long-term care patients diagnosed with the virus in Ontario were taken to hospital (Payne, 2020). The significance of ageism needs to be acknowledged, as does the fact that the staff and residents are predominantly female. The undervaluing of women and women's work must be considered. The consequences of both ageism and sexism are evident in Elizabeth Wettlaufer's murders.

One of the most important pieces of information that came to light during the preliminary investigations into the large percentage of deaths in long-term care had to do with inadequate staffing levels and types. The situation in long-term care institutions during the global pandemic was finally seen to be so dire that the Armed Forces were called in to assist in caregiving. The personnel were largely trained nursing officers and medical technicians (Government of Canada, 2020). The military officers warned of severe problems in infection control, standards of practice, supplies, staffing communication, and inappropriate behaviour (Tumility, 2020). These inadequacies were especially noteworthy in for-profit homes.

Many issues have come to light regarding the functioning of long-term care homes since the start of the COVID-19 pandemic, including the fact that they tend to rely on poorly paid part-time staff (for whom they are not required to pay benefits). Due to this part-time work, many staff members are employed at two or more homes in order to make a living wage, which has meant that staff are more likely to spread the virus from home to home. Additionally, long-term care is in a congregate setting. Some people live in double or quadruple rooms. Usually residents eat and socialize together in communal spaces. These features of congregate living increased the transmission of the virus from resident to resident and would do so with any of many contagious diseases.

## Discussion: How Did Medicine Go Awry in the Case of Elizabeth Wettlaufer?

Did medicalization play a part in Elizabeth Wettlaufer's story? Did the social determinants approach help us to understand the accumulated deaths in people under Wettlaufer's care? Yes. Chief among the causes of the errors in this case are both medical system issues and the social determinants of health. Medical system issues can be concentrated primarily on the disproportionate investment in the acute care medical system, with a focus on high-tech and aggressive medicine. This emphasis on high-tech acute care is a part of medicalization. Medicine usurps investments of health care into the acute care system and at the same time undervalues chronic and long-term care, resulting in underinvestment and privatization in this system. Caring has much less prestige and financial support in general and especially in the care of the elderly who, after all, are going to die and not recover from their condition of being terminally old. Indeed, the elderly in long-term care tend to have several overlapping complex chronic conditions for which heroic medicine is unlikely to be of great benefit. Most of them also have some degree of cognitive decline. Even geriatrics, the medical specialty designed to be responsible for diseases of ageing, has relatively low levels of prestige for doctors-in-training and in the field (Meiboom et al., 2015), possibly because the patients cannot be cured. In fact, geriatrics is seen as a boring and slow branch of medicine and, in consequence, is not favoured by doctors-in-training (Robert Wood Johnson Foundation, 2012).

Both ageism and sexism support the relative neglect of people who live in long-term care. These oppressive social and cultural values lead to a relative neglect of the elderly (mostly women). The current social and economic arrangements tend to overemphasize medicine and cure, and encourage an abandonment of the elderly and an underinvestment in their care. Long-term care facilities are not covered by the Canada Health Act. Thus, the quality and quantity of home care institutions is very much a provincial or territorial matter, as is their oversight, support, and regulation. The services offered and the level and types of care included are highly variable. Funding and oversight of long-term care is a polit-ical matter. Overinvestment in the allopathic medical care system and support for its continuing dominance has meant that fund-ing for long-term and home care, the less medicalized options, has been poor. This situation became eminently clear when, in 2020, the vast majority of the deaths in the country during the COVID-19 pandemic occurred among residents of long-term care institu-tions. Elizabeth Wettlaufer was allowed to continue in the system, in part, because of labour force issues. There were and are insuf-ficient numbers of adequately trained staff working or available to work in institutions. The hardship faced by the staff in this situ-ation, characterized by a lack of resources and a duty to care, is called moral distress. Recent research finds that part of caring for elderly people in long-term care, especially those with dementia, is frequent moral distress (Pijl-Zieber et al., 2018). Staff may know that there is a right thing to do, but they do not have the time or the means to do it. This situation is getting worse over time in Canada (Chamberlain et al., 2019) and is continuing to endanger the health and safety of nurses and others working in the sector (Braedley et al., 2018). Rethinking the division of investment so that more money, thinking, and policy development is directed into alter-nate care models in long-term and home care is imperative for the improvement of the lives of elderly Canadians and their family members.

With respect to the social determinants of health, no one who worked at the nursing homes where the elderly people were mur-dered, nor any family and friends of the victims, noticed that the deaths needed investigation during the eight plus years in which they occurred. Wettlaufer's attempts to confess to the murders and assaults were not heeded by her pastor, a lawyer, co-workers, or her friends. Had she not finally admitted to someone who took her seriously and realized the urgency of the situation, people could still be dying unobserved in nursing homes at the hands of Wet-tlaufer. Many of the issues that contributed to that situation and those results continue today. The lack of attention to sudden, pos-sibly unexpected deaths in nursing homes in a society character-ized by an ageing population without adequate resources for the ageing and their families is one that may have unintentionally fostered the invisible deaths.

## Conclusion

Medicalization is evident in the policies that continue to invest in hospital-based care, even for the elderly who do not require high-tech acute care medicine, at the expense of long-term care institutions. The fact that long-term care institutions are largely populated with elderly females supports this underfunding and lack of assiduous regulation and monitoring. That Elizabeth Wettlaufer, as a particular individual, was a nurse experiencing both addiction and mental health issues and a serial killer in health care cannot be ignored. However, the fact that she was not stopped, that she continued to be employed, even after facing a number of different complaints, speaks to many things, but perhaps chiefly to the lack of available staff and the paucity of monitoring and an effective accountability structure. That the residents were generally old and female may have been significant in the ease with which the deaths were ignored.

# chapter seven

# Dr. Norman Barwin: The Story of the Mixed-Up Sperm

## The Issue

The next story of medical error hits very close to home. About sixteen years ago, close friends of my daughter wanted to start their family. They considered their options and decided that they would try to become pregnant using a sperm donor. There were several alternatives to do this. Two of their friends had advertised in the *New York Times* for a known sperm donor who would want to have some involvement in the life of the child, perhaps as an uncle figure or as a more distantly involved father. It worked out, and a gay guy who lived in a different city agreed to become a sperm donor for two children and to have some involvement in their lives as a known donor. This donor takes care of the children about one weekend a month and also takes the children on a holiday every year. In that case, those involved in the arrangement had a written agreement drawn up by a lawyer, which detailed all their rights and responsibilities over time. In another case, a woman acquaintance acquired the semen from a friend who was willing to provide the sperm but did not want any involvement in the life of the child. This arrangement, too, was written into a legal document, which specified the rights and responsibilities of each person. Of course, there are also other options for building a family outside of the conventional and dominant heterosexual model, including adoption.

My daughter's friends decided that they each wanted to give birth to a child. At the time, they lived near Ottawa. They decided to have their children with the sperm from an anonymous donor. They did not want to have to deal with potential problems in case the known sperm donor changed his mind about any aspects of a potential agreement. Thus, they decided to seek insemination with a well-known and seemingly beloved fertility doctor, Dr. Norman Barwin. He was reputed at the time to be a champion of support for lesbian couples and others with fertility issues. He was sometimes called the "baby god" and had received the Order of Canada for his work in this area of medical practice (Motluk, 2019).

The couple who wanted to conceive decided that they would only consider sperm donors who would be willing to meet with their offspring once the child was sixteen or older. Dr. Barwin gave them a number of files of anonymous donors who fit this stipulation and from whom they could choose. They were told that being this specific cut the field of potential donors substantially, but they still had choice. They were able to learn certain things about the socio-demographic characteristics, the health profiles of family members, and the physical size and colouring of the potential donors. After a great deal of happy excitement, they chose a donor and had six vials of sperm put aside. After a couple of attempts, punctuated by two very early but nevertheless very sad miscarriages, one of the women became pregnant, and the pregnancy lasted until she had a perfectly healthy baby girl in 2005. A couple of years later, they returned to Dr. Barwin and asked to use the same sperm donor (which they had asked be saved) to get pregnant. After several unsuccessful tries, there was no more sperm from that same donor. They selected a different donor, again one who had agreed to meet his offspring when the child turned sixteen, if the child desired. Nine months later, another perfectly healthy baby, this time a boy, was born.

Soon after the pregnancy, this couple began to hear rumours of difficulties in the organization of the practice and the files of Dr. Barwin. But they were busy with their two little ones and wonderfully happy because both children seemed to be healthy. The carelessness in the office did not seem to have affected them. However, as their first child grew, she seemed to be growing increasingly different in appearance from the physical characteristics that they had been told typified the sperm donor. For example, she was tall, and the donor had been described as short. Her skin was an olive hue, and her eyes were dark. The donor had been described as fair. They began to doubt that the sperm donor they had selected was their daughter's biological father. They lived with this uncertainty. It was still a long time before their daughter might want to meet her sperm donor.

The stories about Dr. Barwin and errors in his practice grew. It became increasingly implausible that the young girl could be the child of the sperm donor who had been selected. It wasn't until the women were contacted by the law firm developing a class action suit against Dr. Barwin on account of the numerous mistakes he had made that they decided to try to find out whether their information about the donor was correct. The donor was to be determined by matching the sperm donor's identification number with the numbers that were to have been on file in Dr. Barwin's office. Unfortunately, there was no record of either of the donors who had been selected. There would be no genetically linked donor to contact.

## Dr. Barwin: Decades of "Errors" or Intentional Harms?

This story is just one of many stories that emerged from the decades of medical error at the hands of Dr. Barwin. In 1973, the Ottawa General Hospital hired Dr. Barwin, a general practitioner, to manage a high-risk fertility clinic. Dr. Barwin worked very hard and was a progressive, seemingly feminist, practitioner. He undertook numerous initiatives, including developing a sperm bank at the hospital. He left the hospital about a decade later to establish his own practice, where he continued to offer fertility treatments and associated medical services. He was known for his compassion and warmth, as well as for his focus on women's health and fertility issues. On the surface, things seemed to be going well with his work. However, in 1995, Dr. Barwin was sued by a lesbian couple for (allegedly) using the wrong sperm to inseminate one of the women as they built their family. The case was settled out of court in 1998, and there is no record that the College of Physicians and Surgeons of Ontario (CPSO) was informed of it at the time. By settling out of court, Dr. Barwin managed to avoid public scrutiny for many more years (Payne, 2018).

This error, and even earlier egregious ones, finally, after twenty more years, resulted in the revocation of Dr. Barwin's licence to practice as a doctor. The CPSO issued the decision on 25 June 2019 (CPSO, 2019). The Discipline Committee of the CPSO found that Dr. Barwin had engaged in professional misconduct and had failed to maintain the standards of the profession. Furthermore, the Discipline Committee found Dr. Barwin to be "incompetent, disgraceful, dishonorable or unprofessional" (CPSO, 2019).

Dr. Barwin had arrived in Canada and first been licensed in this country in July 1973. As early as the late 1970s, Dr. Barwin had been implicated in making the types of errors that would come to define his work (CPSO, 2019). After doing a thorough investigation in 2018 and 2019, the CPSO documented the first case on its website, which had occurred in 1975–76. In this case, a couple having trouble conceiving went to Dr. Barwin for his help. The husband provided sperm samples for insertion into his wife. Eventually, the woman became pregnant and delivered twins. They were raised with both the parents and the children believing that they were biologically linked. It was not until the family heard about the numerous errors Dr. Barwin had made that they decided to have DNA tests. They then discovered that the twins could not possibly be the offspring of their father. They were able to determine indirectly, through the similarity of their DNA to two young women who had already been genetically linked to Dr. Barwin, that they too were Barwin's offspring. Not only was Dr. Barwin carelessly mixing up sperm samples, willy-nilly, but he was also using his own sperm.

Even though the errors now documented began in the early seventies and there had already been an out-of-court settlement against Barwin, it was not until 2013 that Dr. Barwin was formally accused of mixing up sperm. In this case, three families lodged complaints with the CPSO. The college responded, and Dr. Barwin was disciplined. He was banned from practice for two months (Lindeman, 2019) and fined $3,650 (CPSO, 2019). In response, he resigned from his position as a recipient of the Order of Canada.

There is now a class action lawsuit against Dr. Barwin, signed by over 150 former patients and their families. The suit originated when one of the first plaintiffs, Rebecca Dixon, became suspicious of her parentage after developing celiac disease, a hereditary disease that neither of her parents had. Dixon and her parents investigated further through blood testing, which indicated that her father could not be her biological father, even though his sperm was supposed to have been used to inseminate her mother. This suspicion was confirmed by a DNA test (Motluk, 2017). Another young woman, Kat Palmer, was searching online for half-siblings after learning that she had been conceived using sperm from a donor. Using an ancestry website, she had traced her DNA to a relative of Dr. Barwin, whom she knew as the fertility doctor who had artificially inseminated her mother (purportedly using her known father's sperm). Palmer contacted the clinic to arrange a paternity test, which confirmed that Dr. Barwin was her biological father. Palmer was then introduced to Rebecca Dixon, and further genetic testing showed that the women were half-sisters, confirming that Dixon had also been conceived using Dr. Barwin's sperm.

Many people who were conceived through Barwin's treatments claim that they are the offspring of the wrong sperm donor. In some cases, the doctor was supposed to have used the sperm of the child's father, but the DNA results indicate that the sperm belonged to an unknown person. The wishes of people who clearly chose sperm from a specific sperm donor for any of a variety of reasons were ignored. In several cases, the parents had chosen a sperm donor because he was willing to meet with the child once the child was sixteen years of age, if the child desired. This violation of patient consent also meant that the family had no knowledge of the particular genetic history or forewarning of potential health issues, such as Dixon's celiac disease (Payne, 2018).

Dr. Barwin had been revered because of his focus on infertility and on hormone treatments for trans people long before such interventions were commonplace (DiManno, 2013). However, despite his apparently progressive stance on women's and trans rights, he grossly violated patient consent throughout his career. We have to question the motivations for his work. Indeed, there are other reasons to question Dr. Barwin's sense of appropriate ethical behaviour, as his disregard for fairness and justice extended beyond his clinic. In 2000, Dr. Barwin was censured by the director of the Boston marathon for taking shortcuts during the race and barred from running it again. Just a year later, he was caught cheating at the National Capital Marathon in Ottawa (DiManno, 2013).

Is the case of Dr. Barwin an example of one "bad apple" or a lack of oversight of medical or fertility clinic practice? Or is it both? Dr. Barwin made numerous "mistakes" over many years. Were these "mistakes" unintentional as he has claimed? Dr. Barwin had an explanation for his own sperm leading to the birth of at least sixteen children. He said that contamination of the instruments used in fertilization must have occurred when he used his sperm to calibrate one instrument, one time. The CPSO hired an expert to examine this assertion and determine whether or not this explanation could have possibly been true. The expert said that the doctor's explanation was completely implausible and that insemination with his sperm could not have been the result of such an accidental occurrence.

## What Is the Harm in This Case?

What is the harm done here? All these parents were able to conceive with the help of Dr. Barwin. The children grew up with parents who wanted them, who had needed to take extra steps to conceive and did. These children are all unique people now, for whom their DNA is just one part of their identity. In fact, that was Dr. Barwin's response when he was confronted by Kat Palmer as she, at twenty-two years of age, was asking for records of her sperm donor (Motluk, 2017). When the identification numbers proved to be missing, she asked if he could name the donor sperm banks with which he had worked. He gave her a shortlist, and she checked them all out. None had ever shipped sperm to Dr. Barwin during and around the time of her conception. She was, as an only child, particularly interested in whether or not she had any half-siblings. She tried another tack and registered at the Donor Sibling Registry, an online portal through which, usually using sperm donor identification numbers, siblings can connect with each another. Kat did not have a sperm donor identification number, but she was able through clever investigation to connect with others from Barwin's clinic. None shared her DNA. Then, using a DNA registry and a mention of being conceived at Dr. Barwin's clinic, she was able to find a linkage between her DNA and a third cousin of Barwin's. She emailed Dr. Barwin about her discovery of her DNA link to him and asked for his phone number. By this time, she was beginning to be suspicious that she and the doctor were biologically related. He sent his phone number to her. When she called, he said he had no idea how there could be a biological link with her unless it had to do with the one time he had used his own sperm to calibrate an instrument in his office. She made an appointment to meet Dr. Barwin and ask him directly for information about her heritage. He was willing to meet but apparently responded as if he had no idea about the potential negative impact of his decisions. She said he seemed charming, but he suggested that her search for her sperm donor might be obsessive, because, after all, she was young, healthy, successful, and talented. Later, he did agree to give her a sample of his DNA. The paternity test confirmed that he was her sperm donor. Palmer turned out to be one of his offspring.

As to the question of harm, the above description of Kat Palmer's search indicates that she spent hours and hours of time and years of anguished searching for a connection to half siblings or to a biological inheritance, which characterized just a small part of her suffering. There were and are many negative consequences to the violations of medical practice that resulted from Dr. Barwin's actions. There are layers upon layers and levels of pain ("Barwin's other casualties," 2018). His actions have had an impact most obviously on the offspring who are biologically linked to Barwin himself, as well as on all of their close family members. All those who have discovered this tie (and there may be more who do not know or who have not yet come forward) have to live with the fact that one of their biological parents acted to harm and deceive others in this harm. All of these offspring were betrayed, as were their parents, grandparents, aunts and uncles, and other significant people in their networks of family and friends. This betrayal will have intergenerational effects.

Some offspring whose sperm donor was not the person chosen by their parents and is unknown because of the sloppy records and absence of accurate sperm identification numbers in Dr. Barwin's office may never find their biological parentage or their biological siblings. Some of the parents have worked long and hard to find answers. They have sought and paid for several DNA tests for their children and themselves. Families have searched various DNA websites. Some may have found the donor. Some offspring have found that they have many, many half-siblings or diblings (donor-conceived siblings). Others are still searching for a connection to their DNA. They are living in the liminal spaces of ambiguity. At the CPSO meeting to assess Dr. Barwin's fitness to practise, some of the parents and offspring of mixed-up sperm delivered victim impact statements. One of the people who gave such a statement was a mother who still had not been able to tell her daughter that she was not related to the man whom she had always believed was both her social and biological father. The mother said that Dr. Barwin had assured her the sperm was her husband's before he inseminated her, showing her the vial he said contained her husband's sperm. "I felt so violated, I felt dirty, almost as though I had been raped," she said. I have heard others report that, in retrospect, the insemination felt like a rape. It was a violation of their bodies. It was against their will (Payne, 2019). Another offspring of Barwin, Rebecca Dixon, said that her very self-identity was "thrown into question" when she learned Barwin was her biological father. She said: "I was in shock. Something inside me shifted. It made me feel like my existence was something to be ashamed of." She said she remains challenged by what she now knows about herself. "What does it mean to be related to somebody who is responsible for creating this harm in other people's lives?" she asks. Dixon has waived her right to anonymity because she wants to make it clear that these actions have had a real and human effect. It is important to note that Dr. Barwin is not the only fertility doctor with a record of mistakes. Even as the fertility industry is growing, there are many more examples of calamitous errors (Kirkey, 2016). Furthermore, in the absence of adequate regulation and oversight, such incidents will continue. Below, we will turn to a discussion of the causes of these errors.

Finally, in 2021, decades after Dr. Barwin's abuse of his power and skill began, there was a settlement in the class action case against Dr. Barwin. All of those named in the settlement were to share 13.3 million dollars (Payne, 2021).

## How Could This Have Happened and for So Long?

### The Power Differential between Doctors and Patients

How could this have happened? How could a man who seemingly has deceived and betrayed his patients by using either his own or the wrong sperm during artificial insemination over so many years continue to do so without patients' awareness? How could he have come to have such a sterling reputation? Apparently, his social and communication skills were excellent. He was considered to be a warm and empathetic practitioner. His interpersonal style did not raise any concerns; in fact, his very cordiality may have spared him from scrutiny and earlier punishment. His reputation as a progressive leader in the field of women's reproductive health, demonstrated by his executive positions in Planned Parenthood and his early care of trans people, could have shielded him from critical eyes. Certainly, his receiving the Order of Canada would have buttressed the esteem in which he was held. The very fact that he was a doctor, a member of a well-regarded professional group, would also have insulated Dr. Barwin from suspicion.

Conventional allopathic medical practitioners have long been considered to be members of the archetypical profession (Friedson, 1988). Medical professionalism is linked to highly desired and respected characteristics such as altruism, "decency, integrity and honesty," as well as the "skill, knowledge and judgment" appropriate to the demands of practice (CPSO, n.d.-d).

As professionals, conventional medical doctors have been granted, by the state, considerable financial wherewithal relative to the average person in the country and most likely in comparison to their patients (Statistics Canada, 2016). For example, the average gross clinical payment in Canada to family medicine physicians during 2016–17 was $277,000. The average gross clinical payment per medical specialist was $357,000, and the average per surgical specialist was $477,000 (CIHI, 2019). As of September 2017, the average wage for Canadian employees was $986 per week – or just over $51,000 per year (Workopolis, 2017). In Ontario, the province with the highest minimum wage, the hourly payment is only $14.00 (Retail Council of Canada, 2019).

Once certified and licensed, doctors have a great deal of autonomy and independence to practise as they will. This freedom may especially be the case with solo general practitioners. Solo practitioners, such as Dr. Barwin, lack some of the potential normative pressures that may affect those working in clinics or with one or more partners. General practitioners may also lack the constraints under which specialists work. Specialists are monitored indirectly by their peers because they are dependent on referrals and hospital access for their work. Although guided by legislation and educated to very high standards in medical schools across Canada and elsewhere, doctors essentially police themselves through bodies dominated by medical practitioners and not citizens. This arrangement is partly because the nature of the knowledge base upon which practising physicians work is somewhat esoteric. Doctors are educated over many years in universities and then undergo a form of apprenticeship when they work as interns. During these years, they learn not only the medical subjects and approach to practice but also the operating norms of different medical communities. Medical practice is, after all, both a science and an art. It is based both on intuition – good informed guesses – and evidence from double-blind scientific studies described in evidence-based sites, as well as on normatively derived guidelines in action. One of the clearest examples of this duality, and one that we have discussed earlier, is the accepted prescription of off-label pharmaceuticals. It is widely viewed as standard to prescribe drugs on the basis of opinion, informal discussion, and physician community norms. That is, drugs, as we discussed in Chapter 3, are sometimes acceptably used experimentally, off-label.

There is a power imbalance between doctors and their patients. The esoteric knowledge and social distance (Turner, 2012) provide doctors will a special status; as Clarke (2016) points out, "the fundamental characteristic of a profession is the ability of the group to impose its perspective and the necessity of its services upon its clients" (p. 282). This status is partly due to the actual complexity and quantity of the medical information held by the physician about the conditions/diagnoses/signs/symptoms of the patient but also because of the many protections held by doctors. Patients are usually alone in the medical consultation (although they may at times be accompanied by family or friends), while the doctor has office or hospital staff to act as a line of defence against access. Doctors have an arcane language that the average patient does not speak. They are protected by their presumed professionalism and the assumption that they have sworn an ethical oath that they maintain. A social distance between doctors and patients often exists. The power differential between doctors and their patients is likely greater when the doctor is male and the patient is female. There is a significant wage gap between men and women in Canada; women make 75 cents per dollar of the average income of men for full-time work (Canadian Women's Foundation, 2018). Indeed, the gender pay gap among Canadian male and female doctors is twice the international average (Grant, 2016).

## The "Bad Apple" Doctor

I have argued that a dramatic change has taken place in the conceptualization of medical error. In the past, error was seen as infrequent and anomalous. If it occurred, it was thought to be the result of a particular individual who was uniquely incompetent, careless, or unethical. Now, the idea of medical error is most often associated with poor systems design or implementation. Most problems, this theory holds, can be eradicated through an emphasis on the design of the system as a whole. The focus on errors as systems problems has had a lot of benefits. For instance, checklists to ensure hand washing before entering a new patient room have been instrumental in the decrease in the spread of infection from patient to patient. However, there are situations in which it is also important to pay attention to the problem individual. There are personalities in the health care system who are or behave as "bad apples" (Shojania & Dixon-Woods, 2013). Some doctors and nurses tend to be repeat offenders. A study of patient complaints in Australia found, for example, that 3 per cent of the medical personnel were responsible for almost half (49 per cent) of the problems, and further, that 1 per cent were responsible for 25 per cent of all patient grievances (Shojania & Dixon-Woods, 2013). Parallel findings have been noted in other research. Together, these studies suggest that a small number of doctors may be recurrent offenders who need to be identified. Concentrating on the very few doctors who are particularly careless and have mental and other health or substance abuse disorders, for example, may go a long way towards increasing patient safety. Focusing on and supporting these doctors as much as possible, on a case-by-case basis, is a necessary intervention, although not a sufficient correction.

Shojania and Dixon-Woods (2013) found that, in 97 per cent of 280 cases studied, the doctor had caused patient harm on more than one occasion, and in 99 per cent of the cases, the doctor had intended to cause harm. Of the cases, 95 per cent were caused by male doctors working in practices in which 89 per cent lacked oversight. The vast majority (95 per cent) were in non-academic settings. More than half of the cases involved a doctor with serious issues such as personality disorders or substance abuse problems. There were no obvious warnings of danger or of problematic practice standards, "no red flags" (p. 16). Yet, there were numerous documented patient harms. While from one point of view, such abuses are rare, another view holds that "documented cases are approximately as common as new incidences of breast cancer and far more common than HIV, and we know that cases of violations are significantly underreported" (Dubois et al., 2019). This research, then, suggests the value of assuming that there will be "bad apples" or repeat offenders in any system and planning accordingly.

## What Were the Systems Level Causes of These Medical "Errors" and How Can They Be Prevented?

### Oversight and Monitoring of Practising Doctors

The first system level problem is the organization of the medical system that allowed this harm to happen and to happen over decades. The regulation and monitoring of medical practice within a medical culture in which doctors have considerable autonomy and are expected to police themselves is complex. Although the egregious errors or intentional harms we now know about began in the early 1970s, it was not until 2013 that families complained to the CPSO about sperm mix-ups (Lindeman, 2019). In response, Dr. Barwin was banned from practice for two months and given a small fine of less than $4,000 (CPSO, 2019). His harmful behaviour continued. It was not until June 2019 that the CPSO finally seriously chastised Dr. Barwin for using his own and the wrong sperm to impregnate women in his clinic. His medical licence was revoked, and he was asked to pay a fine of $10,730 within thirty days of the judgement at his disciplinary hearing (Canadian Press, 2019). While the permanent retraction of his medical licence is an appropriate remedy, I think we need to ask questions about the small fines Dr. Barwin was asked to pay in each case. We need to question whether such small fines are in any way a deterrent in the case of a medical practitioner's probable salary level. The CPSO, as the medical regulator of the province, has a major goal to "provide guidance to Ontario physicians on professionalism and issues relevant to the practice of medicine" (CPSO, n.d.-b). Its primary duty is to ensure that members of the profession are competent in the areas in which they practise (CPSO, n.d.-c).

The CPSO does undertake regular and random assessments of doctors. Its website, under the section directed at doctors, states that the "CPSO has a legislated mandate to ensure quality care is provided by physicians" (CPSO, n.d.-e). The college has a number of potential remedies if it finds the evaluated doctor to be inadequate in any way. These remedies include support and training for improvement but also, ultimately, allow for the possibility of turning to remedies under schedule 2, section 80.2, of the Regulated Health Professions Act for doctors whose practice continues to be inadequate (CPSO, n.d.-a). In that case, possible remedial action may include further education, limits on practice, or disclosure of the name of the doctor to the Inquiries, Complaints and Reports Committee (ICRC) if the Quality Assurance Committee believes that the individual under assessment is incompetent, incapacitated, or has committed an act of professional misconduct. There are also specialist organizations. It must be noted, however, that these rules are not consistent across the country. Furthermore, this inconsistency underscores the fact that, at any time, there will be doctors practising who are incompetent, incapacitated, or fail to fulfil their professional obligations. These are doctors who have not yet been assessed, doctors regarding whom reports of complaints may not have been received, or doctors who have otherwise managed to fly under the radar of investigation.

The other body that offers ongoing support to and monitors the work of doctors is the Canadian Medical Protective Association (CMPA). It provides legal defence, liability protection, and risk management education for Canadian doctors, as well as compensation for patients harmed by negligent practice (see https:// www.cmpa-acpm.ca/en/home). While it is not officially an insurance company, the CMPA charges annual fees, which depend on the professional group's level of risk. Those specialties that are more likely to be sued pay higher annual membership dues. The CMPA invests these annual fees and financially supports doctors who have been sued in cases that it thinks are defensible. In this way, it seems to act as an insurance company.

It should also be noted that there is no record of any of Dr. Barwin's staff reporting any questions or concerns about his practice over the years. It is not clear how much staff member(s) might have known about or contributed to the carelessness in record-keeping or the unhappy patients, such as those who settled out of court in 1998. The role of staff as potential whistle-blowers of incompetent or malfeasant behaviour needs to be clarified.

## The Regulation of Fertility Clinics

Fertility issues are growing in Canada. As many as one in six couples have difficulties with conception (Government of Canada, 2019); 16 per cent of women have difficulty conceiving. The current rate of infertility (defined as unable to get pregnant after six months of trying for women under thirty-five and after one year of trying for women over forty) is double the rate recorded in the 1980s. This increase could be a measurement artefact resulting from more women being willing to come forward to admit to the problem due to greater public knowledge of options available for those who are infertile. It could also be an artefact of more assiduously kept records. For our purposes, the increased rate indicates that more people than ever before are trying to conceive through fertility interventions. There are numerous fertility clinics across the country, both private and public (Government of Canada, 2013). In 2017, thirty-six clinics initiated 33,092 in vitro fertilization (IVF) cycles (Canadian Fertility and Andrology Society, 2018). Many other procedures, however, are undertaken in fertility clinics, and as new technologies develop and spread, additional treatments will be offered. Consequently, the potential for problems such as the ones we are discussing is large. There have been attempts to oversee and manage this new technology, but they have faced both legal and political impediments. For instance, the bill that was passed by the federal government to regulate fertility clinics, the Assisted Human Reproduction Act, was overturned in 2010 because of a Supreme Court challenge (Scotti, 2016). The court successfully argued that the federal act was overstepping its limits because health care is under provincial jurisdiction. As it stands, the provision of fertility services varies from province to province. More or fewer services are covered in different provincial jurisdictions through the federal

Medicare system. The amount of coverage, the numbers of fertility clinics, and other aspects of this service differ across provinces. The regulations, too, are uneven. The federal government has stepped in where it can and is developing regulations for egg and sperm donation (Government of Canada, 2020). However, fertility clinics face uneven oversight, and users have to do diligent research in a situation where the knowledge may not be available. Fertility enhancement and intervention is a multibillion-dollar industry that is inadequately regulated (Payne, 2018). Could the dreadful results from Dr. Barwin's clinic have been prevented? A series of new standards has been adopted to regulate the work of doctors and clinics, and other new regulations are under construction (Canadian Fertility and Andrology Society, n.d.). These standards will help to ensure that the government of Canada through the relevant medical colleges has more jurisdiction over the storage of eggs and sperm, the screening of sperm donors, and the accuracy of information about donors and recipients. Under the new regulations, sperm would be tested for a variety of diseases and even checked to make sure it reflects the DNA of the specific sperm donor identified. Doctors who use their own sperm or mixed-up sperm, therefore, could in the future be criminally charged. However, there are ongoing debates about jurisdiction (Cattapan et al., 2019). One obvious limitation to the legislation is that it is restricted to Canada, and reproductive technologies are increasingly being used in a transnational manner. A great deal of the sperm used in Canada, for instance, comes from the United States. The introduction of new technologies always or almost always precedes the policy framework to manage the new technologies. Further, there is a need to always strike a balance between supporting innovation and ensuring safety or mitigating risk (OECD, n.d.)

## Discussion: How Did Medicine Go Awry in the Case of Dr. Norman Barwin?

The immediate cause of medical error in this case seems to be a serious flaw in the moral compass of this individual doctor. He was publicly praised as a progressive leader in women's rights to health care, in particular, sexual and reproductive health. He was a leader in his attention to transgender people as well. He had been called the "baby god" because of his advocacy for fertility treatment for those who wanted to conceive using medical help. He was often described as warm and compassionate. Despite all of these accolades and strengths, Dr. Barwin wreaked enormous harm on hundreds of people through his ethical vacuum, his carelessness, and his profound betrayal of numerous patients. His ignorance of the needs of others indicated a warped ethical code. The intermittent, or lack of, oversight by his peers reflect organizational inadequacies of the medical system. An explanation is needed as to why his staff did not report potential and noticeable problems, and remedies must be put in place to enable staff members to "whistle blow" without fear of retribution.

Part of the larger context of this case is that of new technologies, which are often introduced before there is sufficient training, planning, or policy. Such innovations can shift the level of education and training required, even while access to the new training is not available. Thus, health care professionals may be caught in a situation in which they are using new equipment even though they lack enough information and practise to do so safely or beneficially. New technology may, at times, require new specialties. It is also a case in which the inevitable degree of autonomy and privacy under which doctors work, especially those in solo practice, should be questioned. Additionally, an absence of sufficient legislation guiding the use of new reproductive technologies may make practitioners particularly vulnerable to slipshod work habits.

The social determinants of health appear to have also played a role in these medical errors in that the immediate subject of the medical intervention was a female who was being inseminated or impregnated by a male doctor. Even though more women are entering medical school across the country in Canada today, the practitioners of medicine and the power brokers in the medical establishment tend to be male, which may have influenced the attitudes of Dr. Barwin towards his patients. Thus, these errors may reflect the gendered nature of medical power and the role of women as reproducers of the species. Indeed, the relative social and economic power of doctors as compared to both the average male and, even more clearly, the average female may have played an underlying but nevertheless important role in the freedom Dr. Barwin felt to continue violating his medical oath. The fact that individual victims did not take their cases to the highest authority, the CPSO, may be related to the respect within which doctors tend to be held in Canada.

## Conclusion

The case of Dr. Barwin points to medicalization in the sense that people readily define infertility as a medical or biological problem that should be solved through intervention at the biological level. People make this choice rather than that of adoption, choosing to live childless, or accepting life as a childless person. The lack of regular monitoring of medical practices is another significant problem in this case. There are also the inevitable problems with new and emerging technologies and specialties developed and introduced before new regulations are in place. The "bad apple theory" fits here. Dr. Barwin did not make just one error. Instead, he maintained an unethical stance towards his patients and failed repeatedly to honour the contracts he made with them. Dr. Barwin's gender and that of most of his clients may be another factor that allowed him to think such egregious behaviour was acceptable, illustrating the role of the social determinants of health in this case. His gender may also have played a role in people burying their suspicions over many years. As in the other cases, error is the result of cultural, social, and medical system errors.

# Conclusion

Medical error is a frequent cause of death, illness, and suffering around the world. Yet for most of the modern history of medicine, medical error has been largely invisible as a cause of death or other distress. When error occurred, it was considered to be anomalous. It was thought to be infrequent. Its measurement is not part of official statistical death reports. In Canada, the United States, and elsewhere in the developed world, causes of death are registered using the World Health Organization's International Statistical Classification of Disease and Related Health Problems (Makary & Daniel, 2016). This code does not include deaths caused by human and system factors such as medical errors.

Thus, there is an absence of official statistics regarding errors that could be used as benchmarks for identification, measurement, or improvement over time. Recently, a number of governments and medical and other organizations have attempted to develop ways to estimate various error rates. There are now many different efforts to approximate the breadth of types of medical errors and their varieties of consequences. The pre-eminent *British Medical Journal* (*BMJ*) published an article that reviewed and assessed a range of different methods for appraising rates of medical error in the United States (Makary & Daniel, 2016). The authors assessed the ratings and concluded that error is the third leading cause of death in hospital. This estimate has been fairly robust across developed countries in recent times. It is noteworthy, however, that these accident figures only include deaths that occur in hospital. They do not include deaths in outpatient offices, clinics, communities, or even long-term care institutions. Official statistics in Canada do not systematically record hospital-based deaths by medical error at all (Statistics Canada, 2020). However, rates similar to the US rates of inadvertent hospital-based deaths have been projected (Finlay, 2015). Neither accidental death nor disability rates for outpatients are recorded in Canada, which makes the overall medical error rates for Canada opaque, impossible to estimate accurately, and underestimated.

Error related to medical treatment became visible in North America in 2000 with the publication of *To Err Is Human* in the United States. This "outing" of medical error as a serious problem resulted in a new and vigorous acknowledgment that the policies and programs in place to manage error had been based on a faulty assumption: that medical error was effectively non-existent. This previous presumption had resulted in a private and small-scale punishment model, also known as the "blame and shame" perspective. In this model, the individual perpetrator of a particular error would be singled out, blamed, and shamed if the adverse event drew notice in the first place. Many, even most, errors were invisible or ignored. After the publication of the report, attention was paid to making errors noticeable and measurable. They were to be considered as a normal cost of medical care and inevitable within the medical care system. This shift in focus resulted in health policy interventions that adopted a systems approach to error identification and diminishment. For example, checklists were developed to ensure that all tools were removed after surgery, and educational campaigns were undertaken promoting handwashing by health care providers. These strategies have made a positive difference, but they have not led to the elimination of error.

The argument of this book extends beyond both the blame and shame and the systems perspectives to demonstrate that medical error will continue to be inevitable and grow further both inside and outside of hospital settings given the relentless and increasing processes of medicalization. This inevitable increase in medical errors is taking place because medicalization expands the definition of what areas of life are relevant to medicine. Medical-ization is associated with a growth of consciousness, beliefs, and behaviours that are considered to be germane to the jurisdiction of medicine (Conrad, 2005). Medicalization's growing relevance to more and more aspects of social life is accompanied by a ready and uncritical acceptance of medicine. Medicine is assumed to be of value for both physical and mental health. Accepting and adopting the dominant allopathic medical model of care and cure is presumed to be fundamental to good citizenship and societal progress. I argue that, while there are innumerable beneficial effects of modern medicine, particularly in the case of acute dis-tress, we need to stay alert to the reality that medicine can also cause harm. Medicine's spread has many negative consequences. The primary threat of medicalization is that it obfuscates the potential problems in the science and practice of the individualiz-ing medical paradigm. It also works to suppress awareness of and investment in community-based solutions to issues. It obscures the powerful potential of health production that would result from attention to mitigating the inequities and oppression evident in the social determinants of health.

This book is based on case studies of medically caused suffer-ing and death. These cases of medical error illustrate and explain the importance of challenging medicalization and being aware of the five fundamental sources of limitations in our everyday use of medical care. Throughout the chapters of this book, I demonstrate the need to understand the inherent, thus unavoidable, limits of (1) medical science, (2) medical practice, (3) medical systems, and (4) pharmaceuticalization. We also need to comprehend how medi-cal error is related to (5) the social determinants of health. In the first place, the social determinants of health powerfully predict the social patterning and the prevalence of disease. They predict the accessibility and acceptability of the medical care system. The social determinants of health also affect the ways in which the sys-tem operates and is organized. As an example, not only are the poor more likely to suffer disease and disability and need care, but they may also be discriminated against because of their poverty as they interact with health care practitioners.

In the next section of this conclusion, I will highlight a few of the most important limitations operating within each case examined. This conclusion is meant as a succinct reminder of the cases and the complex causes of medical errors. After discussion of the cases, I will return to the larger question about what can be done to begin remedying medical error.

## Brian Sinclair

The first case is that of Brian Sinclair, the Indigenous man who died after waiting for thirty-four hours in an emergency room (ER) in a major Winnipeg hospital. He was in the ER because he had a serious but easily treated bladder infection. This infection need not have happened if the home care that was ostensibly in place for Mr. Sinclair had provided the service that was supposed to have occurred. It could have been prevented through the provision of routine hygiene help. Once at the hospital, had he been seen promptly, in the order in which he was supposed to have been triaged, his infection would have been easily managed with antibiotics. Mr. Sinclair would not have been in the hospital at all if he had not been homeless on a cold night in Winnipeg and lost his legs due to freezing temperatures.

In this case, both medical system issues and failures in the social determinants of health contributed to his death. The medical system issues included the lack of adequate home care and the subsequent reliance on an exceptionally busy emergency room. The fact that the staff in charge of the ER did not have clear sight lines to the waiting room was a design problem. Although the nurses had complained, their concerns had not resulted in change, which reflects on the relative lack of power of nurses within the health care system. The overinvestment in costly hospitals and underinvestment in community services, including shelters, reflects the dominance of a medicalized perspective as compared to a social determinants perspective. The everyday use of the ER as a shelter from the cold for poor and disadvantaged people due to a lack of alternatives contributed to Mr. Sinclair's death. The nurses who cared about the indigent First Nations people and others who used the ER, and showed this care by encouraging them to use the space and offering them food and drink, also played a role in Brian Sinclair's death. This very same entrenched benign racism may have led the staff to think Mr. Sinclair was just seeking shelter, and therefore they overlooked Mr. Sinclair's growing distress as he sat in the identical position in his wheelchair over many hours.

## Ashley Smith

The second case is the death of nineteen-year-old Ashley Smith in a federal prison for women. Ashley had been institutionalized essentially from the time she was fifteen years of age because of her norm-violating behaviours and her emotional and mental functioning. She was diagnosed and treated for a number of different and often-contradictory mental illnesses during her time in custody. She spent most of her time in solitary confinement because neither the custodial staff nor the health care providers who were responsible for Ashley could understand, help, or control her. She was tasered, pepper sprayed, and wrapped as punishment. Ashley's case asks us to examine the importance of concepts such as the limits of medical science and medical practice in the face of confusion and uncertainty regarding a diagnosis. These limits are evident in the changing and contradictory diagnoses Ashley Smith received. Medical error is also apparent in the use, despite the lack of assurance concerning validity and reliability, of toxic and sometimes dangerous treatments. Ashley's experiences reflect the imperfect validity and reliability of mental health diagnoses. The case also reflects an aspect of the social determinants of health. That the best option for a teenager who was acting out and causing problems was institutionalization, with a combined medical, punishment, and rehabilitation function, indicates the lack of publicly financed alternative, non-medicalized care for struggling children and adolescents. This case also illustrates the powerful effects of multiple sources of oppression that are possible when uncertain medical diagnosis is the basis for hazardous treatments used as punishment. In this case, we also witness another social determinant factor via the impact of the intersection of power, medicine, brutality, and sexism in prison. Prison guarding is a male-dominated occupation (Correctional Service of Canada, 2015). The predominance of men in prison guard roles in institutions for women may place women prisoners at a higher vulnerability of experiencing sexism and may have sown the seeds for the sexual and other assaults on Ashley Smith.

The Ashley Smith case provides other examples of the limitations in the organization of the medical system. It demonstrates the potentially dangerous and fatal consequences of the lack of integrated care between the community and institutionalization. Furthermore, Ashley was sent from one mental health professional to another and from one institution to another to no avail. There was no one person monitoring Ashley's situation over the duration of the time she was in custody other than, to the limited extent that they were able from a distance, her parents.

## Vanessa Young and Marit McKenzie

Vanessa Young died suddenly at age sixteen after taking a prescribed medication to help prevent vomiting after eating. She was under the care of four doctors at the time, including specialists, and had been taking the pills for about a year. None of the doctors, or the pharmacist who dispensed the medication, advised her against taking this medication. It was, however, specifically contraindicated by several characteristics of Vanessa Young, including her age. To underscore the issues raised above, the case of Marit McKenzie is examined in this chapter as well. Marit McKenzie also died of a reaction to a legitimately prescribed, off-label, medication. Marit had minor acne, but the drug was to be used only for serious acne. She had been on the drug for about a year, although it was indicated to be taken only for a short period of time. These two cases exemplify the importance of pharmaceuticalization issues, in particular off-label prescribing and the lack of sufficient postmarket surveillance. Among the numerous other medical system and pharmaceutical use issues are the relationship between Health Canada and the pharmaceutical industry, and the relative wealth and power of that industry around the world. Medical practice issues are fundamental, including the responsibilities of doctors and pharmacists for knowing about and properly explaining the side effects of various medications.

Furthermore, the social determinants of health played a key role in the deaths of these two young women. These cases highlight the dangers of aspirational medicine. Both Vanessa Young and Marit McKenzie died as the result of prescribed drugs that they may have been using in part because of gender beauty norms. Vanessa apparently had a mild case of vomiting after meals, possibly because of bulimia based on a desire to be slim. Marit's medication may have been used to improve her complexion and, again, to make her a more "attractive" young woman according to beauty norms of the day (Swami et al., 2010). The fact that they were young women may have influenced the careless prescribing of these medications by the doctors (Centre of Excellence for Women's Health, 2015; Morgan, n.d.).

## Amy Tan

The fourth case is that of Amy Tan, who had been living, for more than two decades, with Lyme disease, an illness that for many years had been undiagnosed despite a raft of increasingly serious, changing, and baffling symptoms. It took numerous different doctors and laboratory tests before she was able to get a diagnosis. As is typical with many "new" diseases, it was the Lyme patient, Amy Tan, who was the first person to realize that she had Lyme disease. This chapter illustrates the ironic and potentially harmful effects of medicalization in the case of new and emerging diseases, particularly when patients are the first to observe a new constellation of symptoms. It discusses the problems of diagnoses in diseases first identified by patients, who are then not taken seriously or not believed because their symptoms do not fit textbook models. It suggests one of the limitations of relying only on evidence-based medicine. The chapter also illustrates some limitations in the how the medical system is organized into specialties, which are often based on specific groups of organs, even though chronic and multisystem diseases (across different organ systems at the same time) occur and need diagnosis and treatment. The subjectivity of medical science and practice, and the way that politics and culture infuse medicine, is suggested by the fact that one group of specialists accepted the reality of Lyme, and then chronic Lyme, while other doctors in other locations and specialties repudiated the reality of the condition. The costliness of chronic treatment, coupled with the disputes among various medical specialties, governmental bodies, and health insurance companies, are all issues related to the political and economic ramifications of medical systems under the unquestioned umbrella of medicalization.

The social determinants of health perspective offers additional insight into the medical errors experienced by Amy Tan. For example, Amy Tan's case of Lyme disease might have been recognized earlier had she been male. The evidence suggests that men are less likely to go to doctors than women (Franks & Bertakis, 2003) but they tend to have their symptoms taken more seriously (Wang et al., 2013). However, the fact that Amy Tan was relatively well off meant she could travel from doctor to doctor and pay for different tests. Because she was also relatively well educated and intelligent meant she could relentlessly pursue a diagnosis in the face of contradictory and potentially confusing and discouraging information from different health care providers.

## Dr. Charles Smith

The fifth case is that of Dr. Charles Smith. He was a paediatric forensic pathologist who worked at the Hospital for Sick Children (SickKids) in Toronto. He was responsible for at least a dozen wrongful convictions due to medical errors he made and then attested to as an expert witness in court. We discussed the cases of two wrongfully convicted Indigenous men, William Mullins-Johnson and Richard Brant, in some depth. Dr. Smith had argued that twelve children had died as a result of child abuse. These errors resulted in the lengthy incarceration of innocent parents and caregivers, which had powerful effects not only on those held criminally responsible but also on the family and friends involved with the children who died. The explanations for this series of errors can be found in many medical system limitations. The Dr. Charles Smith case reflects the potential problems of subjectivity or bias in the practice of medicine. It illustrates a way that culture permeates medical practice and may lead to errors. Dr. Smith was practising as a paediatric forensic pathologist at a time when the whole culture demonstrated a reinvigorated concern about the dangers and prevalence of invisible child abuse and sexual abuse (Jenkins, 1998). Smith and his colleagues and supervisors at SickKids seemed to have internalized these cultural emphases and appeared to work to identify more such cases. Additionally, the Dr. Smith case exposes labour force issues in medicine. Medical specialties have continually been expanding over time with sometimes problematic consequences. For example, the definition of the parameters and titles of new specialties may not always be met with an adequately trained labour force of sufficient numbers for practice in the newly designated specialty. Consequently, at any one time, members of new and evolving specialties may be insufficiently prepared for the tasks they are expected to undertake. Furthermore, medical practice in general is not always subject to adequate oversight and monitoring on an ongoing basis, which allows doctors who are making mistakes to remain unobserved over periods of time. The particulars of the lack of monitoring deployed within the paediatric forensic unit at SickKids at the time also played a role in the faulty decisions that led to so many wrongful convictions.

## Elizabeth Wettlaufer

The sixth case documents the murders of eight people in long-term care by their nurse, Elizabeth Wettlaufer. Wettlaufer killed these eight people over a number of years. During this time period, she had confessed to a number of people about what she had done, including her minister, a lawyer, a friend, a student nurse, and a co-member of a Narcotics Anonymous group. Wettlaufer had received ten workplace violations and multiple suspensions over her years of employment as a nurse, but she still kept her job. None of the family members of those who died under her care had ever asked serious questions or demanded answers about why their loved ones had died unexpectedly.

This case is examined from the perspective of the under-resourcing of chronic and long-term care under medicalization, as well as from the standpoint of issues related to the social determinants of health. The overemphasis on high-tech and allopathic medicine within the functioning of the medical care system is associated with insufficient concern for the health care of the elderly and others who may need frequent and sustained assistance. Support of the acute care medical system comes at a cost to those who need chronic care and even long-term institutionalized aid. Labour force issues are evident in that there was a lack of monitoring of Elizabeth Wettlaufer's work and a failure to act on repeated workplace errors. Insulin was so taken for granted as a benign medication that it was not supervised. It was this casual use of a pharmaceutical that killed eight nursing home residents without any remark or notice until Wettlaufer herself confessed.

There are also social determinants of health issues raised by this case. The fact that the people who died unexpectedly were all elderly may also reflect the discrimination and devaluing of the life of the elderly in Canada (Revera Inc. & Sheridan Centre for Elder Research, 2016; Ontario Human Rights Commission, n.d.). According to the Ontario Human Rights Commission, ageism is one of the most socially acceptable forms of discrimination and is reflected both in individual interactions and in system organizations (Ontario Human Rights Commission, n.d.). The Elizabeth Wettlaufer case may illustrate ageism in that no one was suspicious when these elderly people died suddenly and unexpectedly. COVID-19 exposed the understaffed and overcrowded nature of long-term care homes because the majority of Canadians who died of the pandemic disease lived within their walls.

# Dr. Norman Barwin

The seventh and final case is that of Dr. Norman Barwin, the doctor, working as a fertility specialist, who betrayed the trust of many of his patients by using his own sperm and the sperm of random other donors, including some with serious illnesses such as cancer, to impregnate women who had sought his help with artificial insemination. This harmful and unprofessional activity occurred over forty years of practice. It was not until he had been working in this unethical and immoral manner for more than twenty years that there is any record of anyone realizing or acting on his deception. He was sued for using the wrong sperm. This suit was settled out of court, and there is no record of a report of any wrongdoing to the regulating College of Physicians and Surgeons of Ontario (CPSO) until 2013. He was then reported for mixing up sperm, suspended for two months, and fined $3,650 by the college. A few years later, two young women discovered, after much anguish and searching, that they were related through their DNA and that their DNA matched that of Dr. Barwin. There is a recently settled class action lawsuit of more than 13 million dollars against Dr. Barwin (Pfeffer, 2021). The money will be divided among the plaintiffs. Seventeen people, called "Barwin babies," are related by DNA to the doctor. Many others are not able to find their sperm donor because of the negligent record-keeping in the doctor's office. There are more than 200 people whose names are on the suit. The resulting settlement amount was negotiated, which means that Dr. Barwin did not admit that he was guilty.

This case is examined from the perspective of the "bad apple" doctor in an under-regulated system. It is noted that, while the CPSO is the official body charged with oversight, there are severe limitations to its ability or its commitment to fulfil this function. The CPSO is responsible for monitoring medical practice in Ontario, but doctors are only accountable to themselves. There are particular challenges to regulating in a situation in which new technologies and new specialist practices are developing. The challenges related to the enforcement of strong laws in a situation in which provinces are responsible for their own programs and policies in regard to health care provision are also discussed.

There are also social determinants of health issues raised by this case. Those who were harmed were already among the more vulnerable due to their gender, gender identity and sexual orientation, and frequently LGBQ+ status, which may have played a role both in the betrayal and in the lack of proactive complaint in the face of dubious outcomes. That the social and economic status of doctors is greater than that of the average Ontarian may also have played a role in these egregious behaviours and in why they continued unchecked for so many years.

## What Can Be Done?

This book has argued that medical error is inevitable and predictable given our current social arrangements, which include the overwhelming acceptance of the discourses of medicine that characterize medicalization. Each of the case studies illustrates several of the ways that the inherent limits of medical science, medical practice, the organization of the medical care system, pharmaceutical use, and/or the social determinants of health reinforce and contribute to medical error.

This analysis raises many questions. What are the implications of these findings for the future of health and health care? Is error inevitable? Are the documented issues too big to handle? What will happen if we continue to ignore these challenges? What can each of us do to ameliorate this problem? Each case raises different as well as overlapping concerns about social forces within and outside of the health care system. There are numerous social changes and innovations in policies and programs that could be considered in answer to these questions. The discussion of these possible solutions could easily fill another book. Instead, I conclude with an attempt to offer some reflections on the significance of a couple of policy changes for the mitigation of large-scale or population-based error. I very briefly emphasize the value of addressing the social determinants of health and discuss some individual initiatives in which we can

all engage. I end by selecting and briefly explaining just three significant innovations that derive from what we have learned from
the cases in this book about the causes of medical error.

## Examples of Political and Health Policy Changes: Prevention/ Early Detection, Valid Diagnoses, and Pharmaceutical Regulation

Let's think for a moment now about what can or might be done
about the situations documented. How is it possible to minimize
medical error? There are a number of levels of analysis, a number of possible directions for change to consider. Medicine is supported and its jurisdiction is expanded at the widest level through
the political system. In Canada, and in most of the developed
world with the notable exception of the United States, medicine
is a public good. It is therefore paid for largely through tax dollars. Idealistically speaking then, this structure means that we,
the citizens of Canada, need to ask questions of our political can-
didates about the benefits and the efficacy of medicine. We need
to demand answers to questions about, for instance, how reliable
and valid (over the short, medium, and long-term) the research
establishing diagnoses and treatments is before we are willing to
undergo medical intervention. We need to find a way to have our
voices heard when we experience changing symptoms in multiple
organs. We need to measure errors and set ourselves on a course to
their eradication. We need to ask about the potential health costs of
universal pharmacare in a situation lacking adequate safeguards
and monitoring. Individual initiative is necessary to demand systemic change in the medical system. We also need to embark on
continuing serious critiques of the way that we have come to turn
to and frequently overuse medicine for issues that might best be
attended to in community with self-resourcefulness and creativity.

There is a long history of errors and potential errors related to
medical intervention, whether at the stage of prevention/early
detection, diagnosis, or treatment. Each error, however, has been
studied as if it were a unique incident. I will describe just one
example of each.

A widely heralded and publicly supported preventative/early detection measure is the annual mammogram for women to detect breast cancer. Over many years, Anthony B. Miller, an epidemiologist, studied large cohorts of women to evaluate the cost/benefit of mammographic screening. This research was published in the highly regarded *British Medical Journal* (*BMJ*). It was based on results from following more than 89,000 women and concluded that screening for breast cancer does not reduce death for women from forty to fifty-nine years of age (the ages of women in the study). Moreover, 22 per cent of the breast cancers were diagnosed in error and constituted an overdiagnosis of breast cancer (Miller et al., 2014). Not only can screening itself cause some cancers (Kohn et al., 2000), but false positives (diagnosing disease when there is none) can cause painful worry and anxiety. This anxiety or mental suffering is another, frequently ignored, negative consequence of screening (Tosteson et al., 2014). This study suggests that we need to question population-based early detection policies before their widespread adoption. The cautionary principle should prevail until the evidence is available regarding the safety and efficacy of such interventions.

Diagnoses can be wrong. In fact, a wide range of studies has documented a high rate of diagnostic error. You may wonder, as I did at first, how diagnostic error could be investigated. There are actually a variety of methods for studying diagnostic error, including autopsies (which are, of course, only possible if the patient dies), second reviews, patient reporting, voluntary admission by doctors, audits, and malpractice claims, among others (Graber, 2013). Regardless of the method used to estimate diagnostic errors, the conclusion is consistent: too many errors are being made. Graber (2013) estimates that the rate of mistaken diagnosis is over 25 per cent. Evidence-based medicine (EBM) is one serious and important strategy to attempt to reduce the incidence of such errors. But EBM is itself imperfect. For example, as was demonstrated in the case of Amy Tan, EBM does not offer any help to those who have new diseases. It may be that a serious diagnosis, because of the potential for error, needs to trigger a second opinion financed by the medical system. This high rate of misdiagnosis also reflects back the value of self-care to see whether symptoms might disappear without diagnosis and treatment.

Treatment errors are too frequent. For example, the withdrawal of the drug rofecoxib, marketed as Vioxx (also called Ceeoxx or Ceoxx), a non-steroidal anti-inflammatory drug that was prescribed to millions – especially elderly people who were suffering pain from arthritis, younger women with dysmenorrhea, and others with acute pain – is a case in point. Estimates indicate that over eighty million people were prescribed this medication at some point before it was taken off the market. It was introduced to the market in 1999 and withdrawn five years later. It was only withdrawn after numerous complaints concerning its possible fatal side effects, including an increased risk of heart attacks and stroke (Juni et al., 2004). There was significant scientific evidence that it should have been withdrawn much earlier. In the end, between 88,000 and 140,000 people developed serious heart disease during the time rofecoxib was on the market. The current opioid epidemic is, in part, the result of the overprescription of opioids for chronic pain at the insistence of some pharmaceutical companies claiming that opioids were not addictive (see, for instance, DeWeerdt, 2019).

The studies of error discussed above reflect a small fraction of the breadth of medical error in the modern world. Unlike the cases based on the experience of individuals as described in this book, each problem discussed above is just one of many population-based problems. These problems demand political intervention and decision-making. Political change is required to change health policies and programs related to oversight of early detection and prevention policies and the reliability of diagnostics and treatment.

### The Social Determinants of Health

This book has argued that racism, sexism, and ageism were instrumental aspects of the deaths of Brian Sinclair, Ashley Smith, Vanessa Young, Marit McKenzie, and those murdered by Elizabeth Wettlaufer, as well as of the imprisonment of those wrongfully convicted by Dr. Charles Smith. Progress has been made over the past half century on each one of these "isms," but there is still a very long way to go. A number of different strategies need to be implemented in order to continue the small advances that have already occurred. Chief among the deliberate interventions are education at all levels of the school system, including education about discrimination and stereotyping and the damages they do to both the perpetrator and the recipient. Advertising, along with mass campaigns focusing on stories that shed light on the meanings and the negative impacts of such social interactions, could be very powerful tools for cultural change. A guaranteed annual income is another progressive idea that would contribute to the elimination of inequities. There are many other initiatives that could be considered in further detail. The murder of George Floyd in Minneapolis has resulted in worldwide action and a reinvigoration of the global Black Lives Matter movement (Togoh, 2020). In response, major corporations around the world have offered enormous financial support to anti-racist organizations. For example, Home Depot has donated one million dollars to the Lawyers Committee for Civil Rights under the Law (Togoh, 2020). Facebook has pledged ten million dollars to various campaigns dedicated to racial justice. Others have organized to demand changes to police forces, including the Defund the Police Movement (Kelly, 2020). I ask whether this powerful movement in the midst of the global COVID-19 pandemic will result in substantial changes in many areas of inequity and oppression, but particularly in regard to racism and policing.

**Individual Change**

There are also things we can do as individual citizens. Though influenced by culture and the definitional creep of modern medicine, we can use our critical thinking skills to ask whether or not medical intervention is the only or the best choice. Cultural shifts are very important to eliminating medical error. The culture of medicine works to individualize the way we see ourselves. As medical subjects, we tend to focus on ourselves as based in individual bodies that can become faulty and sick, and need the care of a professional health care provider. This emphasis on the self can tend to diminish our sense of community, family connection, and mutual aid. Reaching out to offer help and support when a neighbour or family member is "under the weather" could very well provide the assistance needed for a return to health and without the use of potentially unnecessary drugs such as antibiotics. Another cultural consequence of medicine, and the medical model that undergirds it, is the encouragement to rely on experts if we want to change or get better. Sometimes this individualization and expertization can lead to the overuse of medicine for a quick fix or in an effort to be better than normal. For instance, the rates of cosmetic surgery grew over 132 per cent from 2000 to 2016 (Gould & Mosher, 2017). This statistic refers specifically to surgery not used to repair a problem caused by injury or disease, but to change something for personal improvement. In other words, this surgery is discretionary plastic surgery and includes aspirational interventions such as liposuction, breast augmentation, nose reshaping, and facelifts. Another example of the overuse of medicine that often results from individual decision-making is illustrated by Uscher-Pine and colleagues (2013) in their review of studies of emergency room (ER) use. The authors found a large overuse of the ER for non-urgent conditions in the United States. They also found that this practice leads to excess testing and treatment. The Canadian Institute for Health Information (2014) has done research to corroborate the costly significance of inappropriate use of the ER in Canada. Telehealth is just one option to consider in the face of worrying symptoms when access to a doctor is difficult or impossible.

## Three Specific Changes Derived from the Case Studies

Numerous medical system changes are necessary to minimize medical error in the future. Many of them have been alluded to in this book. I want to end this conclusion by highlighting how small changes could have prevented the errors well documented in this book. Each of these interventions speaks to the mitigation of the power of medicalization. In the cases of both Brian Sinclair and Ashley Smith, a social care associate who would work to ensure that diagnoses and services were coordinated and consistent, and that the rules and regulations were abided by for a client, could have prevented these two deaths. Both individuals were absolutely dependent on the state: Ashley Smith because she was incarcerated and thus had no freedom of movement or decision-making, and Brian Sinclair because of his physical challenges and limitations. They both needed someone in place with an oversight role to track how they were doing and how the medical system was actually functioning to aid their health. Both needed a figure outside of the medical care system who would be able to take the responsibility of ensuring on a daily, weekly, monthly, and yearly basis that the state was providing excellent care. Had someone in this role observed the many changing diagnoses and treatments or the recurrent, although illegal, solitary confinement that Ashley Smith received, these two contributors to her death could have been avoided. Had there been a care associate with an Indigenous background who knew that Brian Sinclair had not had his catheter changed for a long period of time and had the capacity to intervene and ensure this catheter cleaning occurred, Brian Sinclair would not have had to go to the ER in the first place.

The cases of Elizabeth Wettlaufer, Dr. Charles Smith, and Dr. Norman Barwin highlight the significance of ongoing social support, evaluation, and monitoring for medical professionals at all levels. Complaints had been lodged against Ms. Wettlaufer, Dr. Smith, and Dr. Barwin. Ms. Wettlaufer was known to have sought help for her mental health problems, to have been addicted to both drugs and alcohol, and to have confessed her murders to others as she sought help. Had the institutions within which she worked or the overriding regulatory bodies been adequately assiduous in their observations of Wettlaufer's numerous suspensions, they might have found help and support for her before she murdered those she was supposed to be caring for. Dr. Barwin could have been stopped earlier had people not settled out of court and had the CPSO demanded more redress than a two-month suspension and a small fine. Had anyone in the department where Dr. Smith worked taken decisive action in the face of the myriad complaints and findings against him, many of the people who spent time in prison would not have had to do so. Issues related to the adequacy of training for new specialties and labour force availability for these same specialties need to be considered as well.

Changes in the regulation of the pharmaceutical companies, particularly in post-market surveillance and informing prescribers of problems and side effects with drugs as they emerge, could have prevented the deaths of Marit McKenzie and Vanessa Young. Were new, multisystem diseases, often defined first by patients (such as fibromyalgia, chronic fatigue syndrome, environmental allergies and sensitivities), been taken more seriously by the medical system, Amy Tan's decades-long fight for a diagnosis and treatment might not have had to occur. Had new disease definition and diagnosis been more supported with active, well-funded research and training for doctors during medical school, Amy Tan might have been diagnosed and treated more expeditiously. Notwithstanding the promise of these two interpolations, there is a third change I want to address because of its potential to prevent error and enhance well-being.

Investment in the expansion of publicly funded and delivered home, community, and long-term care would have had the potential to have helped both the patients murdered by Elizabeth Wettlaufer, Wettlaufer herself, Ashley Smith, and Brian Sinclair. Long-term care in Canada consists of a mixture of public and private (for-profit) facilities (Centre for Health Services and Policy Research, n.d.). At the present, they make up almost 10 per cent of the health care budget, or 17 billion dollars. Long-term care comprises both medical services, such as administering medications, changing dressings, and the like, and residential services. Residential services are paid for out of a different budget than medical services and largely depend on the financial capacity of the resident, with co-payments from governments as needed. Some evidence shows that these for-profit services can leave residents exposed to harm and inconsistent care (McGregor & Ronald, 2011). There are many different ways of assessing the differences in the quality of care between the two types of homes. For now, one example will suffice. It has been found that the rates of bedsores or pressure ulcers are higher in the for-profit residences. Pressure ulcers are signs that bed-ridden residents are not being turned frequently enough, and the ulcers are both painful and can lead to life-threatening infections.

Notwithstanding the problems with for-profit care homes, there are not enough of either type of facility for the burgeoning population with chronic conditions who need ongoing care (wwhealth-line.ca, 2018). In just one example, Parkwood Mennonite Home in Waterloo, Ontario, has ninety-six beds available for residents. It has 253 people waiting for a basic room (to be shared with others) and 262 people waiting for a single room. Further, nine out of ten people waiting to get into Parkwood have to wait 1,486 days before they are given a place. In the meantime, people who are waiting for appropriate long-term care across the country and their families are often suffering and unsafe. Sometimes they are waiting in the emergency room of a local hospital or in an acute care bed, although they do not need that level of medical care. Sometimes they are being cared for by a highly stressed, ill, or even demented family member. There are clearly needs for a greater number of safe and healthy long-term care homes. The Brian Sinclair case reminds us that some homes must be culturally specific. Brian Sinclair wanted to live with other First Nations people and not with, as he said, white men. The Ashley Smith case reminds us of the importance of housing alternatives for young men and women in precarious situations.

The argument of this book extends beyond both the blame and shame and the medical systems perspectives. It asserts that medical errors will continue to be inevitable given the relentless and expanding processes of medicalization, because medicalization assumes the beneficence of allopathic medicine's goals and functioning. It tends to resist critical thinking and decision-making. The definitional power of medicalization over many aspects of life obfuscates the serious ongoing and challenging limits in medical science, medical practice, medical systems organization, and pharmaceutical use. The dominance of medicalization also obscures the powerful impacts of the social determinants of health, along with the roles of history and culture in health.

# Notes

**Preface**

1 Here are just a few examples of the many I did not include. They have all been observed, noted, and come to the attention of a journalist from one of the major news outlets in Canada. Further, it is important to note that they occurred for a long period of time before they were identified as problematic. For instance, I have excluded Motherisk (Mendleson, 2017), the hair analysis tests that were found to be unreliable and inadequate, and yet were associated with children being removed from their homes and other child protection cases across the country over many years. There have been many cases of misread pathology tests resulting in both false positives, such as a mastectomy in a case where there actually was no breast cancer, and false negatives, resulting in a failure to treat and ignoring a cancer that was present ("Woman sues," 2010). There have been cases of errors leading to hundreds of missed breast cancer diagnoses (Gibb, 2009). There have been a number of pharmaceutical errors too. One important example, because it was so widely prescribed, is Vioxx, the popular drug that was only withdrawn after years of suits against the company that knew of its fatal and serious side effects ("Vioxx," 2005).

2 For instance, the discovery of penicillin was accidental. It was the result of a growth in an unclean dish left in a lab for a time.

3 Brian Sinclair's case is the only one in which racialization is evident. At least two of the wrongful convictions in Dr. Smith's case were against Indigenous men. This is noted in the text. The relationship between

racialization and medicalization is complex and not the subject of discussion except in the cases noted.

4 It needs to be stressed that some people may find some of these cases upsetting to read and think about.

## 3. Vanessa Young and Marit McKenzie

1 The information about Vanessa Young is from the book *Death by Prescription*, written by her father, T.H. Young (2012).

# References

**Preface**

Blackwell, T. (2011, 1 February). Tribunal revokes licence of discredited pathologist Charles Smith. *National Post*. https://nationalpost.com /news/canada/hearing-to-consider-disciplinary-charges-for-discredited -pathologist-charles-smith

Brennan, R.J. (2009, 4 March). Troubled teen died in prison "needlessly." *Toronto Star*. https://www.thestar.com/news/canada/2009/03/04 /troubled_teen_died_in_prison_needlessly.html

Canadian Press, The. (2007, 30 November). Ex-chief coroner knew of issues with pathologist but took little action. *CBC News*. https://www.cbc.ca /news/canada/toronto/ex-chief-coroner-knew-of-issues-with-pathologist -but-took-little-action-1.657302

Canadian Press, The. (2013, 29 August). Housekeeping, but not nurses, called after Brian Sinclair threw up in the Winnipeg ER where he died. *National Post*. https://nationalpost.com/news/canada/housekeeping -but-not-nurses-called-after-brian-sinclair-threw-up-in-the-winnpeg-er -where-he-died

CBC News. (2001, 20 March). Family of teen never told of drug warnings. *CBC News*. https://www.cbc.ca/news/canada/family-of-teen -never-told-of-drug-warnings-1.283

CBC News. (2009, 3 March). Jail cell death of N.B. teen "entirely preventable": Report. *CBC News*. https://www.cbc.ca/news/canada /jail-cell-death-of-n-b-teen-entirely-preventable-report-1.841541

Clarke, J.N. (2016). The underside of medicalisation: The portrayal of medical error over time in North American popular mass magazines. *Health, Risk & Society, 18*(5–6), 270–82. https://doi.org/10.1080/13698575.2016.1241383

Dubinski, K. (2019, 31 July). "Systemic vulnerabilities" let killer nurse Elizabeth Wettlaufer keep on killing – Report. *CBC News*. https://www.cbc.ca/news/canada/london/wettlaufer-inquiry-report-recommendations-woodstock-ontario-1.5231324

Duffy, A. (2010, 14 September). Fertility lawsuits name Ottawa doctor: Two families want to rule out possibility Barwin was sperm donor. *The Ottawa Citizen*, C1.

Geary, A. (2017, 19 September). Ignored to death: Brian Sinclair's death caused by racism, inquest inadequate, group say. *CBC News*. https://www.cbc.ca/news/canada/manitoba/winnipeg-brian-sinclair-report-1.4295996

Gibb, G. (2009, 17 April). Breast cancer misdiagnosis: A sad story in Canada. *Lawyers and Settlements.com*. https://www.lawyersandsettlements.com/features/medical_malpractice/breast-cancer-misdiagnosis.html

Globe and Mail, The. (2009, 10 March). Ashley Smith's inhumane death. *The Globe and Mail*. https://www.theglobeandmail.com/news/national/ashley-smiths-inhumane-death/article4318995/

Johns Hopkins Medicine. (2016, 3 May). Study suggests medical errors now third leading cause of death in the U.S. [Press release]. https://www.hopkinsmedicine.org/news/media/releases/study_suggests_medical_errors_now_third_leading_cause_of_death_in_the_us

Jones, E. (2021, 13 February). "This is what Marit wanted": Calgary teen saved lives by donating organs. *National Post*. https://nationalpost.com/health/this-is-what-marit-wanted-calgary-teen-saved-lives-by-donating-organs

Kanwar, A. (2010, 24 September). Sperm donor mix-up: Where do these two girls come from? *The Globe and Mail*. https://www.theglobeandmail.com/life/parenting/sperm-donor-mix-up-where-do-these-two-girls-come-from/article570411/

Kohn, L.T., Corrigan, J.M., & Donaldson, M.S. (Eds.). (2000). *To err is human: Building a safer health system*. Institute of Medicine (US) Committee on the Quality of Health Care in America. National Academy Press.

Makin, K. (2007, 11 December). Staff was in crisis, chief pathologist testifies. *The Globe and Mail.* https://www.theglobeandmail.com/news/national /staff-was-in-crisis-chief-pathologist-testifies/article699537/

McCoy, J.J. (2003, 12 August). "I am in this for the long haul": Writer Amy Tan's frustrating struggle with Lyme disease highlights the controversy on diagnosis and treatment. *The Washington Post,* A31.

Mendleson, R. (2017, 19 October). Separated by a hair. *Toronto Star.* https:// projects.thestar.com/motherisk/

Pfeffer, A. (2020, 6 January). Disgraced fertility doctor's clinic broke federal rules as far back as 1999, inspection reports reveal. *CBC News.* https://www.cbc.ca/news/canada/ottawa/disgraced-fertility-doctor -s-clinic-broke-federal-rules-as-far-back-as-1999-inspection-reports -reveal-1.5411100

Sims, J. (2017, 24 March). Nurse was fired prior to murder charges; dismissed for misusing drugs, warrant says. *National Post,* A1.

Vioxx: Lessons for Health Canada and the FDA. (2005). *CMAJ, 172*(1), 5. https://doi.org/10.1503/cmaj.045206

Welsh, M. (2016, 25 October). Nurse charged with murdering eight Ontario nursing home residents. *Toronto Star.* https://www.thestar.com/news /canada/2016/10/25/nurse-charged-with-murdering-8-ontario-nursing -home-residents.html

White, P. (2009, 16 June). Homeless man's family feels marginalized at inquest. *The Globe and Mail.* https://www.theglobeandmail.com /news/national/homeless-mans-family-feels-marginalized-at-inquest /article4355550/

Woman sues over mistaken mastectomy (2010, 3 March). *Toronto Star.* https://www.thestar.com/life/health_wellness/2010/03/03/woman _sues_over_mistaken_mastectomy.html

Zlomislic, D. (2013, 19 October). Calgary teen was slowly dying and didn't know it. *Toronto Star.* https://www.thestar.com/life/health _wellness/2013/10/19/calgary_teen_was_slowly_dying_and_didnt _know_it.html

**Introduction**

Abimanyi-Ochom, J., Bohingamu Mudiyanselage, S., Catchpool, M., Firipis, M., Wanni Arachchige Dona, S., & Watts, J.J. (2019). Strategies to reduce diagnostic errors: A systematic review. *BMC Medical Informatics and Decision Making, 19*(1), 174. https://doi.org/10.1186/s12911-019-0901-1

Abraham, J. (2009). The pharmaceutical industry, the state and the NHS. In J. Gabe & M. Calnan (Eds.), *The new sociology of the health service* (pp. 99–120). Routledge.

Abraham, J. (2010a). Pharmaceuticalization of society in context: Theoretical, empirical and health dimensions. *Sociology, 44*(4), 603–22. https://doi.org/10.1177/0038038510369368

Abraham J. (2010b). The sociological concomitants of the pharmaceutical industry and medications. In C. Bird, P. Conrad, A. Fremont, & S. Timmermans (Eds.). *Handbook of medical sociology* (pp. 290–308). Vanderbilt University Press.

Alkureishi, M.A., Lee, W.W., Lyons, M., Press, V.G., Imam, S., Nkansah-Amankra, A. ... Arora, V.M. (2016). Impact of electronic medical record use on the patient-doctor relationship and communication: A systematic review. *Journal of General Internal Medicine, 31*(5), 548–60. https://doi .org/10.1007/s11606-015-3582-1

Almasi, E.A., Stafford, R.S., Kravitz, R.L., & Mansfield, P.R. (2006). What are the public health effects of direct-to-consumer drug advertising? PLos *Medicine, 3*(3), e145. https://doi.org/10.1371/journal.pmed.0030145

American Psychiatric Association. (n.d.). *Diagnostic and statistical manual of mental disorders* (DSM-5). www.psychiatry.org/psychiatrists/practice/dsm

Arout, C.A., Sofuoglu, M., Bastian, L.A., & Rosenheck, R.A. (2018). Gender differences in the prevalence of fibromyalgia and in concomitant medical and psychiatric disorders: A National Veterans Health Administration study. *Journal of Women's Health, 27*(8), 1035–44. https://doi.org/10.1089 /jwh.2017.6622

Ayo, N. (2012). Understanding health promotion in a neoliberal climate and the making of health conscious citizens. *Critical Public Health, 22*(1), 99–105. https://doi.org/10.1080/09581596.2010.520692

Baile, W.F., & Epner, D. (2015). Disclosing harmful medical errors. In A. Surbone & M. Rowe (Eds.), *Clinical oncology and error reduction: A manual for clinicians* (pp. 101–10). Wiley-Blackwell.

Bertakis, K.D. (2009). The influence of gender on the doctor-patient interaction. *Patient Education and Counseling, 76*(3), 356–60. https:// doi.org/10.1016/j.pec.2009.07.022

Blomqvist, A., & Busby, C. (2012). *How to pay family doctors: Why "pay per patient" is better than fee for service* (Commentary no. 365). C.D. Howe Institute. https://doi.org/10.2139/ssrn.2172035

Bolton, D. (2013). Overdiagnosis problems in the DSM-IV and the new DSM-5: Can they be resolved by the distress-impairment criterion? *Canadian Journal of Psychiatry, 58*(11), 612–17. https://doi.org/10.1177/070674371305801106

Bosk, C. (2005). Continuity and change in the study of medical error. The culture of safety on the shop floor. (Unpublished occasional paper of the School of Social Science). University of Pennsylvania. http://citeseerx.ist.psu.edu/viewdoc/download?doi=10.1.1.112.385&rep=rep1&type=pdf

Bryant, T., Raphael, D., Schrecker, T., & Labonte, R. (2011). Canada: A land of missed opportunity for addressing the social determinants of health. *Health Policy, 101*(1), 44–58. https://doi.org/10.1016/j.healthpol.2010.08.022

Budnitz, D.S., Lovegrove, M.C., Shehab, N., & Richards, C.L. (2011). Emergency hospitalizations for adverse drug events in older Americans. *New England Journal of Medicine, 365*(21), 2002–12. https://doi.org/10.1056/NEJMsa1103053

Burns, K.K. (2008). Canadian patient safety champions: Collaborating on improving patient safety. *Healthcare Quarterly, 11*(3 Spec No.), 95–100.

Busfield, J. (2006). Pills, power, people: Sociological understandings of the pharmaceutical industry. *Sociology, 40*(2), 297–314. https://doi.org/10.1177/0038038506062034

Canadian Foundation for Healthcare Improvement. (2011). Myth: Medicare covers all necessary health services. https://web.archive.org/web/20171018022849/http://www.cfhi-fcass.ca/PublicationsAndResources/Mythbusters/ArticleView/11-05-12/dd2b140f-7405-461c-a077-06ad45256fb1.aspx

Canadian Institute for Health Information (CIHI). (2019). National health expenditure trends, 1975 to 2019. https://www.cihi.ca/sites/default/files/document/nhex-trends-narrative-report-2019-en-web.pdf

Canadian Medical Protective Association. (2017). Canadian Medical Protective Association at a glance. https://www.cmpa-acpm.ca/en/connect/media-room/the-canadian-medical-protective-association-at-a-glance

Cecco, L. (2019, 13 December). Canada: Nearly 14,000 people die from opioid overdoses in four years. *The Guardian*. https://www.theguardian.com/world/2019/dec/13/canada-opioids-crisis-overdoses-report

Chang, V.W., & Lauderdale, D.S. (2009). Fundamental cause theory, technological innovation, and health disparities: The case of cholesterol in the era of statins. *Journal of Health and Social Behavior, 50*(3), 245–60. https://doi.org/10.1177/002214650905000301

Charney, W. (2012, 10 May). Do no harm? The epidemic of fatal medical errors in the US and Canada. *Canadian Dimension*. https://canadiandimension.com/articles/view/do-no-harm

Clarke, A.E., Shim, J., Mamo, L., Fosket, J.R., & Fishman, J.R. (2003). Biomedicalization: Technoscientific transformations of health, illness, and US biomedicine. *American Sociological Review, 68*(2), 161–94. https://doi.org/10.2307/1519765

Clarke, J.N. (2016). *Health, illness and medicine in Canada* (7th ed.). Oxford University Press.

Classen, D.C., Resar, R., Griffin, F., Federico, F., Frankel, T., Kimmel, N., … James, B.C. (2011). "Global trigger tool" shows that adverse events in hospitals may be ten times greater than previously measured. *Health Affairs, 30*(4), 581–9. https://doi.org/10.1377/hlthaff.2011.0190

Clearfield, C., & Tilcsik, A. (2018). *Meltdown: Why our systems fail and what we can do about it*. Penguin Press.

Coburn, D. (2006). Medical dominance then and now: Critical reflections. *Health Sociology Review, 15*(5), 432–43. https://doi.org/10.5172/hesr.2006.15.5.432

Conference Board of Canada. (2017). Demand for long-term care beds in Canada could nearly double in little more than 15 years [Press release]. https://www.newswire.ca/news-releases/demand-for-long-term-care-beds-in-canada-could-nearly-double-in-little-more-than-15-years-660240523.html

Conrad, P. (2005). The shifting engines of medicalization. *Journal of Health and Social Behavior, 46*(1), 3–14. https://doi.org/10.1177/002214650504600102

Conrad, P. (2007). *The medicalization of society: On the transformation of human conditions into treatable disorders*. Johns Hopkins University Press.

Conrad, P., & Schneider, J.W. (1980). *The medicalization of deviance: From badness to sickness*. Mosby.

Cowling, T.E., Cecil, E.V., Soljak, M.A., Lee, J.T., Millett, C., Majeed, A., ... Harris, M.J. (2013). Access to primary care and visits to emergency departments in England: A cross sectional, population-based study. *PloS One, 8*(6), e66699. https://doi.org/10.1371/journal.pone.0066699

Donohue, J.M., Cevasco, M., & Rosenthal, M.B. (2007). A decade of direct-to-consumer advertising of prescription drugs. *New England Journal of Medicine, 357*(7), 673–81. https://doi.org/10.1056/NEJMsa070502

Elliott, C. (2004). *Better than well: American medicine meets the American dream.* W.W. Norton.

Enck, G.G. (2014). Pharmaceutical enhancement and medical professionals. *Medical Health Care and Philosophy, 17*(1), 23–8. https://doi.org/10.1007/s11019-013-9507-z

Fang, F.C., Steen, R.G., & Casadevall, A. (2012). Misconduct accounts for the majority of retracted scientific publications. *Proceedings of the National Academy of Sciences, 109*(42), 17028–33. https://doi.org/10.1073/pnas.1212247109

Ferguson, W.J., & Candib, L.M. (2002). Culture, language, and the doctor-patient relationship. Family *Medicine, 34*(5), 353–61. http://hdl.handle.net/10822/1010575

Foucault, M. (1988). *Madness and civilization: A history of insanity in the age of reason* (R. Howard, Trans.). Vintage. (Original work published 1961)

Foucault, M. (1994). The art of telling the truth. In *Critique and power: Recasting the Foucault/Habermas debate* (M. Kelly, Ed.; pp. 139–48). MIT Press.

Foucault, M. (2006). *History of madness* (J. Murphy, Trans.). Routledge. (Original work published 1961)

Fox, N.J., & Ward, K.J. (2009). Pharma in the bedroom ... and the kitchen ... The pharmaceuticalisation of daily life. In S.J. Williams, J. Gabe, & P. Davis (Eds.), *Pharmaceuticals and society: Critical discourses and debates* (pp. 41–53). Blackwell.

Freund, P.E., McGuire, M.B., & Podhurst, L.S. (2003). *Health, illness, and the social body: A critical sociology.* Prentice Hall.

Friedman, M., & Gould, J. (2007). Consumer attitudes and behaviors associated with direct-to-consumer prescription drug marketing. *Journal of Consumer Marketing, 24*(2), 100–9. https://doi.org/10.1108/07363760710773102

Glauser, W. (2013). Pharma influence widespread at medical school: Study. *CMAJ, 185*(13), 1121–2. https://doi.org/10.1503/cmaj.109-4563

Goold, S.D., & Lipkin, M. (1999). The doctor-patient relationship. *Journal of General Internal Medicine, 14*(1), S26–S33. https://doi.org/10.1046/j.1525-1497.1999.00267.x

Gosden, T., Pedersen, L., & Torgerson, D. (1999). How should we pay doctors? A systematic review of salary payments and their effect on doctor behaviour. *QJM: An International Journal of Medicine, 92*(1), 47–55. https://doi.org/10.1093/qjmed/92.1.47

Government of Canada. (2018). Understanding the report on key health inequalities in Canada. https://www.canada.ca/en/public-health/services/publications/science-research-data/understanding-report-key-health-inequalities-canada.html

Government of Canada. (2019, 9 April). Canada's opioid crisis (fact sheet). https://www.canada.ca/en/health-canada/services/publications/healthy-living/canada-opioid-crisis-fact-sheet.html

Gritzer, G., & Arluke, A. (1989) *The making of rehabilitation: A political economy of medical specialization 1890–1980*. University of California Press.

Grohol, J.M. (2013). DSM-5 released: The big changes. PsychCentral. https://psychcentral.com/blog/dsm-5-released-the-big-changes

Hartung, F.M., Sproesser, G., & Renner, B. (2015). Being and feeling liked by others: How social inclusion impacts health. *Psychology & Health, 30*(9), 1103–15. https://doi.org/10.1080/08870446.2015.1031134

Healy, D.I. (2002). Conflicting interests in Toronto: Anatomy of a controversy at the interface of academia and industry. *Perspectives in Biology and Medicine, 45*(2), 250–63. https://doi.org/10.1353/pbm.2002.0028

Hollon, M.F. (2005). Direct-to-consumer advertising: A haphazard approach to health promotion. *JAMA, 293*(16), 2030–3. https://doi.org/10.1001/jama.293.16.2030

Illich, I. (1976). *Medical nemesis: The expropriation of health*. Pantheon Books.

Jain, M. (2013, 27 May). Medical errors are hard for doctors to admit but it's wise to apologize to patients. *The Washington Post*. https://www.washingtonpost.com/national/health-science/medical-errors-are-hard-for-doctors-to-admit-but-its-wise-to-apologize-to-patients/2013/05/24/95e21a2a-915f-11e2-9abd-e4c5c9dc5e90_story.html

James, S.A. (2017). The strangest of all encounters: Racial and ethnic discrimination in US health care. *Cadernos de saude publica, 33*(Suppl 1), e00104416. https://doi.org/10.1590/0102-311X00104416

Jensen, C.B. (2008). Sociology, systems and (patient) safety: Knowledge translations in healthcare policy. *Sociology of Health & Illness, 30*(2), 309–24. https://doi.org/10.1111/j.1467-9566.2007.01035.x

Kaba, R., & Sooriakumaran, P. (2007). The evolution of the doctor-patient relationship. *International Journal of Surgery, 5*(1), 57–65. https://doi.org /10.1016/j.ijsu.2006.01.005

Kanaris, C. (2021). Moral distress in the intensive care unit during the pandemic: The burden of dying alone. *Intensive Care Medicine, 47*(1), 141–3. https://doi.org/10.1007/s00134-020-06194-0

Kohn, L.T., Corrigan, J.M., & Donaldson, M.S. (Eds.). (2000). *To err is human: Building a safer health system.* Institute of Medicine (US) Committee on the Quality of Health Care in America. National Academy Press.

Kudlow, P. (2013). The perils of diagnostic inflation. *CMAJ, 185*(1), E25–6. https://doi.org/10.1503/cmaj.109-4371

Leapfrog Hospital Safety Grade. (2013). Hospital errors are the third leading cause of death in the U.S., and new hospital safety scores show improvements are too slow [Press release]. https://www.hospitalsafety grade.org/newsroom/display/hospitalerrors-thirdleading-causeof deathinus-improvementstooslow

Lexchin, J. (2013). Health Canada and the pharmaceutical industry: A preliminary analysis of the historical relationship. *Healthcare Policy, 9*(2), 22–9. https://doi.org/10.12927/hcpol.2013.23621

Lexchin, J., Mintzes, B., Bero, L., Gagnon, M-A., & Grundy, Q. (2020, 8 October). Canada's COVID-19 Vaccine Task Force needs better transparency about potential conflicts of interest. *The Conversation.* https://theconversation.com/canadas-covid-19-vaccine-task-force-needs -better-transparency-about-potential-conflicts-of-interest-147323

Loughran, J., Smith, K., & Berry, A. (Eds.). (2011). *Scientific literacy under the microscope: A whole school approach to science teaching and learning* (Vol. 11). Springer Science & Business Media.

Makary, M.A., & Daniel, M. (2016). Medical error – The third leading cause of death in the US. *BMJ, 353*, i2139. https://doi.org/10.1136/bmj.i2139

Mamatis, D., Sanford, S., Ansara, D., & Roche, B. (2019). *Promoting health and well-being through social inclusion in Toronto.* Toronto Public Health and Wellesley Institute. https://www.wellesleyinstitute.com/wp-content /uploads/2019/07/Social-Inclusion-Report.pdf

Marmot, M. (2018). Inclusion health: Addressing the causes of the causes (Comment). *The Lancet, 391*(10117), 186–8. https://doi.org/10.1016 /S0140-6736(17)32848-9

Masic, I., Miokovic, M., & Muhamedagic, B. (2008). Evidence based medicine – New approaches and challenges. *Acta Informatica Medica, 16*(4), 219–25. https://doi.org/10.5455/aim.2008.16.219-225

McLeod, C.B., Lavis, J.N., Mustard, C.A., & Stoddart, G.L. (2003). Income inequality, household income, and health status in Canada: A prospective cohort study. *American Journal of Public Health, 93*(8), 1287–93. https:// doi.org/10.2105/ajph.93.8.1287

Mizrahi, T. (1984). Managing medical mistakes: Ideology, insularity and accountability amongst internists-in-training. *Social Science and Medicine, 19*(2), 135–46. https://doi.org/10.1016/0277-9536(84)90280-6

Moynihan, R., & Cassels, A. (2006). *Selling sickness: How drug companies are turning us all into patients.* Nation Books.

Moynihan, R., Heath, I., & Henry, D. (2002). Selling sickness: The pharmaceutical industry and disease mongering (Commentary: Medicalisation of risk factors). *BMJ, 324,* 886. https://www.bmj.com /content/324/7342/886.1

Mozes, A. (2018, 14 May). Opioid prescriptions tied to perks for doctors. *WebMD.* https://www.webmd.com/mental-health/addiction/news /20180514/opioid-prescriptions-tied-to-perks-for-doctors

National Institute on Drug Abuse. (2020). Opioid overdose crisis. https:// www.drugabuse.gov/drug-topics/opioids/opioid-overdose-crisis

OECD (Organisation for Economic Co-operation and Development). (2015). Focus on health spending: OECD health statistics 2015. https://www .oecd.org/health/health-systems/Focus-Health-Spending-2015.pdf

OECD (Organisation for Economic Co-operation and Development). (2018). Health status. https://stats.oecd.org/Index.aspx?DataSetCode= HEALTH_STAT

Ornstein, C., Weber, T., & Grochowski Jones, R. (2019, 17 October). We found over 700 doctors who were paid more than a million dollars by drug and medical device companies. *ProPublica.* https://www.propublica.org /article/we-found-over-700-doctors-who-were-paid-more-than-a-million -dollars-by-drug-and-medical-device-companies

Paget, M. (2004). *The unity of mistakes.* Temple University Press.

Parekh, A., Marcus, R., Roberts, M., & Raisch, D.W. (2012). Risks and benefits of direct to consumer advertising on patient-provider relationships – Report of the ISPOR direct to consumer advertisements working group. *International Society for Pharmacoeconomics and Outcomes Research, 18*, 9–13.

Payer, L. (1992). *Disease-mongers: How doctors, drug companies and insurers are making you feel sick.* Wiley.

Perrow, C. (1984). Normal accidents: Living with high-risk technologies. Basic Books.

Raphael, D. (2002a). *Poverty, income inequality, and health in Canada.* CSJ Foundation for Research and Education.

Raphael, D. (2002b). *Social justice is good for our hearts: Why societal factors – not lifestyles – are major causes of heart disease in Canada and elsewhere.* CSJ Foundation for Research and Education.

Raphael, D. (Ed.). (2016). *The social determinants of health: Canadian perspectives* (3rd ed.) Canadian Scholar's Press.

Rathert, C., Brandt, J., & Williams, E.S. (2012). Putting the "patient" in patient safety: A qualitative study of consumer experiences. *Health Expectations, 15*(3), 327–36. https://doi.org/10.1111/j.1369-7625.2011.00685.x

Rittel, H.W., & Webber, M.M. (1973). Planning problems are wicked problems: Dilemmas in general theory of planning. *Policy Science, 4*, 155–69. https://doi.org/10.1007/BF01405730

Riverin, B.D., Li, P., Naimi, A.I., & Strumpf, E. (2017). Team-based versus traditional primary care models and short-term outcomes after hospital discharge. *CMAJ, 189*(16), E585–93. https://doi.org/10.1503/cmaj.160427

Rose, N. (2003). Neurochemical selves. *Society, 41*(1), 46–59. https://doi.org /10.1007/BF02688204

Rose, N. (2007) Beyond medicalization. *Lancet, 369*, 700–1. https://doi.org /10.1016/S0140-6736(07)60319-5

Roseman, M., Turner, E.H., Lexchin, J., Coyne, J.C., Bero, L.A., & Thombs, B.D. (2012). Reporting of conflicts of interest from drug trials in Cochrane reviews: Cross sectional study. *BMJ, 345*, e5155. https://doi.org/10.1136/bmj.e5155

Saha, S., Arbelaez, J.J., & Cooper, L.A. (2003). Patient–physician relationships and racial disparities in the quality of health care. *American Journal of Public Health, 93*(10), 1713–19. https://doi.org/10.2105/ajph.93.10.1713

Saloner, B., McGinty, E.E., Beletsky, L., Bluthenthal, R., Beyrer, C., Botticelli, M., & Sherman, S.G. (2018). A public health strategy for the opioid crisis.

*Public Health Reports, 133*(1_suppl), 24S–34S. https://doi.org/10.1177
/0033354918793627

Schieber, A.C., Delpierre, C., Lepage, B., Afrite, A., Pascal, J., Cases,
C., ... Kelly-Irving, M., for the INTERMEDE group. (2014). Do gender
differences affect the doctor–patient interaction during consultations in
general practice? Results from the INTERMEDE study. *Family Practice,
31*(6), 706–13. https://doi.org/10.1093/fampra/cmu057

Shnier, A., Lexchin, J., Mintzes, B., Jutel, A., & Holloway, K. (2013). Too few,
too weak: Conflict of interest policies at Canadian medical schools. *PloS
One, 8*(7), e68633. https://doi.org/10.1371/journal.pone.0068633

Sibbald, B. (2004). Rofecoxib (Vioxx) voluntarily withdrawn from market.
*CMAJ, 171*(9), 1027–8. https://doi.org/10.1503/cmaj.1041606

Silversides, A. (2010). Drug safety provisions in US and Europe outshine
Canada. *CMAJ, 182*(1), E23–4. https://doi.org/10.1503/cmaj.109-3102

Smith, B.L. (2012). Inappropriate prescribing. *Monitor on Psychology, 43*(6),
36. http://www.apa.org/monitor/2012/06/prescribing.aspx

Statista. (2018). Global pharmaceutical industry – Statistics & facts. https://
www.statista.com/topics/1764/global-pharmaceutical-industry/

Steen, R.G. (2011). Retractions in the scientific literature: Is the incidence of
research fraud increasing? *Journal of Medical Ethics, 37*(4), 249–53. https://
doi.org/10.1136/jme.2010.040923

Stossel, S. (2016, 7 July). Should we still listen to Prozac? Peter D. Kramer
jumps back into the antidepressant debate. *The New York Times.* https://
www.nytimes.com/2016/07/10/books/review/peter-d-kramer
-ordinarily-well-about-antidepressants.html

Traversy, G., Barnieh, L., Akl, E.A., Allan, G.M., Brouwers, M., Ganache, I., ...
Tonelli, M. (2021). Managing conflicts of interest in the development of health
guidelines. *CMAJ, 193*(2), E49–54. https://doi.org/10.1503/cmaj.200651

Usher, W., & Skinner, J. (2012). EMPIRE and health website
recommendations: Technologies of control. *Social Theory & Health, 10*(1),
20–41. https://doi.org/10.1057/sth.2011.10

van Daalen, K.R., Bajnoczki, C., Chowdhury, M., Dada, S., Khorsand, P.,
Socha, A., ... Rajan, D. (2020). Symptoms of a broken system: The gender
gaps in COVID-19 decision-making. *BMJ Global Health, 5*(10), e003549.
https://doi.org/10.1136/bmjgh-2020-003549

Verlinde, E., De Laender, N., De Maesschalck, S., Deveugele, M., &
Willems, S. (2012). The social gradient in doctor-patient communication.

*International Journal for Equity in Health, 11*, 12. https://doi.org/10.1186/1475-9276-11-12

Villani, J., & Mortensen, K. (2013). Nonemergent emergency department use among patients with a usual source of care. *Journal of the American Board of Family Medicine, 26*(6), 680–91. https://doi.org/10.3122/jabfm.2013.06.120327

Waring, J.J. (2007). Doctors' thinking about "the system" as a threat to patient safety. Health: An Interdisciplinary Journal for the Social Study of Health, *Illness and Medicine, 11*(1), 29– 46. https://doi.org/10.1177/1363459307070801

Weingart, S.N., Pagovich, O., Sands, D.Z., Li, J.M., Aronson, M.D., Davis, R.B., & Phillips, R.S. (2005). What can hospitalized patients tell us about adverse events? Learning from patient-reported incidents. *Journal of General Internal Medicine, 20*, 830–6. https://doi.org/10.1111/j.1525-1497.2005.0180.x

Weisz, G. (2006). *Divide and conquer: A comparative history of medical specialization.* Oxford University Press.

Williams, S.J., Martin, P., & Gabe, J. (2011). The pharmaceuticalization of society? A framework for analysis. *Sociology of Health & Illness, 33*(5), 710–25. https://doi.org/10.1111/j.1467-9566.2011.01320.x

Williams, S.J., Seale, C., Boden, S., Lowe, P., & Steinberg, D.L. (2009). Waking up to sleepiness: Modafinil, the media and the pharmaceuticalisation of everyday/night life. In S.J. Williams, J. Gabe, & P. Davis. (Eds.), *Pharmaceuticals and society: Critical discourses and debates* (pp. 25–40). Blackwell.

Wouters, A., Bakker, A.H., van Wijk, I.J., Croiset, G., & Kusurkar, R.A. (2014). A qualitative analysis of statements on motivation of applicants for medical school. *BMC Medical Education, 14*, 200. https://doi.org/10.1186/1472-6920-14-200

Zaitsu, M., Yoo, B.K., Tomio, J., Nakamura, F., Toyokawa, S., & Kobayashi, Y. (2018). Impact of a direct-to-consumer information campaign on prescription patterns for overactive bladder. *BMC Health Services Research, 18*(1), 325. https://doi.org/10.1186/s12913-018-3147-1

Zelek, B., & Phillips, S.P. (2003). Gender and power: Nurses and doctors in Canada. *International Journal for Equity in Health, 2*(1), 1. https://doi.org/10.1186/1475-9276-2-1

Zola, I.K. (1972). Medicine as an institution of social control. *The Sociological Review, 20*(4), 487–504. https://doi.org/10.1111/j.1467-954X.1972.tb00220.x

## 1. Brian Sinclair

Andermann, A. (2017). Outbreaks in the age of syndemics: New insights for improving Indigenous health. *Canada Communicable Disease Report, 43*(6), 125–32. https://doi.org/10.14745/ccdr.v43i06a02

Bousquet, M.-P. (2021, 14 July). Residential schools: We *must* read the Commission reports. *Policy Options*. https://policyoptions .irpp.org/magazines/july-2021/residential-schools-we-should-read -the-commission-reports/

Brian Sinclair Working Group. (2017). *Out of sight: A summary of the events leading up to Brian Sinclair's death, the inquest that examined it and the interim recommendations of the Brian Sinclair Working Group.* https://www.dropbox .com/s/wxf3v5uh2pun0pf/Out/of/Sight/Final.pdf

Canadian Institute for Health Information (CIHI). (n.d.). Health inequalities. https://www.cihi.ca/en/health-inequalities

Carabez, R., Pellegrini, M., Mankovitz, A., Eliason, M., Ciano, M., & Scott, M. (2015). "Never in all my years ...": Nurses' education about LGBT health. *Journal of Professional Nursing, 31*(4), 323–9. https://doi.org/10.1016/j .profnurs.2015.01.003

Chambers, L.A., Rueda, S., Baker, D.N., Wilson, M.G., Deutsch, R., Raeifar, E., Rourke, S.B., & The Stigma Review Team. (2015). Stigma, HIV and health: A qualitative synthesis. *BMC Public Health, 15*(1), 848. https:// doi.org/10.1186/s12889-015-2197-0

Clarkson, A.F., Christian, W.M., Pearce, M.E., Jongbloed, K.A., ... Spittal, P.M., for the Cedar Project Partnership. (2015). The Cedar Project: Negative health outcomes associated with involvement in the child welfare system among young Indigenous peoples who use injection and non-injection drugs in two Canadian cities. *Canadian Journal of Public Health, 106*(5), 265–70. https://doi.org/10.17269/cjph.106.5026

Currie, C., Wild, T.C., Schopflocher, D., & Laing, L. (2015). Racial discrimination, post- traumatic stress and prescription drug problems among Aboriginal Canadians. *Canadian Journal of Public Health, 106*(6), 382–7. https://doi.org/10.17269/cjph.106.4979

Daiski, I. (2005). The health bus: Healthcare for marginalized populations. *Policy, Politics, & Nursing Practice, 6*(1), 30–8. https://doi.org/10.1177 /1527154404272610

Delgado, R. (1982). Words that wound: A tort action for racial insults, epithets, and name-calling. *Harvard Civil Rights – Civil Liberties Law Review, 17,* 133. https://scholarship.law.ua.edu/fac_articles/360

Dinsmore, A.P. (2012). A small-scale investigation of hospital experiences among people with a learning disability on Merseyside: Speaking with patients and their carers. *British Journal of Learning Disabilities, 40*(3), 201–12. https://doi.org/10.1111/j.1468-3156.2011.00694.x

Eliason, M.J., Dibble, S.L., & Robertson, P.A. (2011). Lesbian, gay, bisexual, and transgender (LGBT) physicians' experiences in the workplace. *Journal of Homosexuality, 58*(10), 1355–71. https://doi.org/10.1080/00918369.2011.614902

Employment and Social Development Canada. (2019, 20 February). *The Government of Canada announces significant investments to address Indigenous homelessness and housing* [News release]. https://www.canada.ca/en/employment-social-development/news/2019/02/the-government-of-canada-announces-significant-investments-to-address-indigenous-homelessness-and-housing.html

First Nations adults more than twice as likely to die from avoidable causes. (2015, 19 August). *CBC News.* https://www.cbc.ca/news/indigenous/first-nations-adults-more-than-twice-as-likely-to-die-from-avoidable-causes-1.3196496

First Nations in Manitoba. (2021, 11 February). *Wikipedia.* https://en.wikipedia.org/wiki/First_Nations_in_Manitoba

Galli, G., Noel, J.P., Canzoneri, E., Blanke, O., & Serino, A. (2015). The wheelchair as a full-body tool extending the peripersonal space. *Frontiers in Psychology, 6,* 639. https://doi.org/10.3389/fpsyg.2015.00639

Garner, R., Carrière, G., Sanmartin, C., & the Longitudinal Health and Administrative Data Research Team. (2010). *The health of First Nations living off-reserve, Inuit, and Métis adults in Canada: The impact of socioeconomic status on inequalities in health* (Working paper). Catalogue no. 82-622-X – No. 004. Statistics Canada, Health Information and Research Division. http://www.statcan.gc.ca/pub/82-622-x/82-622-x2010004-eng.pdf

Geary, A. (2017, 19 September). Ignored to death: Brian Sinclair's death caused by racism, inquest inadequate, group says. *CBC News.* https://www.cbc.ca/news/canada/manitoba/winnipeg-brian-sinclair-report-1.4295996

Gershon, A.S., Khan, S., Klein-Geltink, J., Wilton, D., To, T., Crighton, E.J., ...
Henry, D.A. (2014). Asthma and chronic obstructive pulmonary disease
(COPD) prevalence and health services use in Ontario Métis:
A population-based cohort study. *PLoS One, 9*(4), e95899. https://
doi.org/10.1371/journal.pone.0095899

Gladwell, M. (2005). *Blink: The power of thinking without thinking*. Little
Brown.

Goldner, E.M., Bilsker, D., & Jenkins, E. (2016). *A concise introduction to mental
health in Canada*. Canadian Scholars' Press.

Government of Canada. (2019). Social determinants of health and health
inequalities. https://www.canada.ca/en/public-health/services/health
-promotion/population-health/what-determines-health.html

Graham, J. (2020, 3 June). Survivors of missing, slain indigenous women in
Canada impatient for action. *Thomson Reuters Foundation News*. https://
news.trust.org/item/20200603162150-jy5cx/

Human Rights Watch. (2017, 12 January). Canada: Events of 2016. In *Human
Rights Watch, World Report, 2017: Events of 2016* (pp. 171–4). https://www
.hrw.org/world-report/2017/country-chapters/canada

Hwang, J., & Hopkins, K.M. (2015). A structural equation model of the
effects of diversity characteristics and inclusion on organizational
outcomes in the child welfare workforce. *Children and Youth Services
Review, 50*, 44–52. https://doi.org/10.1016/j.childyouth.2015.01.012

Kirkup, K. (2017, 25 October). Canada's Indigenous population growing 4
times faster than rest of country. *Global News*. https://globalnews.ca
/news/3823772/canadas-growing-indigenous-population/

Kool, N., van Meijel, B., van der Bijl, J., Koekkoek, B., & Kerkhof, A. (2015).
Psychometric properties of the Dutch version of the Attitude Towards
Deliberate Self-Harm Questionnaire. *International Journal of Mental Health
Nursing, 24*(4), 334–41. https://doi.org/10.1111/inm.12131

Kubinec, V.-L. (2013, 13 September). Brian Sinclair observed at least 17 times
by ER staff. *CBC News*. https://www.cbc.ca/news/canada/manitoba
/brian-sinclair-observed-at-least-17-times-by-er-staff-1.182

Leung, M. (2015, 15 December). Aboriginal children at residential
schools often buried in unmarked graves, report reveals. *CTV News*.
https://www.ctvnews.ca/canada/aboriginal-children-at-residential
-schools-often-buried-in-unmarked-graves-report-reveals-1
.2701373

Levasseur, J., & Marcoux, J. (2015, 14 October). Bad water: "Third World" conditions on First Nations in Canada. *CBC News.* https://www.cbc.ca /news/canada/manitoba/bad-water-third-world-conditions-on-first -nations-in-canada-1.3269500

Lewis, S., & Stenfert-Kroese, B. (2010). An investigation of nursing staff attitudes and emotional reactions towards patients with intellectual disability in a general hospital setting. *Journal of Applied Research in Intellectual Disabilities, 23*(4), 355–65. https://doi.org/10.1111 /j.1468-3148.2009.00542.x

Ly, A., & Crowshoe, L. (2015). "Stereotypes are reality": Addressing stereotyping in Canadian Aboriginal medical education. *Medical Education, 49*(6), 612–22. https://doi.org/10.1111/medu.12725

MacDonald, N. (2015, 22 January). Welcome to Winnipeg: Where Canada's racism problem is at its worst. *MacLean's Magazine.* https://www .macleans.ca/news/canada/welcome-to-winnipeg-where-canadas -racism-problem-is-at-its-worst/

Manitoba's Aboriginal population continues to grow. (2013, 8 May). *CBC News.* https://www.cbc.ca/news/canada/manitoba /manitoba-s-aboriginal-population-continues-to-grow-1.1337131

Martens, K. (2019, 17 December). Canada has made "dreadful progress" in fulfilling TRC's calls to action. *APTN National News.* https://www .aptnnews.ca/national-news/canada-has-made-dreadful-progress -in-fulfilling-trcs-calls-to-action/

Meiboom, A., Diedrich, C., Vries, H.D., Hertogh, C., & Scheele, F. (2015) The hidden curriculum of the medical care for elderly patients in medical education: A qualitative study. *Gerontology & Geriatrics Education, 36*(1), 30–44. https://doi.org/10.1080/02701960.2014.966902

Menzies, P. (2020, 25 March). Intergenerational trauma and residential school. *The Canadian Encyclopedia.* https://www.thecanadianencyclopedia .ca/en/article/intergenerational-trauma-and-residential-schools

Monks, R., Topping, A., & Newell, R. (2013). The dissonant care management of illicit drug users in medical wards, the views of nurses and patients: A grounded theory study. *Journal of Advanced Nursing, 69*(4), 935–46. https://doi.org/10.1111/j.1365-2648.2012.06088.x

Morgan, B.D. (2014). Nursing attitudes toward patients with substance abuse disorders in pain. *Pain Management Nursing, 15*(1), 165–75. https:// doi.org/10.1016/j.pmn.2012.08.004

National Collaborating Centre for Aboriginal Health. (2013). An overview of Aboriginal health in Canada. http://www.nccah-ccnsa.ca/Publications /Lists/Publications/Attachments/101/abororiginal_health_web.pdf

National Inquiry into Missing and Murdered Indigenous Women and Girls. (2019). *Reclaiming power and place: The final report of the National Inquiry into Missing and Murdered Indigenous Women and Girls.* https://www.mmiwg -ffada.ca/final-report/

Paradies, Y., Truong, M., & Priest, N. (2014). A systematic review of the extent and measurement of healthcare provider racism. *Journal of General Internal Medicine, 29*(2), 364–87. https://doi.org/10.1007/s11606-013-2583-1

Potvin, L. (2015). Public health and the sad legacy of Indian residential schools. *Canadian Journal of Public Health, 106*(5), e257–60. https://doi .org/10.17269/cjph.106.5264

Provincial Court of Manitoba. (2014). Brian Sinclair Inquest. http://www .manitobacourts.mb.ca/site/assets/files/1051/brian_sinclair_inquest _-_dec_14.pdf

Provincial Implementation Team. (2015). *The Provincial Implementation Team report on the recommendations of the Brian Sinclair Inquest report.* Manitoba Minister of Health. https://www.gov.mb.ca/health/documents/bsi _report.pdf

Puskar, K., Gotham, H.J., Terhorst, L., Hagle, H., Mitchell, A.M., Braxter, B., ... Burns, H.K. (2013). Effects of screening, brief intervention, and referral to treatment (SBIRT) education and training on nursing students' attitudes toward working with patients who use alcohol and drugs. *Substance Abuse, 34*(2), 122–8. https://doi.org/10.1080/08897077.2012 .715621

Razali, S.M., & Ismail, Z. (2014). Public stigma towards patients with schizophrenia of ethnic Malay: A comparison between the general public and patients' relatives. *Journal of Mental Health, 23*(4), 176–80. https:// doi.org/10.3109/09638237.2014.910644

Read, G., & Webb, T. (2012). "The Catholic Mahdi of the North West": Louis Riel and the Metis resistance in transatlantic and imperial context. *Canadian Historical Review, 93*(2), 171–95. https://doi.org/10.3138 /chr.93.2.171

Rollason, K., & Welch, M.A. (2014, 13 December). Inquest report disappoints: Review of Sinclair's ER death fails him, family, doctor says. *Winnipeg Free*

*Press*. https://www.winnipegfreepress.com/local/inquest-report
-disappoints-285702111.html

Rotenberg, C. (2012). *Aboriginal Peoples Survey: The social determinants of
health for the off-reserve First Nations population, 15 years of age and older,
2012*. Catalogue no. 89-653-X2016009. Statistics Canada. http://www
.statcan.gc.ca/pub/89-653-x/89-653-x2016010-eng.pdf

Ryan, C.J., Cooke, M.J., Leatherdale, S.T., Kirkpatrick, S.I., & Wilk, P. (2015).
The correlates of current smoking among adult Métis: Evidence from the
Aboriginal Peoples Survey and Métis Supplement. *Canadian Journal of
Public Health, 106*(5), e271–6. https://doi.org/10.17269/cjph.106.5053

Sanders-Phillips, K., Settles-Reaves, B., Walker, D., & Brownlow, J. (2009).
Social inequality and racial discrimination: Risk factors for health
disparities in children of color. *Pediatrics, 124*(Supplement 3), S176–86.
https://doi.org/10.1542/peds.2009-1100E

Shattock, L., Williamson, H., Caldwell, K., Anderson, K., & Peters, S.
(2013). "They've just got symptoms without science": Medical trainees'
acquisition of negative attitudes towards patients with medically
unexplained symptoms. *Patient Education and Counseling, 91*(2), 249–54.
https://doi.org/10.1016/j.pec.2012.12.015

Silins, E., Conigrave, K.M., Rakvin, C.C., Dobbins, T., & Curry, K. (2007). The
influence of structured education and clinical experience on the attitudes
of medical students towards substance misusers. *Drug & Alcohol Review,
26*(2), 191–200. https://doi.org/10.1080/09595230601184661

Statistics Canada. (2017a). *Focus on geography series, 2016 Census: Canada*.
Statistics Canada Catalogue no. 98–404-X2016001. https://www12.statcan
.gc.ca/census-recensement/2016/as-sa/fogs-spg/Facts-CAN-eng.cfm
?Lang=Eng&GK=CAN&GC=01&TOPIC=9

Statistics Canada. (2017b). *Focus on geography series, 2016 Census: Province
of Manitoba*. Statistics Canada Catalogue no. 98–404-X2016001. https://
www12.statcan.gc.ca/census-recensement/2016/as-sa/fogs-spg/Facts
-PR-Eng.cfm?TOPIC=9&LANG=Eng&GK=PR&GC=46

Statistics Canada. (2018). National Indigenous Peoples Day ... by the
numbers. https://www.statcan.gc.ca/eng/dai/smr08/2018/smr08
_225_2018

Sue, D.W. (2010). *Microaggressions in everyday life: Race, gender and sexual
orientation*. Wiley.

Tang, S.Y., & Browne, A.J. (2008). "Race" matters: Racialization and egalitarian discourses involving Aboriginal people in the Canadian health care context. *Ethnicity and Health, 13*(2), 109–27. https://doi.org /10.1080/13557850701830307

Truth and Reconciliation Commission of Canada (TRC). (2015). *Honouring the truth, reconciling for the future: Summary of the final report of the Truth and Reconciliation Commission of Canada.* http://www.trc.ca/assets /pdf/Honouring_the_Truth_Reconciling_for_the_Future_July_23 _2015.pdf

Union of BC Indian Chiefs. (2015). UN human rights report shows that Canada is failing Indigenous peoples (Joint statement). https://www .ubcic.bc.ca/canadafailingindigenouspeoples

United Nations. (2010). State of the world's Indigenous peoples. [Press release]. https://www.un.org/esa/socdev/unpfii/documents/SOWIP /press%20package/sowip-press-package-en.pdf

Vowel, C. (2016). *Indigenous writes: A guide to First Nations, Metis & Inuit issues in Canada.* Highwater Press.

White, L., & McGrew, J. (2013). Parents served by assertive community treatment: Prevalence, treatment services, and provider attitudes. *Journal of Behavioural Health Services & Research, 40*(3), 263–78. https://doi.org /10.1007/s11414-013-9321-7

## 2. Ashley Smith

Ashley Smith death ruled a homicide by inquest jury. (2013, 19 December). *National Post.* https://nationalpost.com/news/canada/ashley -smith-death-ruled-a-homicide-by-inquest-jury

Ashley Smith inquest: Warden didn't know of guard's confusion about entering cell. (2013a, 30 September). *CTV News.* https://www.ctvnews.ca /canada/ashley-smith-inquest-warden-didn-t-know-of-guard-s -confusion-about-entering-cell-1.1476269

Ashley Smith inquest: Key recommendations from the jury. (2013b, 19 December). *Global News.* https://globalnews.ca/news/1041116 /ashley-smith-inquest-key-recommendations-from-the-jury/

Ashley Smith's sedation in custody unwarranted: Report. (2010, 1 November). *CBC News.* https://www.cbc.ca/news/canada /ashley-smith-s-sedations-incustody-unwarranted-report-1.928740

Black out Ashley Smith evidence: Prison service. (2011, 16 May).
   *CBC News.* https://www.cbc.ca/news/canada/black-out-ashley
   -smith-evidence-prison-service-1.979435
Canadian Medical Protective Association (CMPA). (2021). *Consent:*
   *A guide for Canadian physicians* (4th ed.). https://www.cmpa-acpm.ca/en
   /advice-publications/handbooks/consent-a-guide-for-canadian-physicians
Carlson, K.B. (2013, 19 December). Mother "elated" as Ashley Smith's
   jail death is ruled a homicide. *The Globe and Mail.* https://www
   .theglobeandmail.com/news/national/ashley-smith-inquest
   /article16052548/
Chief Coroner, Province of Ontario. (2013). Coroner's inquest touching the
   death of Ashley Smith. https://www.csc-scc.gc.ca/publications/005007
   -9009-eng.shtml
Citizens Commission on Human Rights. (n.d.). Antipsychotic drug
   side effects. https://www.cchrint.org/psychiatric-drugs/anti
   psychoticsideeffects/
Citizens Commission on Human Rights. (2010). Mood stabilizers: The facts
   about their effects. https://www.cchr.org/sites/default/files/education
   /mood-stabilizers-booklet.pdf
Cocozza, J.J., & Skowyra, K.R. (2000). Youth with mental health disorders:
   Issues and emerging responses. *Juvenile Justice, 7*(1), 3–13. https://www
   .ojp.gov/pdffiles1/ojjdp/178256.pdf
Correctional Service of Canada. (2014). Coroner's inquest touching the death
   of Ashley Smith. https://www.csc-scc.gc.ca/publications/005007-9009
   -eng.shtml
Fazel, S., & Danesh, J. (2002). Serious mental disorder in 23,000 prisoners: A
   systematic review of 62 surveys. *The Lancet, 359,* 545–50. https://doi.org
   /10.1016/S0140-6736(02)07740-1
*Fifth Estate, The.* (2010a, 8 January). Out of control. *CBC.* https://www.cbc
   .ca/fifth/episodes/2009-2010/out-of-control
*Fifth Estate, The.* (2010b, 12 November). Behind the wall. *CBC.* https://www
   .cbc.ca/fifth/episodes/2010-2011/behind-the-wall
*Fifth Estate, The.* (2010c, 12 November). Timeline: The life and death of
   Ashley Smith. *CBC.* https://www.cbc.ca/fifth/blog/the-life-and-death
   -of-ashley-smith
Goffman, E. (1961). *Asylums: Essays on the social situation of mental patient and
   other inmates.* Anchor Books.

Health board criticizes Ashley Smith's prison treatment before death. (2011, 19 July). *Toronto Star*. https://www.thestar.com/news/canada /2011/07/19/health_board_criticizes_ashley_smiths_prison_treatment _before_death.html

Hirschfield, P., Maschi, T., White, H.R., Traub, L.G., & Loeber, R. (2006). Mental health and juvenile arrests: Criminality, criminalization, or compassion? *Criminology, 44*(3), 593–630. https://doi.org /10.1111/j.1745-9125.2006.00058.x

James, D.J., & Glaze, L.E. (2006). Mental health problems of prison and jail inmates. *Bureau of Justice Statistics*. https://www.bjs.gov/index .cfm?ty=pbdetail&iid=789

Kaba, F., Lewis, A., Glowa-Kollisch, S., Hadler, J., Lee, D., Alper, H., ... Venters, H. (2014). Solitary confinement and risk of self-harm among jail inmates. *American Journal of Public Health, 104*(3), 442–7. https://doi .org/10.2105/AJPH.2013.301742

Kilty, J.M., & LeBlanc, N. (2012). Ashley Smith (1988–2007): A predictable death. *Policy Options*. https://policyoptions.irpp.org/magazines /talking-science/kilty-leblanc/

Larocque, R. (2017). *Segregation in Ontario: Segregation literature review*. Prepared for the Independent Review of Ontario Corrections, Ministry of the Solicitor General of Ontario. https://www.mcscs.jus.gov.on.ca /english/Corrections/IndependentReviewOntarioCorrections /SegregationOntarioLiteratureReview.html

Martel, J. (2006). Les femmes et l'isolement cellulaire au Canada: un défi de l'esprit sur la matière [Women and solitary confinement in Canada: Mind over matter]. *Canadian Journal of Criminology and Criminal Justice, 48*(5), 781–801. https://doi.org/10.3138/cjccj.48.5.781

Mendez, J. (2011, 18 October). Solitary confinement should be banned in most cases, UN expert says. *UN News*. https://news.un.org/en /story/2011/10/392012-solitary-confinement-should-be-banned-most -cases-un-expert-says

Office of the Correctional Investigator. (2014). Backgrounder: "A preventable death." https://www.oci-bec.gc.ca/cnt/rpt/oth-aut/oth-aut20080620info -eng.aspx

Office of the Provincial Advocate for Children and Youth of Ontario. (2015). *It's a matter of time: Systemic review of secure isolation in Ontario youth justice facilities*. https://www.publications.gov.on.ca/its-a-matter

-of-time-systemic-review-of-secure-isolation-in-ontario-youth-justice-facilities

Ombudsman and Child Youth Advocate. (2008). *The Ashley Smith report.* Office of the Ombudsman and Youth Advocate. https://www.ombudnb .ca/site/images/PDFs/AshleySmith-e.pdf

Perkel, C. (2013, 18 April). RCMP pilot defends decision to duct tape Smith during prison death inquest. *Global News.* https://globalnews.ca /news/491210/rcmp-pilot-to-testify-at-teens-prison-death-inquest/

Perreault, S. (2012). Police-reported crime statistics in Canada, 2012. Statistics Canada. https://www150.statcan.gc.ca/n1/pub/85-002-x /2013001/article/11854-eng.htm

Razack, S.H. (2014). Racial terror: Torture and three teenagers in prison. *Borderlands, 13*(1), 1–26. https://www.thefreelibrary.com /Racial+terror%3A+torture+and+three+teenagers+in+prison -a0383981192

Seglins, D. (2011, 4 May). Ashley Smith's family settles $11 million suit. *CBC News.* https://www.cbc.ca/news/canada/ashley-smith -family-settles-11m-suit-1.1003660

Shelton, D. (2002). Failure of mental health policy – Incarcerated children and adolescents. *Pediatric Nursing, 28*(3), 278.

Statistics Canada. (2013). Canadian community health survey: Mental health, 2012. https://www150.statcan.gc.ca/n1/daily-quotidien/130918 /dq130918a-eng.htm

Stout, B.D., & Holleran, D. (2012). The impact of mental health services implementation on juvenile court placements: An examination of New Jersey's SOC initiative. *Criminal Justice Policy Review, 23*(4), 447–64. https://doi.org/10.1177/0887403411414408

Taylor-Butts, A., & Bressan, A. (2008). Youth crime in Canada, 2006. *Juristat, 28*(3), 1. https://www150.statcan.gc.ca/n1/pub/85-002-x/2008003 /article/10566-eng.htm

Templin, L.A., Abram, K.M., McClelland, G.M., Dulcan, M.K., & Mericle, A.A. (2002). Psychiatric disorders in youth juvenile detention. *Archives of General Psychiatry, 59*(12), 1133–43. https://doi.org/10.1001 /archpsyc.59.12.1133

Ullman S.E. (2016). Sexual revictimization, PTSD, and problem drinking in sexual assault survivors. *Addictive Behaviors, 53*, 7–10. https://doi.org /10.1016/j.addbeh.2015.09.010

Vincent, D. (2013a, 25 March). Did Ashley Smith belong in prison
at all? *Waterloo Regional Record*. https://www.waterloochronicle.ca
/news-story/2629164-did-ashley-smith-belong-in-prison-at-all-/

Vincent, D. (2013b, 17 April). Ashley Smith inquest: Ex-investigator slams
"culture of intimidation at Saskatoon prison." *Toronto Star*. https://
www.thestar.com/news/canada/2013/04/17/ashley_smith_inquest
_exinvestigator_slams_culture_of_intimidation_at_saskatoon_prison.html

Vincent, D. (2013c, 8 May). Ashley Smith given five injections of drugs in
seven hours at Quebec prison, inquest told. *Toronto Star*. https://www
.thestar.com/news/canada/2013/05/08/ashley_smith_given_five
_injections_of_drugs_in_seven_hours_at_quebec_prison_inquest_told
.html

Waddell, C., Lavis, J.N., Abelson, J., Lomas, J., Shepherd, C.A., Bird-Gayson,
T., ... Offord, D.R.D. (2005). Research use in children's mental health
policy in Canada: Maintaining vigilance amid ambiguity. *Social Science &
Medicine, 61*(8), 1649–57. https://doi.org/10.1016/j.socscimed.2005.03.032

Whitaker, R.H. (2001). *Mad in America: Bad science, bad medicine and the
enduring mistreatment of the mentally ill*. Basic Books.

Whitaker, R.H. (2010). *Anatomy of an epidemic: Magic bullets, psychiatric
drugs, and the astonishing rise of mental illness in America*. Crown
Publishers.

Zlomislic, D. (2009, 10 October) From generous girl to "caged animal."
*Toronto Star*. https://www.thestar.com/news/canada/2009/10/10/from
_generous_girl_to_caged_animal.html

Zlomislic, D., & Vincent, D. (2013, 15 December). Excerpt: The life and
death of Ashley Smith. *Toronto Star*. https://www.thestar.com/news
/canada/2013/12/15/excerpt_the_life_and_death_of_ashley_smith.html

## 3. Vanessa Young and Marit McKenzie

AllTrials. (n.d.). What does all trials registered and reported mean? https://
www.alltrials.net/find-outmore/all-trials/

American Society of Plastic Surgeons. (2019, 10 April). Americans spent more
than $16.5 billion on cosmetic plastic surgery in 2018 [Press release].
https://www.plasticsurgery.org/news/press-releases/americans
-spent-more-than-16-billion-on-cosmetic-plastic-surgery-in-2018

Belzak, L., & Halverson, J. (2018). Evidence synthesis – The opioid crisis in Canada: A national perspective. *Health Promotion and Chronic Disease Prevention in Canada: Research, Policy and Practice, 38*(6), 224–33. https:// doi.org/10.24095/hpcdp.38.6.02

Blum, L.M., & Stracuzzi, N.F. (2004). Gender in the Prozac nation: Popular discourse and productive femininity. *Gender & Society, 18*(3), 269–86. https://doi.org/10.1177/0891243204263108

Budnitz, D.S., Lovegrove, M.C., Shehab, N., & Richards, C.L. (2011). Emergency hospitalizations for adverse drug events in older Americans. *New England Journal of Medicine, 365*(21), 2002–12. https://doi.org/10.1056 /NEJMsa1103053

Canadian Foundation for Healthcare Improvement. (2010, 1 October). Myth: If a drug makes it to the market it is safe for everyone. https://web .archive.org/web/20171018040746/http://www.cfhi-fcass.ca /PublicationsAndResources/Mythbusters/ArticleView/2010/10/01 /f1ca3fcf-f9aa-4dcb-a64c-a95f2bbadd8d.aspx

Canadian Foundation for Healthcare Improvement. (2013, 13 March). Myth: When it comes to drugs and devices, newer is always better. https:// web.archive.org/web/20171017234755/http://www.cfhi-fcass.ca /PublicationsAndResources/Mythbusters/ArticleView/13-03 -13/7081e550-fed8-4c8c-84c6-bfd360e48f19.aspx

Canadian Institute for Health Information. (2014). *Bariatric surgery in Canada.* https://secure.cihi.ca/free_products/Bariatric_Surgery _in_Canada_EN.pdf

Clarke, J.N. (2009). Women's work, worry and fear: The portrayal of sexuality and sexual health in US magazines for teenage and middle-aged women, 2000–2007. *Culture, Health & Sexuality, 11*(4), 415–29. https:// doi.org/10.1080/13691050902780776

Clarke, J.N. (2013). Medicalisation and changes in advice to mothers about children's mental health issues 1970 to 1990 as compared to 1991 to 2010: Evidence from Chatelaine magazine. *Health, Risk & Society, 15*(5), 416–31. https://doi.org/10.1080/13698575.2013.802295

Clarke, J.N. (2016). The underside of medicalisation: The portrayal of medical error over time in North American popular mass magazines. *Health, Risk & Society, 18*(5–6), 270–82. https://doi.org/10.1080/13698575 .2016.1241383

Clarke, J.N., & Miele, R. (2016). Trapped by gender: The paradoxical portrayal of gender and mental illness in anglophone North American magazines: 1983–2012. *Women's Studies International Forum, 56,* 1–8. https://doi.org/10.1016/j.wsif.2016.01.002

Coleman, J.J., & Pontefract, S.K. (2016). Adverse drug reactions. *Clinical Medicine Journal* (London), *16*(5), 481–5. https://doi.org/10.7861 /clinmedicine.16-5-481

Collins, R.L. (2011). Content analysis of gender roles in media: Where are we now and where should we go? *Sex Roles, 64*(3–4), 290–8. https:// doi.org/10.1007/s11199-010-9929-5

DATAC. (2018, 13 February). Health Canada switches to mainly pharmaceutical funding. https://datac.ca/health-canada -switches-mainly-pharmaceutical-funding/

Donella, L. (2019, 6 February). Is beauty in the eyes of the colonizer? *NPR.* https://www.npr.org/sections/codeswitch/2019/02/06/685506578 /is-beauty-in-the-eyes-of-the-colonizer

Dresser, R., & Frader, J. (2009). Off-label prescribing a call for heightened governmental and professional oversight. *Journal Law & Medical Ethics,* *37*(3), 476–86. https://doi.org/10.1111/j.1748-720X.2009.00408.x

Ellis, E. (2013, 25 April). Diet industry expands right along with North America waistlines. *Global News.* https://globalnews.ca/news/519060 /diet-industry-expands-right-along-with-north-america-waistlines/

Evans, A., & Riley, S. (2013). Immaculate consumption: Negotiating the sex symbol in postfeminist celebrity culture. *Journal of Gender Studies, 22*(3), 268–81. https://doi.org/10.1080/09589236.2012.658145

FDA (US Food and Drug Administration). (2018). Preventable adverse drug reactions: A focus on drug interactions. https://www.fda.gov /drugs/drug-interactions-labeling/preventable-adverse-drug-reactions -focus-drug-interactions

Glauser, W. (2013). Pharma influence widespread at medical school: Study. *CMAJ, 185*(13), 1121–2. https://doi.org/10.1503/cmaj.109-4563

Government of Canada. (2011). Obesity in Canada. https://www.canada .ca/en/public-health/services/health-promotion/healthy-living/obesity -canada.html

Government of Canada. (2018). Prescription drug pricing and costs. https:// www.canada.ca/en/health-canada/services/health-care-system /pharmaceuticals/costs-prices.html

Hajli, M.N. (2014). A study of the impact of social media on consumers. *International Journal of Market Research, 56*(3), 387–404. https://doi.org /10.2501/IJMR-2014-025

Hazel L., & Shakir, S.A. (2006). Under-reporting of adverse drug reactions: A systematic review. *Drug Safety, 29*(5), 385–96. https://doi.org/10.2165 /00002018-200629050-00003

Health Canada. (2000). Cisapride (Prepulsid): Interactions. *Canadian Adverse Reaction Newsletter.* https://www.canada.ca/en/health-canada/services /drugs-health-products/medeffect-canada/health-product-infowatch /published-canadian-adverse-reaction-newsletters.html

Health Canada. (2014). Health Canada's review of Diane-35 supports current labelling and use. https://healthycanadians.gc.ca/recall-alert-rappel -avis/hc-sc/2013/29283a-eng.php

Hunt, K., Adamson, J., Hewitt, C., & Nazareth, I. (2011). Do women consult more than men? A review of gender and consultation for back pain and headache. *Journal of Health Services Research & Policy, 16*(2), 108–17. https:// doi.org/10.1258/jhsrp.2010.009131

International Society of Aesthetic Plastic Surgery. (2019, 3 December). Top 10 surgical cosmetic procedures worldwide in 2019 [Graph]. *Statista.* https://www.statista.com/statistics/293437/leading -surgical-cosmetic-procedures/

Jamieson, D.G. (2006). Literacy in Canada. *Paediatrics & Child Health, 11*(9), 573–4. https://doi.org/10.1093/pch/11.9.573

Jureidini, J.N., Doecke, C.J., Mansfield, P.R., Haby, M.M., & Menkes, D.B. (2004). Efficacy and safety of antidepressants for children and adolescents. *BMJ, 328,* 879–83. https://doi.org/10.1136/bmj.328.7444.879

Kashubeck-West, S., & Huang, H. (2013). Social class relations with body image and eating disorders. In W.M. Liu (Ed.), *The Oxford handbook of social class in counseling* (pp. 197–217). Oxford University Press.

Kravitz, R.L., Epstein, R.M., Feldman, M.D., Franz, C.E., Azari, R., Wilkes, M.S., ... Franks, P. (2005). Influence of patients' requests for direct-to-consumer advertised antidepressants: A randomized controlled trial. *JAMA, 293*(16), 1995–2002. https://doi.org/10.1001/jama.293.16.1995

Lexchin, J. (2006). Relationship between pharmaceutical company user fees and drug approval in Canada and Australia: A hypothesis generating study. *Annals of Pharmatherapy, 40*(12), 2216–22. https://doi.org/10.1345 /aph.1H117

Lexchin, J. (2009). Drug safety and Health Canada: Going, going … gone? Canadian Centre for Policy Alternatives. http://www.policyalternatives .ca/sites/default/files/uploads/publications/National_Office_Pubs/2009 /Drug_Safety_and_Health_Canada.pdf

Lexchin, J. (2014). How safe are new drugs? Market withdrawal of drugs approved in Canada between 1990 and 2009. *Open Medicine, 8*(1), e14–19.

Manteuffel, M., Williams, S., Chen, W., Verbrugge, R.R., Pittman, D.G., & Steinkellner, A. (2014). Influence of patient sex and prescribing alignment with guidelines. *Journal of Women's Health, 23*(2), 112–19. https://doi.org /10.1089/jwh.2012.3972

McIver, S., & Wyndam, R. (2013). *After the error: Speaking out about patient safety to save lives.* ECW Press. (See excerpt: Sudden cardiac death: Vanessa's story, posted on the $R_x isk$ blog, https://rxisk.org /sudden-cardiac-death-vanessas-story/).

Minksy, A. (2017, 17 August). Health Canada "gutting" law to detect dangerous medicines, with possible deadly consequences, advocates warn. *Global News.* https://globalnews.ca/news/3674979/dangerous -medicine-prescription-drugs-vanessaslaw-health-canada-gutting/

Mintzes, B. (2004). Drug regulatory failure in Canada: The case of Diane-35. *Women and Health Protection.* http://www.whp-apsf.ca/en/documents /diane35.html

Mintzes, B., Barer, M.L., Kravitz, R.L., Bassett, K., Lexchin, J., Kazanjian, A., … Marion, S.A. (2003). How does direct-to-consumer advertising (DTCA) affect prescribing? A survey in primary care environments with and without legal DTCA. *CMAJ, 169*(5), 405–12. https://www.cmaj.ca /content/169/5/405

Mintzes, B., Barer, M.L., Kravitz, R.L., Kazanjian, A., Bassett, K., Lexchin, J., … Marion, S.A. (2002). Influence of direct to consumer pharmaceutical advertising and patients' requests on prescribing decisions: Two site cross sectional survey. *BMJ, 324*(7332), 278–9. https://doi.org/10.1136 /bmj.324.7332.278

Morgan, S., & Kennedy, J. (2010, June). Prescription drug accessibility and affordability in the United States and abroad. *Issues in International Health Policy,* Commonwealth Fund publication 1408. https://www .commonwealthfund.org/sites/default/files/documents/___media_files _publications_issue_brief_2010_jun_1408_morgan_prescription_drug _accessibility_us_intl_ib.pdf

Moride, Y., Haramburu, F., Requejo, A.A., & Begaud, B. (1997). Underreporting of adverse drug reactions in general practice. *British Journal of Clinical Pharmacology, 43*(2), 177–81. https://doi.org/10.1046/j.1365-2125.1997.05417.x

National Institute of Diabetes and Kidney and Digestive Diseases. (2020). Weight-loss surgery side effects: What are the side effects of bariatric surgery? https://www.niddk.nih.gov/health-information/weight-management/bariatric-surgery/side-effects

National Institute on Aging. (2020). What are clinical trials and studies? https://www.nia.nih.gov/health/what-are-clinical-trials-and-studies#four

NPD Group. (2019, 21 November). Lighting the path to growth in Canada beauty. [Infographic]. https://www.npd.com/news/infographics/2019/lighting-the-path-to-growth-in-canada-beauty/

Odette, F. (2013). Body beautiful/body perfect: Where do women with disabilities fit in? In M. Hobbs & C. Rice (Eds.), *Gender and women's studies in Canada: Critical terrain* (pp. 414–16). Canadian Scholar's Press.

OECD (Organisation for Economic Co-operation and Development). (2020). Pharmaceutical spending (indicator). https://data.oecd.org/healthres/pharmaceutical-spending.htm

Office on Women's Health. (2017). Bulimia nervosa. U.S. Department of Health and Human Services. https://www.womenshealth.gov/mental-health/mental-health-conditions/eating-disorders/bulimia-nervosa

Orbach, S. (1986). *Hunger strike: The anorectic's struggle as a metaphor for our age*. Faber.

Parliament of Canada. (2014). Bill C-17. https://www.parl.ca/DocumentViewer/en/41-2/bill/C-17/royal-assent

Patented Medicine Prices Review Board. (2020). Mandate and jurisdiction. http://pmprb-cepmb.gc.ca/about-us/mandate-and-jurisdiction

Pimentel, C.B., Donovan, J.L., Field, T.S., Gurwitz, J.H., Harrold, L.R., Kanaan, A.O., ... Briesacher, B.A. (2015). Use of atypical antipsychotics in nursing homes and pharmaceutical marketing. *Journal of the American Geriatrics Society, 63*(2), 297–301. https://doi.org/10.1111/jgs.13180

Prayle, A.P., Hurley, M.N., & Smyth, A.R. (2012). Compliance with mandatory reporting of clinical trial results on ClinicalTrials.gov: Cross sectional study. *BMJ, 344*, d7373. https://doi.org/10.1136/bmj.d7373

Prieler, M., & Choi, J. (2014). Broadening the scope of social media effect research on body image concerns. *Sex Roles, 71*(11–12), 378–88. https://doi.org/10.1007/s11199-014-0406-4

Radley, D.C., Finkelstein, S.N., & Stafford, R.S. (2006). Off-label prescribing among office-based physicians. *Archives of Internal Medicine, 166*(9), 1021–6. https://doi.org/10.1001/archinte.166.9.1021

Review Chatter. (2017, 27 June). Fitness & exercise industry statistics, facts & history. https://www.reviewchatter.com/statistics-facts-history/fitness

Rice, C. (2013). Exacting beauty: Exploring women's body projects and problems in the 21st century. In M. Hobbs & C. Rice (Eds.), *Gender and women's studies in Canada: Critical terrain* (pp. 390–410). Canadian Scholar's Press Inc.

Rice, C. (2014). *Becoming women: The embodied self in image culture*. University of Toronto Press.

Rosenbloom, D., & Wyne, C. (1999). Detecting adverse drug reactions. *CMAJ, 16*(3), 247–8. https://www.cmaj.ca/content/161/3/247

Rotermann, M., Sanmartin, C., Hennessy, D., & Arthur, M. (2015). Prescription medication use by Canadians aged 6 to 79. *Statistics Canada*. https://www150.statcan.gc.ca/n1/pub/82-003-x/2014006/article/14032-eng.htm

Sawler, S. (n.d.). Health Canada's post-market surveillance program: Update on new and ongoing initiatives [PowerPoint presentation]. Health Canada. https://www.chpcanada.ca/sites/default/files/scott_sawler.pdf

Shield, K.D., Ialomiteanu, A., Fischer, B., Mann, R.E., & Rehm, J. (2011). Non-medical use of prescription opioids among Ontario adults: Data from the 2008/2009 CAMH Monitor. *Canadian Journal of Public Health /Revue Canadienne de Santé Publique, 102*(5), 330–5. https://doi.org/10.1007/bf03404171

Singh, S., & Wooltorton, E. (2005) Increased mortality among elderly patients with dementia using antipsychotics. *CMAJ, 173*(3), 252. https://doi.org/10.1503/cmaj.050478

Smith, B.L. (2012). Inappropriate prescribing. *Monitor on Psychology, 43*(6), 36. https://www.apa.org/monitor/2012/06/prescribing

Solomon Facial Plastic. (n.d.). Price list: Cosmetic facial plastic surgery. https://www.solomonfacialplastic.com/about-us/price-list/

Song, F., Parekh, S., Hooper, L., Loke, Y.K., Ryder, J., Sutton, A.J., ... Harvey, I. (2010). Dissemination and publication of research findings: An updated review of related biases. *Health Technology Assessment, 14*(8), 1–193. http://doi.org/10.3310/hta14080

Swami, V., Coles, R., Wyrozumska, K., Wilson, E., Salem, N., & Furnham, A. (2010). Oppressive beliefs at play: Association among beauty ideals and practices and individual differences in sexism, objectification of others, and media exposure. *Psychology of Women Quarterly, 34*(3), 365–79. https://doi.org/10.1111/j.1471-6402.2010.01582.x

Talamas, S.N., Mavor, K.I., & Perrett, D.I. (2016). Blinded by beauty: Attractiveness bias and accurate perceptions of academic performance. *PloS One, 11*(2), e0148284. https://doi.org/10.1371/journal.pone.0148284

Tan, J.O.A., & Koelch, M. (2008). The ethics of psychopharmacological research in legal minors. *Child and Adolescent Psychiatry and Mental Health, 2*, 39–63. https://doi.org/10.1186/1753-2000-2-39

Tannenbaum, C., & Tsuyiki, R.T. (2013). The expanding scope of pharmacy in practice: Implications for physicians. *CMAJ, 185*(14), 1228–32. https://doi.org/10.1503/cmaj.121990

Weeks, C. (2010, 30 April). Health Canada report: Adverse drug reports up 35 per cent in 2009. *The Globe and Mail.* https://www.theglobeandmail.com/life/health-and-fitness/health-canada-report-adverse-drug-reports-up-35-per-cent-in-2009/article4317042/

Whitaker, R. (2001). *Mad in America: Bad science, bad medicine, and the enduring mistreatment of the mentally ill.* Basic Books.

Whitaker, R. (2010). *Anatomy of an epidemic: Magic bullets, psychiatric drugs, and the astonishing rise of mental illness in America.* Crown Publishers.

Wittich, C.M., Burkle, C.M., & Lanier, W.L. (2012). Ten common questions (and their answers) about off-label drug use. *Mayo Clinic Proceedings, 87*(10), 982–90. https://doi.org/10.1016/j.mayocp.2012.04.017

Wolf, N. (1990). *The beauty myth: How images of beauty are used against women.* Random House.

World Economic Forum. (2017). The global gender gap report: 2017. http://www3.weforum.org/docs/WEF_GGGR_2017.pdf

Young, T.H. (2012). *Death by prescription.* Key Porter Books.

Zlomislic, D. (2013a, 19 October). Calgary teen was slowly dying and didn't know it. *Toronto Star.* https://www.thestar.com/life/health_wellness/2013/10/19/calgary_teen_was_slowly_dying_and_didnt_know_it.html

Zlomislic, D. (2013b, 19 October). Health Canada review of controversial acne drug kept secret. *Toronto Star*. https://www.thestar.com/news /gta/2013/10/19/health_canada_review_of_controversial_acne_drug _kept_secret.html

## Chapter 4. Amy Tan

Adams, C. (2017, 22 September). Shania Twain was "shattered" by divorce as she battled Lyme disease: "I never thought I would sing again." *People*. https://people.com/country/shania-twain-lyme-disease-60-minutes/

Ali, A., Vitulano, L., Lee, R., Weiss, T.R., & Colson, E.R. (2014). Experiences of patients identifying with chronic Lyme disease in the health care system: A qualitative study. *BMC Family Practice, 15*, 79. https:// doi.org/10.1186/1471-2296-15-79

Auwaerter, P.G., Bakken, J.S., Dattwyler, R J., Dumler, J.S., Halperin, J.J., McSweegan, E., ... Wormser, G.P. (2011). Antiscience and ethical concerns associated with advocacy of Lyme disease. *The Lancet Infectious Diseases, 11*(9), 713–19. https://doi.org/10.1016/S1473-3099(11)70034-2

Ballantyne, C. (2008). The chronic debate over Lyme disease. *Nature Medicine, 14*(11), 1135–9. https://doi.org/10.1038/nm1108-1135

Berende, A., ter Hofstede, H.J., Vos, F.J., van Middendorp, H., Vogelaar, M.L., Tromp, M., ... Kullberg, B.J. (2016). Randomized trial of longer-term therapy for symptoms attributed to Lyme disease. *New England Journal of Medicine, 374*(13), 1209–20. https://doi.org/10.1056/NEJMoa1505425

Cameron, D.J. (2009). Insufficient evidence to deny antibiotic treatment to chronic Lyme disease patients. *Medical Hypotheses, 72*(6), 688–91. https:// doi.org/10.1016/j.mehy.2009.01.017

CanLyme (Canadian Lyme Disease Foundation). (n.d.-a). Common misdiagnoses. https://canlyme.com/just-diagnosed/testing /common-misdiagnoses/

CanLyme (Canadian Lyme Disease Foundation). (n.d.-b). Lyme basics. https://canlyme.com/lyme-basics/

Centers for Disease Control and Prevention (CDC). (2015). Post-treatment Lyme disease syndrome. https://www.cdc.gov/lyme/postlds/index.html

Centers for Disease Control and Prevention (CDC). (2021). How many people get Lyme disease? https://www.cdc.gov/lyme/stats/humancases.html

Clarke, J.N., & Miele, R. (2016). Trapped by gender: The paradoxical portrayal of gender and mental illness in anglophone North American magazines: 1983–2012. *Women's Studies International Forum, 56*, 1–8. https://doi.org/10.1016/j.wsif.2016.01.002

Connolly, L.E., Edelstein, P.H., & Ramakrishnan, L. (2007). Why is long-term therapy required to cure tuberculosis? *PLoS Medicine, 4*(3), e120. https://doi.org/10.1371/journal.pmed.0040120

Connor, D.M. (2015, 21 October, 30 October, 10 November). Is Lyme disease the new AIDS? (3 Parts). *HuffPost* blog. Part 1: What you need to know, https://www.huffpost.com/entry/lyme-disease-_b_8262536; Part 2: Life with Lyme and controversies, https://www.huffpost.com/entry/is-lyme-the-new-aids-part_b_8345566; Part 3: A caution to gay men, https://www.huffpost.com/entry/is-lyme-the-new-aids-part_b_8345566

European Centre for Disease Prevention and Control. (n.d.). Borreliosis. https://www.ecdc.europa.eu/en/borreliosis

Feder Jr., H.M., Johnson, B.J., O'Connell, S., Shapiro, E.D., Steere, A.C., Wormser, G.P., & the Ad Hoc International Lyme Disease Group. (2007). A critical appraisal of "chronic Lyme disease." *New England Journal of Medicine, 357*(14), 1422–30. https://doi.org/10.1056/NEJMra072023

Frketich, J. (2013, 28 June). Canadians trapped in Lyme disease limbo. *The Hamilton Spectator.* https://www.thespec.com/news/hamilton-region/2013/06/28/canadians-trapped-in-lyme-disease-limbo.html

Glauser, W., Taylor, M., & Tierney, M. (2016, 7 July). Is Lyme disease underdiagnosed or overestimated? *Healthy Debate.* https://healthydebate.ca/2016/07/topic/lyme-disease-testing-underdiagnosed-elisa/

Government of Canada. (2015). National Lyme disease surveillance in Canada 2009–2012. https://www.canada.ca/en/public-health/services/publications/diseases-conditions/national-lyme-disease-surveillance-canada-2009-2012.html

Government of Canada. (2021a). Lyme disease surveillance: Preliminary annual report 2018. https://www.canada.ca/en/public-health/services/publications/diseases-conditions/lyme-disease-surveillance-report-2018.html

Government of Canada. (2021b). Surveillance of Lyme disease. https://www.canada.ca/en/public-health/services/diseases/lyme-disease/surveillance-lyme-disease.html

Green Party of Canada. (2014, 12 December). Senate unanimously passes Elizabeth May's Federal Framework on Lyme Disease Act. https://www .greenparty.ca/en/media-release/2014-12-12/senate-unanimously-passes -elizabeth-may's-federal-framework-lyme-disease

Gregson, D., Evans, G., Patrick, D., & Bowie, W. (2015). Lyme disease: How reliable are serologic results? *CMAJ, 187*(16), 1193–4. https://doi.org /10.1503/cmaj.150874

Haines, A., Kovats, R.S., Campbell-Lendrum, D., & Corvalán, C. (2006). Climate change and human health: Impacts, vulnerability and public health. *Public Health, 120*(7), 585–96. https://doi.org/10.1016/j .puhe.2006.01.002

Halperin, J.J., Baker, P., & Wormser, G.P. (2013). Common misconceptions about Lyme disease. *The American Journal of Medicine, 126*(3), 264-e1. https://doi.org/10.1016/j.amjmed.2012.10.008

Hatchette, T., Davis, I., & Johnston, B. (2014). Lyme disease: Clinical diagnosis and treatment. *Canada Communicable Disease Report, 40*(11), 194–208. https://doi.org/10.14745/ccdr.v40i11a01

Kingston, A. (2014, 24 March). The truth about Lyme disease. *Maclean's.* https://www.macleans.ca/society/health/the-truth-about-lyme -disease/

Kugeler, K.J., Schwartz, A.M., Delorey, M.J., Mead, P.S., & Hinckley, A.F. (2021). Estimating the frequency of Lyme disease diagnoses, United States, 2010–2018. *Emerging Infectious Diseases, 27*(2), 616–19. https:// wwwnc.cdc.gov/eid/article/27/2/20-2731_article

Kumbhare, D., Ahmed, S., & Watter, S. (2018). A narrative review on the difficulties associated with fibromyalgia diagnosis. *Therapeutic Advances in Musculoskeletal Disease, 10*(1), 13–26. https://doi.org/10.1177/17597 20X17740076

Loevinger, B.L., Shirtcliff, E.A., Muller, D., Alonso, C., & Coe, C.L. (2012). Delineating psychological and biomedical profiles in a heterogeneous fibromyalgia population using cluster analysis. *Clinical Rheumatology, 31*(4), 677–85. https://doi.org/10.1007/s10067-011-1912-1

Lyme Maze, The. (n.d.). Find a Lyme-literate doctor. https://thelymemaze .blogspot.com/p/find-lyme-literate-doctor.html

Malat, J. (2001). Social distance and patients' rating of healthcare providers. *Journal of Health and Social Behavior, 42*(4), 360–72. https://doi.org/10.2307 /3090184

Maloney, E.L. (2009). The need for clinical judgment in the diagnosis and treatment of Lyme disease. *Journal of American Physicians and Surgeons, 14*(3), 82–9. https://www.jpands.org/vol14no3/maloney.pdf

Marshall McNagny, K. (2017, 9 August). Innovative science research in Canada is dying a silent death. *Maclean's.* https://www.macleans.ca /opinion/innovative-science-research-in-canada-is-dying-a-silent-death/

Mayer, A. (2014, 26 February). Touched by Lyme: What does the CDC's 300,000 number really mean? *Lymedisease.org.* https://www.lymedisease .org/alix-mayer-cdc-2/

Mervis, H. (2017, 9 March). Data check: U.S. government share of basic research funding falls below 50%. *Science.* https://www.sciencemag .org/news/2017/03/data-check-us-government-share-basic-research -funding-falls-below-50

Ogden, N.H., Bouchard, C., Badcock, J., Drebot, M.A., Elias, S.P., Hatchette, T.F., … Webster, D. (2019). What is the real number of Lyme disease cases in Canada? *BMC Public Health, 19*(1), 849. https://doi.org/10.1186 /s12889-019-7219-x

Ogden, N.H., Maarouf, A., Barker, I.K., Bigras-Poulin, M., Lindsay, L.R., Morshed, M.G., … Charron, D.F. (2006). Climate change and the potential for range expansion of the Lyme disease vector *Ixodes scapularis* in Canada. *International Journal for Parasitology, 36*(1), 63–70. https://doi.org /10.1016/j.ijpara.2005.08.016

Ogden, N.H., Radojevic, M., Wu, X., Duvvuri, V.R., Leighton, P.A., & Wu, J. (2014). Estimated effects of projected climate change on the basic reproductive number of the Lyme disease vector *Ixodes scapularis. Environmental Health Perspectives, 122*(6), 631–8. https://doi.org/10.1289/ehp.1307799

Oxtoby, K. (2013). Where to draw the line in relationships with patients. *BMJ, 346,* f2848. https://doi.org/10.1136/bmj.f2848

Patz, J.A., Olson, S.H., Uejio, C.K., & Gibbs, H.K. (2008). Disease emergence from global climate and land use change. *Medical Clinics of North America, 92*(6), 1473–91. https://doi.org/10.1016/j.mcna.2008.07.007

Payne, E. (2016, 16 May). Medical community failing Lyme patients, Calgary doctor says. *CanLyme.* http://canlyme.com/2016/05/21 /medical-community-failing-lyme-patients-calgary-doctor-says/

Radcliffe, S. (2020, 14 January). Justin Bieber's reveal shows why Lyme disease is often misdiagnosed. *Healthline.* https://www.healthline.com /health-news/justin-bieber-lyme-disease

Rebman, A.W., & Aucott, J.N. (2020). Post-treatment Lyme disease as a model for persistent symptoms in Lyme disease. *Frontiers in Medicine, 7,* 57. https://doi.org/10.3389/fmed.2020.00057

Schwartz, A.M., Kugeler, K.J., Nelson, C.A., Marx, G.E., & Hinckley, A.F. (2021). Use of commercial claims data for evaluating trends in Lyme disease diagnoses, United States, 2010–2018. *Emerging Infectious Diseases, 27*(2), 499–507. https://wwwnc.cdc.gov/eid/article/27/2/20-2728_article

Singh, S.K., & Girschick, H.J. (2004). Lyme borreliosis: From infection to autoimmunity. *Clinical Microbiology and Infection, 10*(7), 598–614. https://doi.org/10.1111/j.1469-0691.2004.00895.x

Specter, M. (2015, 15 January). A new front in the Lyme wars. *The New Yorker.* https://www.newyorker.com/news/daily-comment/new-front-lyme-wars

Stricker, R.B., & Johnson, L. (2014). Lyme disease: Call for a "Manhattan Project" to combat the epidemic. *PLoS Pathogens, 10*(1), e1003796. https://doi.org/10.1371/journal.ppat.1003796

Tan, A. (n.d.). Lyme disease: How a tiny speck changed my life forever. http://www.amytan.net/lyme-disease.html

Telling, G. (2015, 1 April). Avril Lavigne opens up about her health crisis: "I was bedridden for 5 months." *People.* https://people.com/celebrity/avril-lavigne-lyme-disease-singer-was-bedridden-for-5-months/

Turcotte, M. (2015). Women and health. *Statistics Canada.* https://www150.statcan.gc.ca/n1/pub/89-503-x/2010001/article/11543-eng.htm

Unravelling the mystery of Lyme disease: Why Canada needs to do more. (n.d.). *Hospital News.* https://hospitalnews.com/unravelling-the-mystery-of-lyme-disease-why-canada-needs-to-do-more/#comment-116194

Wilske, B. (2005). Epidemiology and diagnosis of Lyme borreliosis. *Annals of Medicine, 37*(8), 568–79. https://doi.org/10.1080/07853890500431934

Zarzour, K. (2015, 18 June). Lyme sufferers desperate for answers, treatment. *Toronto.com.* https://www.toronto.com/news-story/5683615-lyme-sufferers-desperate-for-answers-treatment/

## Chapter 5. Dr. Charles Smith

Boyle, T. (2015, 28 February). Doctors who supervised disgraced pathologist Charles Smith never faced disciplinary hearing. *Toronto Star.* https://www.thestar.com/news/gta/2015/02/28/doctors

-who-supervised-disgraced-pathologist-never-faced-disciplinary
-hearing.html

Canadian Institute for Health Information (CIHI). (2020). Summary report: Physicians in Canada, 2019. https://www.cihi.ca/sites/default/files /document/physicians-in-canada-report-en.pdf

Canadian Medical Association. (2019). CMA physician workforce survey. https://surveys.cma.ca/

Canadian Medical Protective Association (CMPA). (n.d.). Canadian Medical Protective Association at a glance. https://www.cmpa-acpm .ca/en/connect/media-room/the-canadian-medical-protective -association-at-a-glance

Canadian Medical Protective Association (CMPA). (2018). Addressing physician disruptive behaviour in healthcare institutions. https:// www.cmpa-acpm.ca/en/advice-publications/browse-articles/2013 /addressing-physician-disruptive-behaviour-in-healthcare-institutions

Canadian Medical Protective Association (CMPA). (2020). A five-year trend of CMPA's medico-legal services. In *2020 annual report: A year in numbers.* https://www.cmpa-acpm.ca/static-assets/pdf/about/annual -report/2020/20-annual-report-by-the-numbers-5yr-trend-e.pdf

Chorneyko, K., & Butany, J. (2008). Canada's pathology. *CMAJ, 178*(12), 1523–4. https://doi.org/10.1503/cmaj.080710

Cochrane Canada. (n.d.). About us. https://canada.cochrane.org/about-us

College of Physicians and Surgeons of Ontario. (n.d.). What we do. https:// www.cpso.on.ca/About/What-we-do

College of Physicians and Surgeons of Ontario. (2014). *2014 annual report.* https://view.joomag.com/annual-report-2014/0266839001438971379? short

Cordner, S., Ehsani, J., Bugeja, L., & Ibrahim, J. (2008). Pediatric forensic pathology: Limits and controversies. Commissioned by Inquiry into Pediatric Forensic Pathology, Ontario, Canada. https://www .attorneygeneral.jus.gov.on.ca/inquiries/goudge/policy_research/pdf /Limits_and_Controversies-CORDNER.pdf

Dr. Charles Smith: The man behind the public inquiry. (2009, 8 December). *CBC News.* https://www.cbc.ca/news/canada/dr-charles-smith-the -man-behind-the-public-inquiry-1.864004

Eddy, D.M. (1984). Variations in physician practice: The role of uncertainty. *Health Affairs, 3*(2), 74–89. https://doi.org/10.1377/hlthaff.3.2.74

Eggertson, L. (2008). Goudge: "Systemic failings" in Ontario coroner's office. *CMAJ, 179*(10), 995. https://doi.org/10.1503/cmaj.081625

Elston, M.A., & Gabe, J. (2016). Violence in general practice: A gendered risk? *Sociology of Health & Illness, 38*(3), 426–41. https://doi.org /10.1111/1467-9566.12373

Gelles, R.J. (1975). The social construction of child abuse. *American Journal of Orthopsychiatry, 45*(3), 363–71. https://doi.org/10.1111/j.1939-0025.1975 .tb02547.x

Gottlieb, L. (2015). "Lactivism," by Courtney Jung. *The New York Times.* https://www.nytimes.com/2015/12/20/books/review/lactivism-by -courtney-jung.html

Goudge, S.T. (2008). *Inquiry into pediatric forensic pathology in Ontario* (4 Vols.). Ontario Ministry of the Attorney General. https://www.attorneygeneral .jus.gov.on.ca/inquiries/goudge/report/

Hall, J.A., Roter D.L., & Rand, C.C. (1981). Communication of affect between patient and physician. *Journal of Health and Social Behaviour, 22*(1), 18–32. https://doi.org/10.2307/2136365

Harland-Logan, S. (n.d.). William Mullins-Johnson. https://innocence canada.com/exonerations/william-mullins-johnson/

Kinney, H.C., & Thach, B.T. (2009). The sudden infant death syndrome. *New England Journal of Medicine, 361*(8), 795–805. https://doi.org/10.1056 /NEJMra0803836

Lang, S. (2015). *Report of the Motherisk hair analysis independent review.* Ontario Ministry of the Attorney General. http://www.m-hair.ca /docs/default-source/default-document-library/motherisk_enbfb30 b45b7f266cc881aff0000960f99.pdf

Library of Congress, Law Library. (2007). Canada. In *Children's rights: International and national laws and practices* (pp. 51–60). www.loc.gov/law /help/child-rights/canada.php

Mahoney, J., & Bonoguore, T. (2010). 14 cases tainted by Charles Smith evidence. *The Globe and Mail.* https://www.theglobeandmail.com /news/national/14-cases-tainted-by-charles-smiths-evidence /article562711/

McRae, K.N., Cameron, A., Ferguson, C.A., Loadman, E., Longstaffe, S., & Snyder, R. (1984). The forensic pediatrician as a child advocate. *Journal of Developmental & Behavioral Pediatrics, 5*(5), 259–62. https://doi.org /10.1097/00004703-198410000-00007

Milne, V., Pendharkar, S., & Nolan, M. (2014, 20 November). Is Canada's medical malpractice system working? *Healthy Debate*. https:// healthydebate.ca/2014/11/topic/cmpa-medical-malpractice/

Mullins-Johnson happy after AG calls for acquittal. (2007, 27 April). *CBC News*. https://www.cbc.ca/news/canada/toronto/mullins-johnson -happy-after-ag-calls-for-acquittal-1.654177

Newbury-Birch, D., White, M., & Kamali, F. (2000). Factors influencing alcohol and illicit drug use amongst medical students. *Drug and Alcohol Dependence, 59*(2), 125–30. https://doi.org/10.1016/s0376-8716(99)00108-8

Newman-Toker, D.E., Wang, Z., Zhu, Y., Nassery, N., Saber Tehrani, A.S., Schaffer, A.C., Yu-Moe, C.W., Clemens, G.D., Fanai, M., & Siegal, D. (2021). Rate of diagnostic errors and serious misdiagnosis-related harms for major vascular events, infections, and cancers: Toward a national incidence estimate using the "Big Three." *Diagnosis, 8*(1), 67–84. https:// doi.org/10.1515/dx-2019-0104

Parton, N. (1979). The natural history of child abuse: A study in social problem definition. *The British Journal of Social Work, 9*(4), 431–51. https:// doi.org/10.1093/oxfordjournals.bjsw.a057117

Payer, L. (1992). *Disease mongers: How doctors, drug companies, and insurers are making you feel sick.* Wiley.

Royal College of Physicians and Surgeons of Canada. (n.d.). Information by discipline. www.royalcollege.ca/rc

Singh, H., Meyer, A.N., & Thomas, E.J. (2014). The frequency of diagnostic errors in outpatient care: Estimations from three large observational studies involving US adult populations. *BMJ Quality and Safety, 23*, 727–31. https://doi.org/10.1136/bmjqs-2013-002627

Smith, R. (2014). Medical research – still a scandal. *British Medical Journal Blog*. https://blogs.bmj.com/bmj/2014/01/31/richard-smith-medical -research-still-a-scandal/

Tuteur, A. (2016, 15 April). Why have we pathologized mother-infant boding? *Psychology Today*. https://www.psychologytoday.com/intl/blog /push-back/201604/why-have-we-pathologized-mother-infant-bonding

United Nations. (2017). World Day against child labour, 12 June. https:// www.un.org/en/observances/world-day-against-child-labour

Vijaykumar, M. (2018). A crisis of conscience: Miscarriages of justice and indigenous defendants in Canada. *University of British Columbia Law Review, 51*(1), 161–227.

Wrongfully convicted Ont. man gets $4.25M. (2010, 21 October). *CBC News.* https://www.cbc.ca/news/canada/toronto/wrongfully -convicted-ont-man-gets-4-25m-1.967978

## Chapter 6. Elizabeth Wettlaufer

Berendonk, C., Kaspar, R., Bär, M., & Hoben, M. (2017). Improving quality of work life for care providers by fostering the emotional well-being of persons with dementia: A cluster randomized trial of a nursing intervention in German long-term care settings. *Dementia, 18*(4), 1286– 1309. https://doi.org/10.1177/1471301217698837

Braedley, S., Owusu, P., Przednowek, A., & Armstrong, P. (2018). We're told, "Suck it up": Long-term care workers' psychological health and safety. *Ageing International, 43*(1), 91–109. https://doi.org/10.1007 /s12126-017-9288-4

Canadian Association for Long Term Care. (2017). *Caring for Canada's seniors: Recommendations for meeting the needs of an aging population.* https://caltc .ca/wordpress/wp-content/uploads/2017/01/Caring-for-Canadas -Seniors_CALTC.pdf

Canadian Foundation for Healthcare Improvement. (2011, February). Mythbusters: The aging population is to blame for rising health care costs. https://web.archive.org/web/20171018040740/http:// www.cfhi-fcass.ca/PublicationsAndResources/Mythbusters /ArticleView/2011/02/22/f20f6cb8-bfd0-453e-b470-6fb63c93 a629.aspx

Canadian Institute for Health Information. (2017). Commonwealth Fund survey, 2017. https://www.cihi.ca/en/commonwealth-fund-survey-2017

Canadian Institute of Health Research. (2016). *How Canada compares: Results from the Commonwealth Fund 2015 international health policy survey of primary care physicians.* https://www.cihi.ca/sites/default /files/commonwealth_fund_2015_pdf_en_0.pdf

Canadian Medical Association. (2016). *The state of seniors health care in Canada.* https://www.cma.ca/sites/default/files/2018-11/the-state-of -seniors-health-care-in-canada-september-2016.pdf

Canadian Mental Health Association. (2021, 19 July). Fast facts about mental health and mental illness. https://cmha.ca/brochure /fast-facts-about-mental-illness/

Canadian Nurses Association. (2018). Nursing statistics. https://www
.cna-aiic.ca/en/nursing-practice/the-practice-of-nursing/health-human
-resources/nursing-statistics

Cares, A., Pace, E., Denious, J., & Crane, L.A. (2015). Substance use and
mental illness among nurses: Workplace warning signs and barriers to
seeking assistance. *Substance Abuse, 36*(1), 59–66. https://doi.org/10.1080
/08897077.2014.933725

CBC News. (2017, 1 June). "She's a monster": Families of those killed by
ex-nurse Elizabeth Wettlaufer struggling to forgive. https://www.cbc.ca
/news/canada/windsor/she-s-a-monster-families-of-those-killed-by-ex
-nurse-elizabeth-wettlaufer-struggling-to-forgive-1.4141435

Centre for Addiction and Mental Health (CAMH). (n.d.). Mental illness and
addiction: Facts and statistics. https://www.camh.ca/en/driving-change
/the-crisis-is-real/mental-health-statistics

Chamberlain, S.A., Hoben, M., Squires, J.E., Cummings, G.G., Norton, P., &
Estabrooks, C.A. (2019). Who is (still) looking after mom and dad? Few
improvements in care aides' quality-of-work life. *Canadian Journal on
Aging, 38* (1), 35–50. https://doi.org/10.1017/S0714980818000338

Department of Justice, Government of Canada. (2015). *Crime and abuse against
seniors: A review of the research literature with special reference to the Canadian
situation.* https://www.justice.gc.ca/eng/rp-pr/cj-jp/fv-vf/crim/sum-som.html

Fitzpatrick, M. (2017a, 3 June). Health-care killers "statistically rare" but
difficult to spot. *CBC News.* https://www.cbc.ca/news/canada/wettlaufer
-health-care-killers-1.4143174

Fitzpatrick, M. (2017b, 26 July). Caressant Care and Ontario College of
Nurses at odds over serial killer Wettlaufer's firing. *CBC News.* https://
www.cbc.ca/news/canada/caressant-care-and-ontario-college-of-nurses
-at-odds-over-serial-killer-wettlaufer-s-firing-1.4222735

Fraser, L. (2017, 2 June). Here's what ex-nurse Elizabeth Wettlaufer confessed
about killing 8 patients. *CBC News.* https://www.cbc.ca/news/canada
/toronto/Elizabeth-wettlaufer-confession-1.4142647

Gillese, E.E. (2019). *Public inquiry into the safety and security of residents in the
long-term care homes system* (4 vols.). https://longtermcareinquiry.ca/en
/final-report/

Government of Canada. (2020). Operation LASER. https://www.canada.ca
/en/department-national-defence/services/operations/military
-operations/current-operations/laser.html

Hawes, C. (2003). Elder abuse in residential long-term care settings: What is known and what information is needed? In R.J Bonnie & R.B Wallace (Eds.), *Elder mistreatment: Abuse, neglect, and exploitation in an aging America* (pp. 446–500). National Academies Press.

Hawes, C., & Kimbell, A.M. (2010). *Detecting, addressing, and preventing elder abuse in residential care facilities.* Report to the National Institute of Justice, U.S. Department of Justice. School of Rural Public Health, Texas A & M Health Science Center.

Health Canada. (2014). Canadian alcohol and drug use monitoring survey: Summary of results for 2012. Government of Canada. https://www .canada.ca/en/health-canada/services/health-concerns/drug -prevention-treatment/drug-alcohol-use-statistics/canadian-alcohol -drug-use-monitoring-survey-summary-results-2012.html

Health Quality Ontario. (2019). Measuring up 2019: Value and efficiency. https://www.hqontario.ca/System-Performance/Yearly-Reports /Measuring-Up-2019/Value-and-Efficiency

Hildebrandt, A. (2013). Nearly 25% of Canadian nurses wouldn't recommend their hospital. *CBC News.* https://www.cbc.ca/news /health/nearly-25-of-canadian-nurses-wouldn-t-recommend-their -hospital-1.1304601

Hoben, M., Knopp-Sihota, J.A., Nesari, M., Chamberlain, S.A., Squires, J.E., Norton, P.G., … Estabrooks, C.A. (2017). Health of health care workers in Canadian nursing homes and pediatric hospitals: A cross-sectional study. *CMAJ Open, 5*(4), E791–9. https://doi.org/10.9778/cmajo.20170080

Hochschild, A.R. (1990). Ideology and emotion management: A perspective and path for future research. In T.D. Kemper (Ed.), *Research agendas in the sociology of emotions* (pp. 117–42). State University of New York Press.

Ireton, J. (2020, 10 June). COVID-19: Majority of region's long-term care deaths occurred in for-profit homes. *CBC News.* https://www.cbc.ca /news/canada/ottawa/for-profit-nursing-homes-83-percent-of-covid -deaths-eastern-ontario-1.5604880

Kelly, A. (2017, 15 June). One in ten older adults has been abused in the last month. *CBC News.* https://www.cbc.ca/news/canada/british-columbia /one-in-ten-older-adults-has-been-abused-in-the-last-month-1.4162551

Kunyk, D. (2015). Substance use disorders among registered nurses: Prevalence, risks and perceptions in a disciplinary jurisdiction. *Journal of Nursing Management, 23*(1), 54–64. https://doi.org/10.1111/jonm.12081

Levy, B., & Banaji, M.R. (2002) Implicit ageism. In T. Nelson (Ed.), *Ageism, stereotyping and prejudice against older persons* (pp. 49–75). MIT Press.

Loreto, N. (2020, 29 May). Canada's coronavirus crisis exposes the deadly issues in long-term care. *The Washington Post*. https://www.washington post.com/opinions/2020/05/29/canadas-coronavirus-crisis-exposes -deadly-issues-long-term-care/

Lupton, A. (2017). Wettlaufer inquiry begins with investigators promising families input priority. *CBC News*. https://www.cbc.ca/news/canada /london/wettlauferprobe-gillese-1.4233591

MacCharles, T. (2020, 7 May). 82% of Canada's COVID-19 deaths have been in long-term care, new data reveals. *Toronto Star*. https://www.thestar .com/politics/federal/2020/05/07/82-of-canadas-covid-19-deaths-have -been-in-long-term-care.html

MacDonald, G. (2015). The social aspects of aging. In L. Tepperman & P. Albanese (Eds.), *Sociology: A Canadian perspective* (4th ed., pp. 286–312). Oxford University Press.

Mancini, M., Pedersen, K., & Ouellet, V. (2018, 26 January). "It's a horror movie": Nursing home security footage provides raw picture of resident violence problem. *CBC News*. https://www.cbc.ca/news/health /long-term-care-marketplace-1.4501795

McQuigge, M. (2017, 2 June). If you ever do this again, we'll turn you in, pastor told killer nurse. *Toronto Star*. https://www.thestar.com/news /canada/2017/06/02/if-you-ever-do-this-again-well-turn-you-in-pastor -told-killer-nurse.html

Meiboom, A.A., de Vries, H., Hertogh, C.M., & Scheele, F. (2015). Why medical students do not choose a career in geriatrics: A systematic review. BMC *Medical Education, 15*(1), 101. https://doi.org/10.1186 /s12909-015-0384-4

Mezey, M., & Fulmer, T. (2002). The future history of gerontological nursing. *The Journals of Gerontology Series A: Biological Sciences and Medical Sciences, 57*(7), M438–41. https://doi.org/10.1093/gerona/57.7.M438

National Council of State Boards of Nursing. (2011). *Substance use disorder in nursing: A resource manual and guidelines for alternative and disciplinary monitoring programs*. https://www.ncsbn.org/SUDN_11.pdf

National Research Council (US) Panel to Review Risk and Prevalence of Elder Abuse and Neglect. (2003). *Elder mistreatment: Abuse, neglect, and*

*exploitation in an aging America* (R.J. Bonnie & R.B. Wallace, Eds.). National
Academies Press.

Norris, S. (2020, 22 October). Long-term care homes in Canada – How are
they funded and regulated? *HillNotes*. https://hillnotes.ca/2020/10/22
/long-term-care-homes-in-canada-how-are-they-funded-and-regulated/

Ontario Long Term Care Association. (n.d.). The role of long-term care.
https://www.oltca.com/oltca/OLTCA/LongTermCare/OLTCA/Public
/LongTermCare/FactsFigures.aspx

Ontario Long Term Care Association. (2018). *More care. Better care: 2018
budget submission.* https://www.oltca.com/OLTCA/Documents/Reports
/2018OLTCABudgetSubmission-MoreCareBetterCare.pdf

Payne, E. (2020, 8 June). Only 13% of Ontario's long-term care COVID
patients went to hospital; advocates want to know why. *Ottawa Citizen*.
https://ottawacitizen.com/news/local-news/only-13-of-ontarios
-long-term-care-covid-patients-went-to-hospital-advocates-want
-to-know-why

Payscale. (2018a). Average personal support worker (PSW) hourly pay in
Canada. https://www.payscale.com/research/CA/Job=Personal
_Support_Worker_(PSW)/Hourly_Rate

Payscale. (2018b). Average registered practical nurse (RPN) hourly pay in
Canada. https://www.payscale.com/research/CA/Job=Registered
_Practical_Nurse_(RPN)/Hourly_Rate

Pearson, P. (2021, 8 June). When healers do harm: Women serial killers
in the health care industry. *The Walrus*. https://thewalrus.ca/when
-healers-do-harm-women-serial-killers-in-the-health-care-industry/

Pedersen, K., Mancini, M., & Ouellet, V. (2018, 18 January). Staff
-to-resident abuse in long-term care homes up 148% from 2011. *CBC News*.
https://www.cbc.ca/news/business/elderly-care-violence-marketplace
-investigates-1.4493215

Pijl-Zieber, E.M., Awosoga, O., Spenceley, S., Hagen, B., Hall, B., & Lapins, J.
(2018). Caring in the wake of the rising tide: Moral distress in residential
nursing care of people living with dementia. *Dementia, 17*(3), 315–36.
https://doi.org/10.1177/1471301216645214

Registered Nurses Association of Ontario. (2007). *Staffing and care standards
for long-term care homes.* https://rnao.ca/sites/rnao-ca/files/storage
/related/3163_RNAO_submission_to_MOHLTC_--_Staffing_and_Care
_Standards_in_LTC_-_Dec_21_20071.pdf

Revera Inc. & International Federation on Ageing. (n.d). *Revera report on ageism: A Look at gender differences.* https://www.ageismore.com /getmedia/4130a0e3-c35e-44b2-b297-55ea6ca1db01/Revera-Report _Gender-Differences.pdf.aspx?ext=.pdf

Revera Inc. & Sheridan Centre for Elder Research. (2016). *Revera report on ageism: Independence and choice as we age.* https://www.ageismore.com /research/revera-report-on-ageism-independence-and-choice-a

Robert Wood Johnson Foundation. (2012, 13 March). Health care providers with geriatric training in demand. *Culture of Health Blog.* https://www .rwjf.org/en/blog/2012/03/health-care-providers-with-geriatric-training -in-demand.html

Rzeszut, S.M. (2017). The need for a stronger definition: Recognizing abandonment as a form of elder abuse across the United States. *Family Court Review, 55*(3), 444–57. https://doi.org/10.1111/fcre.12295

Sibbald, B. (2017). Workplace violence is not part of a doctor's job. *CMAJ, 189*(5), E184. https://doi.org/10.1503/cmaj.170086

Tonelli, M., Wiebe, N., Straus, S., Fortin, M., Guthrie, B., James, M. T., … Hemmelgarn, B. (2017). Multimorbidity, dementia and health care in older people: A population-based cohort study. *CMAJ Open, 5*(3), E623–31. https://doi.org/10.9778/cmajo.20170052

Trinkoff, A.M., Storr, C.L., & Wall, M.P. (1999). Prescription-type drug misuse and workplace access among nurses. *Journal of Addictive Diseases, 18*(1), 9–17. https://doi.org/10.1300/J069v18n01_02

Tumility, R. (2020, 28 May). Companies managing troubled Ontario long-term care homes run dozens more, make millions in profits. *National Post.* https://nationalpost.com/news/companies-managing-troubled-ontario -long-term-care-homes-run-dozens-more-make-millions-in-profits

## 7. Dr. Norman Barwin

Barwin's other casualties. (2018, 16 October). *Hey Reprotech.* https:// heyreprotech.substack.com/p/barwins-other-casualties

Canadian Fertility and Andrology Society. (n.d.). CFAS clinical practice guidelines. https://cfas.ca/clinical-practice-guidelines.html

Canadian Fertility and Andrology Society. (2018). Canadian assisted reproductive technologies register plus (CARTR Plus). Canadian Fertility and Andrology Society 64th Annual Meeting, 13–15 September, 2018,

Montreal, PQ. https://cfas.ca/_Library/cartr_annual_reports/CFAS
-CARTR-Plus-presentation-Sept-2018-FINAL-for-CFAS-website.pdf

Canadian Institute for Health Information (CIHI). (2019). *Physicians in Canada, 2017*. https://secure.cihi.ca/free_products/Physicians_in _Canada_2017.pdf

Canadian Press, The. (2019, 25 June). Fertility doctor's licence revoked after he used own sperm to inseminate patients. *CBC News*. https:// www.cbc.ca/news/canada/toronto/fertility-norman-barwin -disciplinary-hearing-1.5183711

Canadian Women's Foundation. (2018). The facts about the gender pay gap in Canada. https://canadianwomen.org/the-facts/the-gender-pay-gap/

Cattapan, A., Gruben, V., & Cameron, A. (2019, 15 April). New reproductive technology regulations don't go far enough: The safety regulations covering fertility clinics and sperm and egg donations must be more rigorous, with regular inspections and enforcement mechanisms. *Policy Options*. https://policyoptions.irpp.org/magazines/april-2019 /new-reproductive-technology-regulations-dont-go-far-enough/

Clarke, J.N. (2016). *Health, illness and medicine in Canada* (7th ed.). Oxford University Press.

College of Physicians and Surgeons of Ontario (CPSO). (n.d.-a).Peer and practice assessment. https://www.cpso.on.ca/Physicians/Your-Practice /Quality-Management/Assessments/Peer-Assessment

College of Physicians and Surgeons of Ontario (CPSO). (n.d.-b). Policies. https://www.cpso.on.ca/Physicians/Policies-Guidance/Policies

College of Physicians and Surgeons of Ontario (CPSO). (n.d.-c). Professionalism and practice program. https://www.cpso.on.ca /Physicians/Policies-Guidance/Professionalism-Practice-Programs

College of Physicians and Surgeons of Ontario (CPSO). (n.d.-d). Requirements. https://www.cpso.on.ca/Physicians/Registration /Requirements

College of Physicians and Surgeons of Ontario (CPSO). (n.d.-e). What we do. https://www.cpso.on.ca/About/What-we-do

College of Physicians and Surgeons of Ontario (CPSO). (2019). Barwin, Bernard Norman. https://doctors.cpso.on.ca/DoctorDetails /Barwin-Bernard-Norman/0023874-28666

DiManno, R. (2013, 4 February). Wrong-sperm doctor Barwin took shortcuts in career and races, too: DiManno. *The Toronto Star*. https://www.thestar

.com/news/gta/2013/02/04/wrongsperm_doctor_barwin_took
_shortcuts_in_career_and_races_too_dimanno.html

DuBois, J.M., Anderson, E.E., Chibnall, J.T., Mozersky, J., & Walsh, H.A. (2019). Serious ethical violations in medicine: A statistical and ethical analysis of 280 cases in the United States from 2008–2016. *The American Journal of Bioethics, 19*(1), 16–34. https://doi.org/10.1080/15265161.2018.1544305

Freidson, E. (1988). *Profession of medicine: A study in the sociology of applied Knowledge.* University of Chicago Press.

Government of Canada. (2013). Fertility treatment options. https://www .canada.ca/en/public-health/services/fertility/fertility-treatment -options.html

Government of Canada. (2019). Fertility. https://www.canada.ca/en /public-health/services/fertility/fertility.html

Government of Canada. (2020). Donating and using third-party sperm or ova (eggs) for assisted human reproduction. https://www.canada .ca/en/health-canada/services/drugs-health-products/compliance -enforcement/assisted-human-reproduction/donating-using.html

Grant, T. (2016, 7 March). Women still earning less money than men despite gains in education: study. *The Globe and Mail.* https://www .theglobeandmail.com/news/national/women-still-earning-less -money-than-men-despite-gains-in-education-study/article 29044130/

Kirkey, S. (2016, 30 July). Switched embryos and wrong sperm: IVF mix-ups lead to babies born with "unintended parentage." *The National Post.* https://nationalpost.com/health/ivf-mix-ups-lead-to-babies -born-with-unintended-parentage

Lindeman, T. (2019, 26 June). Canada IVF doctor loses licence for using wrong sperm – including his own. *The Guardian.* https://www.the guardian.com/world/2019/jun/26/norman-barwin-canada-ivf-doctor -loses-licence-wrong-sperm

Motluk, A. (2017, 7 March). Uncommon ancestry. *Hazlitt.* https://hazlitt.net /longreads/uncommon-ancestry

Motluk, A. (2019, 24 January). The search. Episode of *The Current. CBC Radio One.* https://www.cbc.ca/radiointeractives/thecurrent/the-search

OECD (Organisation for Economic Co-operation and Development). (n.d.). *Regulatory reform and innovation.* https://www.oecd.org/sti/inno /2102514.pdf

Payne, E. (2018, 3 May). Timeline: A look at the story of Dr. Norman Barwin. *Ottawa Citizen*. https://ottawacitizen.com/news/local-news/timeline-a-look-at-the-story-of-dr-norman-barwin

Payne, E. (2019, 25 June). "Beyond reprehensible": College of physicians revokes Barwin's licence, fines him. *Saltwire*. https://www.saltwire.com/nova-scotia/news/beyond-reprehensible-college-of-physicians-revokes-barwins-licence-fines-him-326672/

Payne, E. (2021, 29 July). Former Barwin patients, children will share in proposed $13.3-million settlement. *Ottawa Citizen*. https://ottawacitizen.com/news/local-news/former-barwin-patients-children-will-share-in-proposed-13-3-million-settlement

Retail Council of Canada. (2019). Minimum wage by province. https://www.retailcouncil.org/resources/quick-facts/minimum-wage-by-province/

Scotti, M. (2016, 23 November). Oversight of fertility clinics still lacking across Canada. *Global News*. https://globalnews.ca/news/3070555/oversight-of-fertility-clinics-still-lacking-across-canada/

Shojania, K.G., & Dixon-Woods, M. (2013). "Bad apples": Time to redefine as a type of systems problem? *BMJ Quality and Safety, 22*(7), 528–31. https://doi.org/10.1136/bmjqs-2013-002138

Statistics Canada. (2016). Data tables, 2016 Census. https://www12.statcan.gc.ca/census-recensement/2016/dp-pd/dt-td/Index-eng.cfm

Turner, B.S. (2012). *Medical power and social knowledge* (online ed.). Sage Publications. http://dx.doi.org/10.4135/9781446250426

Workopolis. (2017, 22 December). The average Canadian salaries by industry and region. https://careers.workopolis.com/advice/how-much-money-are-we-earning-the-average-canadian-wages-right-now/

## Conclusion

Canadian Institute for Health Information. (2014). *Sources of potentially avoidable emergency department visits*. https://secure.cihi.ca/free_products/ED_Report_ForWeb_EN_Final.pdf

Centre for Health Services and Policy Research. (n.d.). Evidence and perspectives on funding healthcare in Canada: Long-term care. University of British Columbia. http://healthcarefunding.ca/long-term-care/

Centre of Excellence for Women's Health. (2015). Women, girls, and prescription medication. https://bccewh.bc.ca/wp-content/uploads/2015/09/CRISM-Report-21-Aug-2015.pdf

Conrad, P. (2005). The shifting engines of medicalization. *Journal of Health and Social Behavior, 46*(1), 3–14. https://doi.org/10.1177/002214650504600102

Correctional Service Canada. (2015). Forum on corrections research. https://www.csc-scc.gc.ca/research/forum/e061/e061l-eng.shtml

DeWeerdt, S. (2019, 11 September). Tracing the US opioid crisis to its roots. *Nature.* https://www.nature.com/articles/d41586-019-02686-2

Finlay, K. (2015, 24 October). Preventable medical error is Canadian healthcare's silent killer. *Huffington Post.* https://www.huffingtonpost.ca/kathleen-finlay/medical-error-deaths_b_8350324.html

Franks, P., & Bertakis, K.D. (2003). Physician gender, patient gender, and primary care. *Journal of Women's Health, 12*(1), 73–80. https://doi.org/10.1089/154099903321154167

Gould, S., & Mosher, D. (2017, 22 May). Americans spent $8 billion on plastic surgery in 2016 – Here's the work they got done. *Business Insider.* https://www.businessinsider.com/plastic-surgery-growth-statistics-facts-2016-2017-5

Graber, M.L. (2013). The incidence of diagnostic error in medicine. *BMJ Quality and Safety, 22*, ii21–7. https://doi.org/10.1136/bmjqs-2012-001615

Jenkins, H. (Ed.). (1998). *The children's culture reader.* NYU Press.

Jüni, P., Nartey, L., Reichenbach, S., Sterchi, R., Dieppe, P.A., & Egger, M. (2004). Risk of cardiovascular events and rofecoxib: Cumulative meta-analysis. *The Lancet, 364*(9450), 2021–9. https://doi.org/10.1016/S0140-6736(04)17514-4

Kelly, J. (2020, 9 June). The movement to defund or disband the police: Here's what you need to know now. *Forbes.* https://www.forbes.com/sites/jackkelly/2020/06/09/the-movement-to-defund-or-disband-police-heres-what-you-need-to-know-now/

Kohn, L.T., Corrigan, J.M., & Donaldson, M.S. (Eds.). (2000). *To err is human: Building a safer health system.* Institute of Medicine (US) Committee on the Quality of Health Care in America. National Academy Press.

Makary, M.A., & Daniel, M. (2016). Medical error – The third leading cause of death in the US. *BMJ, 353*, i2139. https://doi.org/10.1136/bmj.i2139

McGregor, M., & Ronald, L. (2011, 24 January). For-profit facilities leave seniors vulnerable. *The Globe and Mail*. https://www.theglobeandmail .com/opinion/for-profit-facilities-leave-seniors-vulnerable/article562963/

Miller, A.B., Wall, C., Baines, C.J., Sun, P., To, T., & Narod, S.A. (2014). Twenty-five year follow-up for breast cancer incidence and mortality of the Canadian National Breast Screening Study: Randomised screening trial. *BMJ, 348*, g366. https://doi.org/10.1136/bmj.g366

Morgan, S. (n.d.). Elderly women more likely to be overprescribed prescription drugs: UBC study. University of British Columbia. https:// www.spph.ubc.ca/elderly-women-more-likely-to-be-overprescribed -prescription-drugs-ubc-study/

Ontario Human Rights Commission. (n.d.). Ageism and age discrimination (fact sheet). http://www.ohrc.on.ca/en/ageism-and-age-discrimination -fact-sheet

Pfeffer, A. (2021, 28 July). Disgraced fertility doctor agrees to $13M settlement with families, including 17 "Barwin babies." *CBC News*. https://www.cbc.ca/news/canada/ottawa/disgraced-fertility -doctor-agrees-to-13m-settlement-with-families-including-17-barwin -babies-1.6119754

Revera Inc. & Sheridan Centre for Elder Research. (2016). Revera report on ageism: Independence and choice as we age. https://www.ageismore .com/getmedia/6daed059-2e80-443a-8e71-717de14a5b03/Independence _and_Choice_Report_2016.pdf.aspx

Statistics Canada. (2020). Leading causes of death, total population, by age group. Table 13-10-0394-01. https://www150.statcan.gc.ca/t1/tbl1/en /tv.action?pid=1310039401

Swami, V., Coles, R., Wilson, E., Salem, N., Wyrozumska, K., & Furnham, A. (2010). Oppressive beliefs at play: Association among beauty ideals and practices and individual differences in sexism, objectification of others, and media exposure. *Psychology of Women Quarterly, 34*(3), 365–79. https://doi.org/10.1111%2Fj.1471-6402.2010.01582.x

Togoh, I. (2020, 3 June). Corporate donation tracker: Here are the companies giving millions to anti-racism efforts. *Forbes*. https://www.forbes.com /sites/isabeltogoh/2020/06/01/corporate-donations-tracker-here-are-the -companies-giving-millions-to-anti-racism-efforts/

Tosteson, A.N., Fryback, D.G., Hammond, C.S., Hanna, L.G., Grove, M.R., Brown, M., … Pisano, E.D. (2014). Consequences of false-positive screening mammograms. *JAMA Internal Medicine, 174*(6), 954–61. https://doi.org/10.1001/jamainternmed.2014.981

Uscher-Pines, L., Pines, J., Kellermann, A., Gillen, E., & Mehrotra, A. (2013). Deciding to visit the emergency department for non-urgent conditions: A systematic review of the literature. *The American Journal of Managed Care, 19*(1), 47–59.

Wang, Y., Hunt, K., Nazareth, I., Freemantle, N., & Petersen, I. (2013). Do men consult less than women? An analysis of routinely collected UK general practice data. *BMJ Open, 3*(8), e003320. https://doi.org/10.1136/bmjopen-2013-003320.

wwhealthline.ca. (n.d.). Long-term care home wait time information. https://www.wwhealthline.ca/libraryContent.aspx?id=20564

# Index